BSAVA Manual of Veterinary Nursing

Editor:

Margaret Moore MA VN CertEd FETC MIScT

Cerberus Training & Consultancy, Yewgate Cottage,
Remenham Hill, Henley-on-Thames, Oxfordshire RG9 3ES

Series Editor for BSAVA Manuals of Veterinary Nursing

Gill Simpson BVM&S MRCVS

Rose Cottage, Edgehead,
Midlothian EH37 5RL

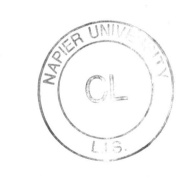

Published by:
British Small Animal Veterinary Association
Woodrow House, 1 Telford Way, Waterwells Business Park,
Quedgeley, Gloucester GL2 4AB, United Kingdom

A company limited by guarantee in England.
Registered company no. 2837793.
Registered as a charity.

The publishers and contributors cannot take responsibility for information
provided on dosages and methods of application of drugs mentioned in
this publication. Details of this kind must be verified by individual users
from the appropriate literature.

Typeset by: Fusion Design, Fordingbridge, Hampshire.

Printed by: Lookers, Upton, Poole, Dorset.

Other titles in the BSAVA Manuals of Veterinary Nursing series:

Manual of Veterinary Care
Edited by Sue Dallas

Manual of Advanced Veterinary Nursing
Edited by Alasdair Hotston Moore

Other BSAVA manuals:

Manual of Canine and Feline Emergency and Critical Care
Manual of Canine and Feline Gastroenterology
Manual of Canine and Feline Nephrology and Urology
Manual of Canine and Feline Wound Management and Reconstruction
Manual of Companion Animal Nutrition and Feeding
Manual of Canine Behaviour
Manual of Exotic Pets
Manual of Feline Behaviour
Manual of Ornamental Fish
Manual of Psittacine Birds
Manual of Raptors, Pigeons and Waterfowl
Manual of Reptiles
Manual of Small Animal Anaesthesia and Analgesia
Manual of Small Animal Arthrology
Manual of Small Animal Clinical Pathology
Manual of Small Animal Dentistry, 2nd edition
Manual of Small Animal Dermatology
Manual of Small Animal Diagnostic Imaging
Manual of Small Animal Endocrinology, 2nd edition
Manual of Small Animal Fracture Repair and Management
Manual of Small Animal Neurology, 2nd edition
Manual of Small Animal Oncology
Manual of Small Animal Ophthalmology
Manual of Small Animal Reproduction and Neonatology

Contents

Contributors

Sally Anne Argyle MVB CertSAC MRCVS
Department of Veterinary Clinical Studies, University of Glasgow Veterinary School, Bearsden Road,
Bearsden, Glasgow G61 1QH

Wendy Busby VN
Edinburgh's Telford College, Crewe Toll, Edinburgh EH4 2NZ

Sue Dallas VN CertEd
Rodbaston College, Rodbaston, Penkridge, Staffordshire ST19 5 TH

Cathy Garden VN DipAVN(Surgical)
Novartis Animal Health UK Ltd, Whittlesford, Cambridge CB2 4XW

Sarah Heath BVSc MRCVS
Behavioural Referrals, 11 Cotebrook Drive, Upton, Chester CH2 1RA

Alasdair Hotston Moore MA VetMB CertSAC CertVR MRCVS
Division of Companion Animals, Department of Clinical Veterinary Science, University of Bristol,
Langford House, Langford, Bristol BS40 5DU

Margaret Kane VN
Waltham Centre for Pet Nutrition, Freeby Lane, Waltham-on-the-Wolds, Near Melton Mowbray, Leicestershire LE14 4RT

Claire Knottenbelt BVSc DSAM MRCVS
Flat 2F4, 7 Albert Street, Leith, Edinburgh EH7 5HL

George Malynicz BVetMed MRCVS
22 Coolgardie Avenue, Chigwell, Essex IG7 5AY

Annaliese Morgan VN
Hird & Partners, 10 Blackwell, Halifax HX1 2BE

Kate Nichols VN
Royal Veterinary College, Hawkshead Lane, North Mymms, Hatfield, Herts AL9 7TA

Linda Oxley VN
Royal Veterinary College, Hawkshead Lane, North Mymms, Hatfield, Herts AL9 7TA

Janet Parker MA VetMB MRCVS
Novartis Animal Health UK Ltd, Whittlesford, Cambridge CB2 4XW

Jane Pocklington VN
Waltham Centre for Pet Nutrition, Freeby Lane, Waltham-on-the-Wolds, Near Melton Mowbray, Leicestershire LE14 4RT

Freda Scott-Park BVM&S PhD MRCVS
Portnellan Trian, Gartocharn, Alexandria, Dunbartonshire G83 8NL

James W. Simpson BVM&S SDA MPhil MRCVS RCVS Specialist Inernal Medicine
Department of Veterinary Clinical Studies, RDSVS, Hospital for Small Animals, Easter Bush Veterinary Centre,
Roslin, Midlothian EH25 9RG

Deborah J. Smith BVSc DVR CertSAS MRCVS
PDSA, 1 Shamrock St, Glasgow G4 9JZ

Garry Stanway BVSc CertVA MRCVS
Hird & Partners, 10 Blackwell, Halifax HX1 2BE

Kit Sturgess MA VetMB CertVR DSAM MRCVS
Department of Clinical Veterinary Science, University of Bristol, Langford House, Langford, Bristol BS40 5DU

Kate Wiggins VN DipAVN(Surg)
Davies White, Manor Farm Business Park, Higham Gobion, Hitchin, Herts SG3 3HR

Foreword

This trilogy of veterinary nursing manuals marks another significant landmark in the history of BSAVA Publications. The rise in status of the veterinary nurse within companion animal practice together with the new syllabus under the S/NVQ training scheme has meant that, after three editions spanning 15 years, *Practical Veterinary Nursing* has reached the end of its useful life. However, it was felt that there still was a need for a publication to complement the established textbook *Veterinary Nursing* (formerly Jones's Animal Nursing) published by Butterworth Heinemann on behalf of the BSAVA.

Based on the extremely successful BSAVA Manual formula of a logical, user-friendly approach, this exciting new series of three manuals caters for all levels of staff working with animals, whether it be in veterinary practice or other areas of animal care.

The editors of each of the manuals, Sue Dallas, Margaret Moore and Alasdair Hotston Moore, together with the series editor Gill Simpson, are to be congratulated on bringing together a wide range of talented contributors, both veterinary surgeons and veterinary nurses, to write individual chapters in an impressively easy-to-read format. They have succeeded in the difficult task of maintaining a continuity of style throughout. Each chapter opens with a summary of the information contained therein. The liberal use of tables and illustrations adds to the appeal of the layout, making the information accessible and highly practical in nature.

The *Manual of Veterinary Care* is a perfect introduction to those wishing to pursue a career working with animals. The *Manual of Veterinary Nursing* is written for student veterinary nurses studying for the new vocational qualification. The *Manual of Advanced Veterinary Nursing* has been designed for qualified veterinary nurses who are already working in practice and who either wish to take the Diploma in Advanced Veterinary Nursing (Surgical) or (Medical) or who just wish to expand their knowledge and further their education. There is, at present, no textbook that deals with the advanced course. This book provides both the necessary theoretical background and practical information, all in an easy-to-read style.

This three-volume series is certain to become an essential addition to the libraries of veterinary practices, training colleges and a wide range of animal care establishments.

P. Harvey Locke BVSc MRCVS
BSAVA President 1999–2000

Series preface

The veterinary profession has developed rapidly in recent years and the role of the ancillary staff in the small animal veterinary practice has increased in importance and diversity. Small animal practice in the new millennium will focus on the team approach to total animal care. Within this team should be adequately and appropriately trained personnel.

The aim of the BSAVA Manuals of Veterinary Nursing is to assist in the training and education of staff who are responsible for the care of animals, either within the veterinary practice or in other establishments which have responsibility for the welfare of animals. The series has been produced for the use of animal care personnel through to veterinary nurses studying for Advanced Diploma but the books fundamentally address the requirements for good nursing care.

The first book, the *Manual of Veterinary Care*, acts as an introduction to the care of small animals kept as pets, exploring the opportunities available for employment with animals, then progressing to describe basic animal care techniques. The second volume, the *Manual of Veterinary Nursing*, aims to assist those student veterinary nurses who are training for a formal qualification. It has been compiled with the needs of the Vocational Qualification in Veterinary Nursing in mind. With the development of veterinary nursing as a profession in its own right the remit of the qualified veterinary nurse is expanding. The objective of the *Manual of Advanced Veterinary Nursing* is to aid qualified veterinary nurses in developing their knowledge and skills. The inclusion of more advanced techniques should assist these nurses in fulfilling their essential role in the modern veterinary practice.

Multiple authors, both veterinary surgeons and veterinary nurses, have been involved in writing these books. Indeed, many sections have been co-written by veterinary surgeons and veterinary nurses working together to give a comprehensive approach to subject areas. Where appropriate, authors have contributed to more than one book, which gives continuity of content and style.

Having been associated with the education and training of veterinary nurses for some years, I am delighted to have been involved with these publications. I am grateful to all the authors who have contributed. Many thanks to Marion Jowett from BSAVA for directing the project and to the volume editors who have worked extremely hard to ensure these manuals are succinct and well presented. In particular I should like to thank BSAVA, who have supported the concept and publication of these manuals with the aim not only to improve the education of veterinary nurses but to improve animal care at all levels.

Gill Simpson
August 1999

Preface

Of the few books available on the applied aspects of veterinary nursing, none offers the truly practical approach as is adopted in this series of manuals. The goal of the authors contributing to the *Manual of Veterinary Nursing* has been to present each subject with the greatest possible practical slant. Detailed hands-on guidance is provided on many of the skills set out in the national standards of the veterinary nursing training scheme. Practical skills, for example in emergency nursing, anaesthesia, radiography, surgical nursing and placement, and care related to feeding tubes are described, many in step-by-step easy-to-follow figure boxes. The book is therefore an ideal resource for student veterinary nurses and for those who are responsible for their training and assessment.

The book also deals with important aspects relating to the responsibilities and high public profile that veterinary nurses have, in the chapters on legal aspects and advising clients.

This volume is a long-awaited technical and practical guide to the veterinary nursing profession and has been written by veterinary nurses and veterinary surgeons, all of whom are experienced in their fields.

As a teacher and trainer of veterinary nurses for over twenty years, I am convinced that this series will successfully fill the gap in the literature currently available. Although this book is written primarily with the student veterinary nurse in mind, qualified nurses wishing to refresh their knowledge will also find it invaluable as a source of reference.

Finally, I would like to take this opportunity to thank the authors for all of their dedicated hard work, my fellow volume editors and the series editor for their suggestions and support over the two years it has taken to produce this book, and of course the BSAVA for making the whole series possible.

Margaret C. Moore
August 1999

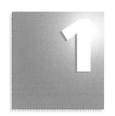

Management of the inpatient

Sue Dallas and Kate Wiggins

This chapter is designed to give information on:

- The area that makes up the hospital environment in the context of patient care
- The basic criteria required to enhance recovery
- The need for basic hygiene
- The requirements for good barrier nursing and isolation
- Provision of care for the hospitalized patient
- Monitoring of standard parameters
- Practical approaches to restraint for routine procedures
- Bandaging techniques
- Casting materials and techniques

The inpatient environment

Animals are hospitalized in order to:

- Be observed
- Be operated on
- Be treated
- Be nursed
- Have samples collected from them.

In order for veterinary staff to do this, the environment must be correct. To ensure a high standard of care, there must be adequate facilities, equipment and human resources.

Locations within the practice for the care of patients include:

- Consultation rooms
- Operating theatre (see Chapter 7)
- Preparation/triage rooms
- Recovery area
- Kennels
- Grooming area
- Exercise areas
- Kitchen/food preparation room.

General considerations for the inpatient include:

- Environmental temperature
- Hygiene and cleaning
- Light, heat, ventilation, noise and security.

More detailed information on animal housing, bedding and hygiene is given in *BSAVA Manual of Veterinary Care* (Chapter 5).

Environmental temperature

In most mammals and birds, body temperature is regulated within the ideal range. This varies between species to allow for the working of the internal body environment of each, and the balance attained is known as homeostasis.

Reptiles (for example, snakes, lizards and tortoises) and amphibians interact with their environmental temperature to maintain a body temperature that is optimal for the particular species, given the opportunity to do so. Thus monitoring of the body temperature of reptiles is not always necessary.

However, all species, by whatever means they control their own body temperature, sometimes need help. When an animal is conscious and healthy, its internal mechanisms are functioning; but when it is ill or injured, it may need assistance from the nursing environment.

In most clinical situations, it is usually desirable to maintain an animal's normal body temperature. Patients in the veterinary clinic that are unable, for a variety of reasons, to maintain their own body temperature within normal limits will benefit – often dramatically – when the environmental temperature is either raised or lowered to suit their special needs.

Methods of assisting patients to raise their body temperature include:

- Under-heat pads
- Bubble wrap

- Water-circulating pads
- Incubators
- Hot-water bottles (well wrapped)
- Ceramic heat lamps (especially for reptiles)
- Lightweight blankets
- Space blankets
- Synthetic fleece
- Beanbags.

Methods used to lower body temerature include:

- Cool pads
- Fans
- Air conditioning

Hygiene and cleaning

The hospital environment may house high concentrations of microorganisms that are potentially pathogenic (i.e. can cause disease). When patients are injured or diseased, they are even more at risk because of a decreased resistance to infection. Every effort must be made to decrease the microbe population in order to safeguard patients.

The aims are to:

- Eliminate or control sources of disease
- Prevent transmission of disease
- Increase host resistance to disease.

Methods of achieving these aims include:

- Isolation and quarantine
- Vaccination
- Improved diet
- Hygiene
- Chemotherapeutic agents
- Euthanasia of animals with uncontrollable infections.

Sources and transmission of disease can be controlled by:

- Improved ventilation
- Physical cleaning
- Chemical disinfectants and antiseptics
- The use of protective clothing (plastic disposable aprons and gloves).

Standards will be adjusted according to the area of the hospital. Chapter 5 of *BSAVA Manual of Veterinary Care* describes in detail how to disinfect surfaces and dispose of waste.

General cleaning

In the case of general cleaning equipment, the level of care is standard. If mops are used for washing floors, the following rules apply:

- Mop heads should be washed daily in the washing machine and dried
- If used more than once daily, they should be soaked for 30 minutes in a bucket of disinfectant
- They should never be left standing in soaking solution for any longer than 30 minutes
- They should be wrung out thoroughly before use on the floors.

To clean a floor with a mop:

- The mop should be moved from left to right across the body; it should never be pushed back and forth in front of the operator
- The mop head should be agitated in the disinfectant solution and wrung out before proceeding to clean
- The operator should start with the area furthest from the door
- When the area immediately around the operator has been cleaned, they should move and repeat the mop rinsing for a new area
- No one should be allowed to walk on the floor until it is dry
- The disinfectant solution should be changed between rooms, or more frequently if heavily soiled
- A separate mop or other cleaning equipment should be used in areas where high standards of clinical cleanliness are important.

Different inpatient areas

Consultation rooms

These rooms form the outpatient, examination and consultation zone (Figure 1.1). They are normally decorated in similar warm tones to the clinic reception area.

It is important to maintain a high standard of repair and hygiene here because this is where the client will spend the greatest amount of time. Excessive fittings are normally avoided; those that are in place are necessary for the purposes of examination of patients.

Fixtures might include:

- Examination table (either floor-mounted or cantilevered from the wall)
- Wall-mounted shelf (with drawers for equipment)
- Hand wash-basin
- Wall-mounted antiseptic solution dispenser
- Paper-towel dispenser
- Bin for waste
- X-ray viewer
- Wall-mounted ophthalmoscope/auriscope.

It is in the consultation room that the client and veterinary surgeon meet, often for the first time. It is important that everything required for a thorough examination is to hand and has been cleaned and disinfected between patients. For this reason, the ideal design allows the veterinary surgeon to use two consultation rooms, with a separate dispensary (Figure 1.2).

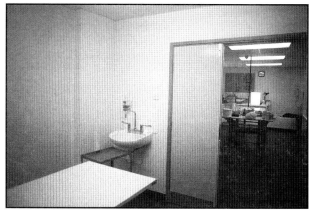

1.1 *The consultation room, with a wide door leading to the treatment area.*
Photo: Sue Dallas.

This type of layout enables each soiled room in turn to be thoroughly cleaned between clients (Figure 1.3) without hindering consultations.

Preparation and triage area

This central area is one of the most important rooms in a modern veterinary clinic (Figure 1.4). It is a non-sterile area, but because of the variety of patients passing through the room it is essential to maintain a high level of hygiene.

Triage (examination and rapid classification of a case) may also take place here; it is a multipurpose room in which patients from the ward, kennels and consultation rooms will:

- Receive medication and treatment
- Have samples collected for diagnostic procedures
- Be examined
- Have bandages, splints or casts removed or changed
- Be prepared for surgical procedure.

It is important that this is a secure area, ideally with a double self-closing door system to be passed through before escape is possible. Instructions to all staff about the opening and closing of these doors are usually displayed on a nearby wall.

- Surfaces in the preparation/triage area must be of a high standard, allowing easy disinfection and excellent hygiene
- The walls should be covered with durable low-maintenance material, allowing regular wiping down
- Floors have to withstand constant traffic (staff and patients) and frequent cleaning
- Considerable storage space is required for both large equipment and disposable materials
- Due to the many functions of this area, it is frequently up to four times the size of the clinic's operating theatre
- Preparation for surgical procedures (anaesthetic induction and clipping up) requires a gas scavenging system, an oxygen supply, an anaesthetic machine and a vacuum facility to collect hair
- Good lighting is essential
  - Fluorescent lights inset into the ceiling with diffuser panels for general room light are an alternative to normal daylight
  - Spotlights (with a dimmer facility) over the treatment tables ensure good light levels in the key work areas of the room
- Ventilation systems, via air conditioning using forced intake and extraction of atmosphere, should be installed; they will also provide constant temperature and humidity
- Windows should not be present, unless escape-proof and with blinds
- In order to reduce noise levels, high-set windows should be double-glazed; purpose-lagged wall panels and fire doors should be kept shut to prevent the transfer of sound through the clinic or outside the clinic.

The preparation/triage room is always sited near the theatre suite for easy movement of patients. Also nearby are:

- Surgical team's scrub-up area
- Sterilizers
- Instrument cleaning and packing facility.

Due to the many roles that this area plays in the work of the clinic, it is essential that order and organization of equipment and disposable materials are well established.

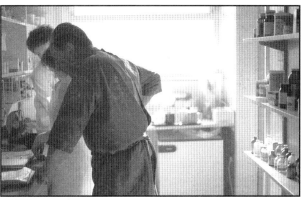

 Dispensary area between two consultation rooms. Photo: Sue Dallas.

1.3 Cleaning routines for consultation rooms

Between clients:

- Clean and disinfect the surface of the examination table
- Spot-clean other surfaces if soiled
- Check and clean soiled instruments
- Collect up and remove soiled dressings or bandage materials
- Sweep up any excess hair/coat
- Use deodorizer spray.

Between consultation surgeries:

- Clean and disinfect all surfaces (morning, afternoon and evening)
- Collect used instruments and sterilize or clean them
- Dispose of all waste
- Empty and disinfect bins
- Restock:
  - Selection of curved and straight scissors
  - Dressings and bandages
  - Cotton wool
  - Antiseptic solution (should be changed and remade between consultation surgeries)
  - Stethoscope
  - Thermometer
  - Selection of forceps.

Disinfectant for cleaning of surfaces:

Cetavolon/Savlon, 10 ml in 100 ml water.

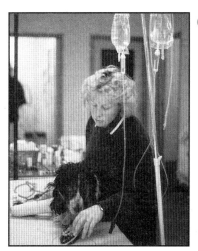

1.4 Setting up fluids in the preparation area. Photo: Sue Dallas.

Systems include:

- Good shelving
- Cupboards and cabinets with obvious labels concerning equipment and use
- Sterilizing dates and equipment named on all packs
- Stock lists required, with quantities.

Cleaning routines are outlined in Figure 1.5.

1.5 Cleaning routines for the preparation/triage area

Between patient preparations or treatments:

- Dispose of waste materials and body fluids as clinical waste
- Clean the clipper blades and clippers
- Check the walls, surfaces, worktops and treatment table and spot-clean with dilute disinfectant
- Check the vacuum collection bag or container and empty it if necessary
- Spot-clean the floor
- Check levels of disposables.

After preparation/treatment sessions:

- Dispose of all waste material; disinfect bins and fit new liners
- Wipe down all surfaces with dilute disinfectant
- Restock cupboards
- Check equipment (e.g. clippers and blades)
- Refill dispensers for hand-cleaners and antiseptics
- Clean all sinks
- Replace towels and paper-towel rolls.

Recovery area

On completion of surgical procedures, patients recover consciousness in an area where staff are able to monitor and observe them (Figure 1.6). These animals should not be disturbed by cleaning routines.

However, it is essential to allow a thorough cleaning routine to take place at some point in each day, when patients have been moved to the ward kennels.

Patients in the recovery stage may vomit, defecate, urinate or salivate. These body fluids must be removed immediately, and disposed of in the correct manner (see Chapter 5 in *BSAVA Manual of Veterinary Care*) by staff wearing protective clothing.

Cleaning should include the following routines:

- Dispose of waste; disinfect bins and replace plastic liners
- Wipe down all surfaces and equipment such as drip stands

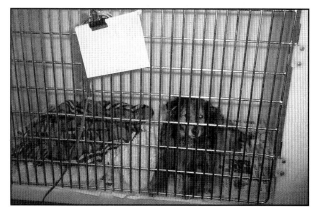

1.6 *Recovery kennel, allowing good patient observation. Photo: Sue Dallas.*

- Clean and disinfect recovery areas
- Check supplies of disposable materials and restock
- Clean floor.

Kennels and wards

Patients move from the recovery area to the inpatient wards (Figure 1.7). These wards are normally situated as far as possible from the consulting and reception areas of the clinic.

- Kennel wards must:
  - Be durable
  - Be secure
  - Be easy to clean
  - Retain heat
  - Allow good observation of the patient
- Kennels must be of the correct size for the type of patient housed and should be made of a material that is non-permeable and is easy to clean and disinfect
- Heating and ventilation are important to assist in maintaining a patient's body temperature, while providing good oxygen levels in the room atmosphere
- For further improvement of the atmosphere, a combination of air conditioning and scavenging systems may be used
- Noise from inpatients is controlled by good soundproofing. Materials used to isolate the noise in the animal ward area include:
  - Acoustic tiles fitted to ceiling and floor
  - Walls well insulated and lagged
  - Double-glazing fitted to any window
  - Self-closing internal doors.

Sick and recovering animals often cannot control urination and defecation; therefore more frequent attention to and cleaning of a soiled kennel is required (Figure 1.8).

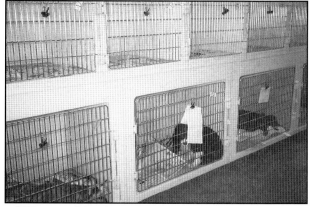

1.7 *Tiered clinic kennels for temporary holding. Photo: Sue Dallas.*

1.8 Daily cleaning routine for kennels and wards

- Remove waste from all bins; replace the plastic liner
- Clean and disinfect walls
- Spot-clean surfaces, doors, cupboard doors, light fixtures, drip stands and any other items routinely kept in this area
- Check and restock any disposable materials
- Clean and disinfect the sink (if any)
- Clean and disinfect the floor
- Disinfect and store cleaning equipment
- Launder all used bedding.

Before disposal of waste materials, check that a sample is not required. If a sample has been requested by the attending veterinary surgeon, it should be collected in an appropriate container, sealed/labelled and refrigerated. There should be a note on the case card that collection has taken place.

Grooming facilities

Grooming facilities may be attached to the clinic as an additional customer service and to enable patients to be groomed before discharge. A bath tub, grooming table and dryers are required. The grooming clippers, combs and brushes are stored and cared for here. For more detail on grooming, see *BSAVA Manual of Veterinary Care* (Chapters 2, 3 and 6).

Exercise run

For reasons of security, exercise areas are adjacent to the kennel wards and there are escape-proof fences or walls between the two (Figure 1.9). The run area is often located within an insulated area of the clinic for control of environmental temperature and noise levels. For details of cleaning and disinfection (Figure 1.10), see Chapter 5 in *BSAVA Manual of Veterinary Care*.

Kitchen/food preparation area

The kitchen is where food is stored and prepared for inpatients.

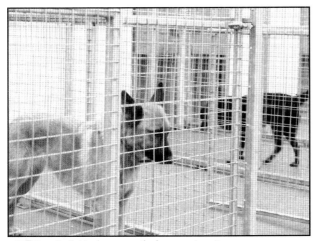

1.9 *Individual run areas for long-stay inpatients. Photo: Sue Dallas.*

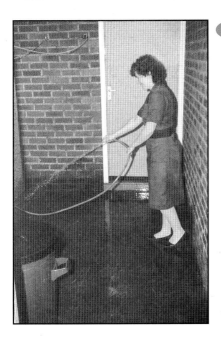

1.10 *Cleaning the run areas. Photo: Sue Dallas.*

- With a variety of species being catered for, a range of tinned, dry and fresh foods needs to be stored
  - The dry foods must be stored in dry rodent-proof containers and labelled for content
  - A storage area is needed for the various types of tinned food, with easy viewing for stock control
  - A refrigerator should be available for the storage of part-used tinned foods, perishables and fresh foods
- The work/preparation surfaces must be durable and easy to clean and disinfect
- There should be a good-sized sink unit, with drainer, for the preparation and washing of fresh leafy foods
- There needs to be a sufficient area of work surfaces to accommodate the washing up, drying and storage of bowls and containers.

Isolation and barrier nursing

If an animal in the practice hospital shows signs of ill health that could be transmitted to other patients, then it should be moved immediately to the isolation unit so that other patients are not exposed and put at risk. For various reasons (disease, stress, injury or not yet vaccinated) these other patients are considered to be susceptible hosts.

The methods used to control the transmission of microorganisms shed by a patient will vary:

- Good ventilation of the isolation area is essential in the control of airborne disease; therefore isolation units need to have a separate air-handling system from the rest of the clinic
- A range of environmental disinfectants is kept in the isolation unit, providing choice in the elimination of specific microbes
- Antiseptic hand-cleaners for use between patients and the wearing of disposable gloves when handling patients are essential
- Although a surgical mask may not be needed routinely, its wearing is recommended when nursing animals with airborne zoonoses (e.g. birds with psittacosis)
- Use of disposable paper towels for hand-washing and cleaning will further reduce transmission of infection
- No visitors should be allowed in the isolation unit – only key nursing staff
- The presence of all disease vectors such as flies, fleas and lice should be actively investigated and eliminated
- Any reusable materials or equipment should be autoclaved within the isolation area before being used on other patients.

The following rules apply to the isolation unit.

- The unit must be totally self-contained, with all its own equipment for feeding, nursing and cleaning
- One nurse should be allocated to this area and should have no other duties in the animal areas
- A foot bath should be used and clothing changed on entering and leaving the unit
- There should be a supply of disposable protective clothing
- Effective and appropriate disinfectants should be used
- Personal and environmental hygiene should be strict
- All waste from the unit should be disposed of safely

- The patient should have no contact with other animals
- Cages, kennels and runs should be contained within the unit
- The unit should have its own sink/kitchen area (with hot and cold water)
- There should be a treatment table and medical supplies
- There must be a good ventilation system (to deal with airborne microbes).

If the unit is well designed its entrance will be separate from that of the main hospital. This enables patients with suspected contagious diseases to be taken directly to isolation.

All soiled cage papers and bedding, also other body discharges such as blood, saliva, urine, faeces and eye and nasal discharges, should be disposed of in the normal way (i.e. as clinical waste). For details on correct disposal methods, see Chapter 5 in *BSAVA Manual of Veterinary Care*.

 Apart from possible transfer of microorganisms to other patients, there may also be the risk of the transfer of zoonoses to the nursing staff.

In certain cases, the owners of a patient discharged from isolation should be informed that their pet may shed the infectious microorganism responsible for its disease for some time. Therefore they should limit contact with other animals during that period and be aware of hygiene issues in the case of diseases transmissible to humans (e.g. leptospirosis).

Care and monitoring of the inpatient

Nursing care is one of the most important duties of the veterinary nurse. Attending to the patients' well-being and monitoring vital signs are paramount in providing good nursing care.

It is important to consider the individual patient. Quite often in a busy veterinary establishment, where there may be an urgency to 'get the job done', it is easy to forget the simple approaches to caring for the patient. It is important to monitor standard parameters of hospitalized patients on a regular basis and record the findings. Early detection of abnormalities permits rapid intervention, preventing deterioration of the individual patient.

Standard parameters

Temperature
Temperature in the conscious patient is monitored per rectum using a veterinary mercury thermometer (Figure 1.11).

1.11 **Taking a rectal temperature**

1. Have the patient suitably restrained (see later)
2. Shake the thermometer to return the mercury to the bulb
3. Lubricate the bulb with a lubricating jelly
4. Insert into the rectum with a gentle rotation movement
5. Leave in place for 1 minute
6. Remove and wipe without handling the bulb end of the thermometer
7. Read and record the temperature.

Normal values are:

- **Dog:** 38.3–38.7°C
- **Cat:** 38.0–38.5°C.

Abnormalities in body temperature are described as follows:

- Hyperthermia – general term for elevation of body temperature above the normal range
  Causes include: heat stroke, exercise, seizures, heat pads.
- Fever (pyrexia) – elevation in body temperature
  Causes include: bacterial or viral infection, pain.
- Hypothermia – reduction of body temperature below the normal range
  Causes include: hypovolaemic shock, general anaesthesia; can commonly occur in neonatal, geriatric or compromised patients, impending parturition.
- Diphasic – fluctuating temperature
  Causes include: canine distemper and other infections.

Pulse
Blood pumped into the aorta during ventricular contraction creates a wave that travels from the heart to the peripheral arteries. This wave is referred to as a pulse.

The pulse is palpated by lightly placing the index and middle fingers on a part of the body where an artery crosses bone or firm tissue. The most common pulse points assessed in the conscious patient are the femoral and dorsal pedal arteries.

Normal values are:

- **Dog:** 60–140 beats per minute (size-dependent – very small and young animals have higher pulse rates)
- **Cat:** 110–180 beats per minute.

Abnormalities:

- Raised rate
  Causes include: pain, fever, early shock, exercise
- Lowered rate
  Causes include: unconsciousness, debilitating disease, sleep, anaesthesia
- Weak
  Causes include: poor peripheral perfusion, hypovolaemia
- Irregular
  Causes include: cardiac dysrhythmias.

Mucous membrane colour
Non-pigmented mucous membranes should be pink. The colour depends upon blood haemoglobin concentration, tissue oxygen levels and peripheral capillary blood flow.

Mucous membrane colour is most commonly assessed at the gums. The conjunctiva of the eye or membranes of the vulva or penis can also be used.

Abnormalities in mucous membrane colours are shown in Figure 1.12.

Capillary refill time
Capillary refill time (CRT) is a measure of blood flow to the capillary beds of the membranes. This flow depends on cardiac output.

To determine capillary refill time, pressure is applied by the index finger to a non-pigmented area of the mucous membranes and then released. The time required for colour to return to the blanched area is recorded as the capillary refill time. The normal value is 1–2 seconds.

1.12 Abnormalities in mucous membrane colours

Pale – decreased haemoglobin concentration, poor perfusion
Causes include: anaemia, shock.

Blue (cyanosis) – inadequate oxygenation of tissues
Causes include: hypoxaemia.

Brick red – hyperdynamic perfusion, vasodilatation
Causes include: early shock, hyperexcitability, sepsis, fever.

Yellow (icteric/jaundiced) – bilirubin accumulation
Causes include: hepatic–biliary disorders.

Red/brown spotting (petechiation) – clotting or bleeding disorders
Causes include: platelet disorder, warfarin poisoning.

Abnormalities:

- Prolonged time (> 2 seconds) – poor peripheral perfusion
  Causes include: later stages of shock, severe vasodilation or vasoconstriction, pericardial effusion, heart failure.

- Rapid time (< 1 second)
  Causes include: anxiety, compensatory shock, fever, pain.

Respiration

Respiration is the exchange of oxygen and carbon dioxide between the air and tissue. The rate and pattern of breathing and the effort required to breathe are controlled by the brain and respiratory muscles.

To monitor respiration requires observation of movements of the thoracic wall or placing the hands lightly on either side of the ribs. The respiratory rate is assessed by counting the expansions of the ribs.

The normal values are:

- **Dog**: 10–30 breaths per minute
- **Cat**: 20–30 breaths per minute.

Abnormalities in respiration are listed in Figure 1.13.

1.13 Abnormalities in respiration

Increased rate (tachypnoea)
Causes include: pain, fever, trauma to the brain or chest, anxiety, heat, exercise.

Decreased rate (bradypnoea)
Causes include: trauma to the brain or spinal cord, low blood carbon dioxide levels, drugs (e.g sedatives), sleep.

Noisy loud breathing (stridor or stertor) – may be present with the following:
- **Difficulty breathing in** (inspiratory dyspnoea)
  Causes include: diseases of the nasal passages, larynx, pharynx or trachea (e.g elongated soft palate, laryngeal paralysis, tumours)
- **Difficulty breathing out** (expiratory dyspnoea)
  Causes include: collapsing intrathoracic trachea
- **Rapid shallow breathing**
  Causes include: disease of the pleural space (air or fluid accumulation, e.g pneumothorax, pneumonia)
- **Laboured breathing** on inspiration and expiration
  Causes include: pulmonary oedema, contusions
- **Coughing** – harsh and dry, or fluid and productive, or blood (haemoptysis)
  Causes include: congestive heart failure, kennel cough, bronchitis, pneumonia.

Demeanour

The general well-being of the patient should be monitored and recorded. Although the hospital environment is not the normal surrounding for patients, observations should be made for abnormal behaviour – for example, a normally placid dog being nervous and exhibiting signs of aggression or fear. It is important to become familiar with each individual animal: time spent talking, fussing and grooming will usually improve the patient's general demeanour. Visits from the owner and familiar-smelling bedding or toys may also be beneficial for the hospitalized patient.

Walking a patient outdoors may improve demeanour. General assessment is often easier away from the hospital environment. Normal and abnormal demeanours are listed in Figure 1.14.

1.14 Patient demeanour

Normal	Abnormal
• Alert	• Dull
• Bright	• Depressed
• Responsive	• Unresponsive
• Relaxed	• Tense
• Comfortable	• Restless

Posture

Positional changes of the patient may indicate an abnormality.
Abnormalities:

- Lameness – scored 1 to 10 (slight to non-use); assess limbs for pain, heat, swelling

- Praying position – sternal recumbency with the forelimbs extended and slight elevation of the abdomen
  Causes include: abdominal pain.

- Reluctance to lie down
  Causes include: pain, anxiety, dyspnoea.

- Paraplegia – loss of use of two limbs (generally hind)

- Quadriplegia – loss of use of all four limbs
  Causes include: spinal cord disease or injury.

Appetite

Appetite is a significant parameter when caring for the hospitalized patient. Careful observation, measurement and recording of the amount and type of food consumed are important. Recording body weight daily, or even twice daily, will indicate the efficiency of the nutritional support. Good nutritional support is essential for the recovering or ill animal, to provide energy and additional support for the demands of the immune system, for wound healing and for cell division and growth.

Changes in enviroment and diet may affect the patient's willingness to eat and it may be neccessary to encourage free-choice eating. In animals reluctant to eat, free-choice intake can be improved through good nursing techniques such as hand-feeding, petting and positive reinforcement while the animal is eating, and through improving palatability and aroma by warming the food.

Loss of appetite is an early parameter indicating that the animal is unwell and it should be investigated immediately, before the condition of the animal deteriorates. There are many causes for loss of appetite, such as dental infections, pharyngitis, nasal congestion, azotaemia and pyrexia.

Abnormalities include:

- Anorexia – absence of appetite
- Coprophagia – eating of faeces
- Pica – indiscriminate eating of non-nutritious or harmful substances (e.g grass, stones, clothing)
- Voracious – eating large quantities.

Fluid intake

Water is one of the non-energy-producing nutrients that animals require in the largest amounts. Fresh drinking water should always be available to patients, unless contraindicated.

Requirements for normal dogs average from 50–60 ml/kg body weight/day varying with the size of dog. Animals may drink significantly more depending on diet, exercise and environmental factors. Cats require 50 to 60 ml/kg/day.

Abnormalities:

- Adipsia – absence of thirst
- Polydipsia – increased thirst
  Causes include: diabetes mellitus, diabetes insipidus, pyometra.

Urine output

Measuring urinary output is a useful means of assessing hydration and renal function. Urine output can be monitored casually by observation; accurate measurement requires indwelling urinary catheterization.

Normal urine output is 1–2 ml/kg body weight/hour.

The act of urination (micturition) should be carefully observed and any difficulty recorded. Assessment of colour, smell and clarity should be recorded.

Hospitalized patients should be given regular opportunities to urinate and defecate. The majority of dogs will not soil indoors and may become distressed and uncomfortable if unable to go outside. Cats should be provided with clean litter trays.

Abnormalities in urine output and urination are listed in Figure 1.15.

1.15 Abnormalities in urine output and urination

Oliguria – urine output of less than 0.5 ml/kg/hour
Causes include: dehydration, renal disease, urinary obstruction.

Dysuria – difficult or painful urination

Haematuria – presence of blood in the urine

Anuria – total absence of urination
Causes include: urinary calculi, prostatic enlargement, acute renal failure.

Polyuria – increased urine production (generally associated with polydipsia)
Causes include: diabetes mellitus, diabetes insipidus.

Defecation

The amount and frequency of faecal material passed should be monitored and recorded. The faeces should be assessed for texture, colour and smell.

Abnormalities:

- Constipation – passing small amounts of hard faeces
  Causes include: rectum or colon obstructions (tumours, foreign bodies); dehydration; environmental factors such as kennel confinement, soiled litter trays; prostatic enlargement; ingested bones.
- Diarrhoea – frequent passage of abnormally soft or liquid faeces
  Causes include: unsuitable diet or changes in diet; bacterial infection; canine parvovirus; colitis.
- Dyschezia – pain on defecation
  Causes include: rectal/anal disease; back pain.

Vomiting

Vomiting (emesis) refers to a forceful ejection of gastric contents through the mouth. This occurs during a forceful sustained contraction of the abdominal muscles. It is generally accompanied by nausea, hypersalivation and heaving. Serious consequences of vomiting include aspiration pneumonia and fluid/electrolyte depletion.

Induction of vomiting may be used to empty the stomach contents, generally to eliminate poisonous substances following accidental ingestion. Emesis is contraindicated in cases of corrosive poisoning or for unconscious or convulsing patients.

Regurgitation should be differentiated from vomiting: it is the retrograde movement of ingested material, usually before it reaches the stomach. Regurgitation is the passive returning of food.

It is important to assess and monitor the volume, frequency and contents of vomitus.

Normally the stomach is completely empty 4–6 hours after eating.

- Vomiting immediately after eating
  Causes include: food intolerance, overeating, stress, excitement, gastritis, hiatal disorder
- Vomiting more than 6 hours after eating
  Causes include: gastric motility disorder, gastric outlet obstruction.

Contents of the vomitus:

- Observe whether either undigested food or clear fluid is present
- **Bile** – bilious vomit
  Causes include: inflammatory bowel disease, intestinal foreign bodies, pancreatitis
- **Blood** – haematemesis
  Causes include: gastric mucosal disorders, poisons.

Type of vomiting:

- **Projectile vomiting** – forceful ejection of stomach contents
  Causes include: gastric or proximal bowel obstruction.
- **Intermittent chronic vomiting** – cyclic
  Causes include: chronic gastritis, inflammatory bowel disease.

DAY PATIENTS					
GEN. DEF LABEL			DATE: VET: PROCEDURE:		

TIME:	T=0		T+1	T+3		T+6
Temperature:						
Pulse rate:						
Respiratory rate:						
MM/CRT:						
Quality of Recovery:						
Pain Score & Demeanour:						
Analgesics given? ☐~ in pre-med ☐~ at surgery ☐~ post operatively:						
Comments and Consumables used:						
Intravenous fluid rate: Fluid:						

Treatments to be given out at discharge:	Start giving:	Given to client?

POPC: .... At: .... Outcome: ....
Recovery Sheet ☐ *Given?* ☐   Itemised Bill ☐ *Given?* ☐
Discharge Appointment: ☐~ Vet ☐~ Nurse ☐~ VHA ☐~ Staying In
Follow-up Appointment in .... days with ☐~ Vet ☐~ VHA

LONG TERM HOSPITAL PATIENTS										
Patient name .... Case No.							VET: CLINICAL SUMMARY			
Owner .... Weight										
Tel. No. .... Date of admission										
Species/breed .... Age .... MALE/FEMALE										

DATE:										
TIME:										
Temperature										
Pulse/heart rate/min										
Respiratory rate/min										
Vomit										
Faeces										
Urine										
Demeanour										
Appetite										
Water intake										
TREATMENT:										
q										
q										
q										
q										
q										
q										
NUTRITION:										
COMMENTS AND CONSUMABLES USED										
HOSP FEE CHARGED:										

1.16 *Examples of kennel record cards.*

Daily care

The frequency and type of monitoring depends upon the individual patient. Figure 1.16 shows examples of kennel record cards.

- Temperature, pulse and respiration should be assessed at least twice daily in the hospitalized patient
- Where abnormal values have been detected, more frequent and regular checks should be made
- Abnormal discharges from nose, ears, eyes, vulva and prepuce should also be observed and recorded
- Water should be available at all times, unless contraindicated (e.g. vomiting cases, or patients being prepared for general anaesthesia)
- Feeding the hospitalized patient will depend upon the individual but twice-daily feeding is preferable to once a day
- Exercise and toileting should be adapted to each individual case
  - The majority of dogs will not urinate or defecate indoors and should be taken outside at least three or four times a day
  - Dogs receiving intravenous fluids or drugs that may increase urine production should be allowed frequent opportunities to urinate outside the hospital environment
  - Cats require clean litter trays
- Daily grooming and frequent contact will enhance the patient's well-being and provide general impressions of a patient's overall demeanour.

Handling and restraint for routine procedures

Reasons for restraint

- Physical examination
- Blood sampling
- Administering treatment
- Application of dressings
- Clinical examination.

Application

Patients require restraint to prevent injury both to themselves and to the handlers. The majority of patients can be restrained with the minimum of force – heavy handling can often exacerbate the situation. Time taken to become familiar with each individual animal can assist in the restraint procedure.

General restraint

Dogs

- Use a suitable slip lead or collar and lead
- Have the patient in a standing position

- Hold the head gently but firmly on either side of the neck. Alternatively, place an arm under the neck, encircling and gently drawing the patient's head towards the handler's body. The latter technique is more suited to large dogs, or medium-sized to large dogs being restrained on an examination table.

Cats

- Always transport cats in a cage
- Check that doors and windows are closed
- Take time to speak to and stroke the cat in the cage before lifting it out
- If the cat responds in a friendly manner it can be lifted out of the cage: place a hand under the thorax and hold the two front legs between the fingers, with the other hand supporting the hindquarters
- To carry a cat:
  - Place one hand over the back of the head
  - Place the other hand under the thorax and grasp the forelimbs between the fingers
  - Lift into the handler's body, positioning the cat's hindquarters under the handler's elbow
  - The cat is supported in sternal recumbency along the handler's forearm
- The majority of cats do not like to be scruffed and so gentle but firm handling should be exercised – light restraint by placing the hand over the top of the neck may be all that is required for a physical examination
- Aggressive cats require more forceful restraint, and scruffing may be necessary: hold the scruffed cat in lateral recumbency with the hindlimbs drawn away from the body and firmly held between the fingers.

Restraint for blood sampling

Jugular venepuncture

Dogs

- The dog should be placed in a sitting position
  - Small and medium-sized dogs are easily restrained on a non-slip examination table
  - Larger breeds are better restrained on the floor with their backs against a solid surface
- Place a hand under the dog's chin and extend the head upwards
- Take the other arm over the dog's shoulders, pulling the dog's body into the handler's body; place the fingers between the forelimbs and hold firmly. (This technique is not always possible in larger breeds: the hand can be placed around the front of the forelimbs)
- A second handler may be required to support the hindquarters of a larger dog to prevent reversing.

Cats
It is possible to restrain cats in the same manner as small dogs. If a towel is used to cover the cat's body and limbs, the handler has better control and is less likely to get scratched.

Another method of control and restraint for jugular venepuncture is to position the cat with all four limbs and body wrapped in a towel or 'catbag', upside down on the handler's lap, extending the head and neck away from the handler.

Cephalic venepuncture

Dogs

- Place the dog in a sitting position or in sternal recumbency
- Place an arm under the dog's neck and gently draw the dog's head towards the handler's body; restrain firmly
- The other arm is taken over the dog's shoulder to hold the dog's elbow in the palm of the hand. Place the thumb over the radius to compress the vein (Figure 1.17)
- A second handler may be required to support the hindquarters of a larger dog to prevent reversing.

Cats
Cats can be restrained for cephalic venepuncture in the same manner as small dogs. Instead of placing the arm around the neck, place the hand over the top of the neck, turning the head into the handler's body.

Scruffing should only be instituted if the cat becomes difficult to handle.

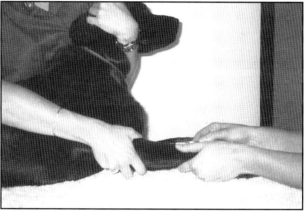

1.17 *Restraint for cephalic venepuncture.*
Photo: Kate Wiggins.

Restraint for the administration of treatment
This is introduced in Chapter 6 of *BSAVA Manual of Veterinary Care*.

Injections
For subcutaneous and intramuscular injections the patient should be restrained in a manner that protects the handler and administrator from being bitten or scratched.

- The animal's head should always be firmly held in any of the positions described above
- Dogs can be positioned either sitting or standing
- Cats should always be restrained on a non-slip examination table, placed in sternal recumbency, with restraint at the head and hindquarters. The person administering the injection can assist with the restraint, by restraining the front or back (depending upon the injection site).

Oral treatment

Dogs

- Place the patient in a sitting position
- Support the head by firmly holding either side of the neck
- The person administering the oral treatment should approach from behind, or from one side of the patient, and take a firm hold of the maxilla with one hand, gently

pulling upwards and slightly backwards. This causes the lower jaw to drop, enabling oral treatment to be placed into the mouth
- Try to place the treatment at the back of the tongue
- Close the mouth, keeping the nose elevated
- Gently massage the pharyngeal area to encourage swallowing.

Cats

- Cats can be restrained in the same manner as described above, with additional restraint of the fore limbs
- The head is drawn back by placing a hand around the back of the neck and holding below the ears. This encourages the bottom jaw to drop, enabling oral treatment to be administered in the same manner as described above.

Restraint for the application of dressings

Bandaging the limbs
The easiest position of restraint for the application of limb dressings in the conscious patient is lateral recumbency (Figure 1.18). A fleece or similar placed on the table will provide a comfortable surface on which to position the patient. The limb to be bandaged is positioned uppermost. Two handlers are usually necessary for bandaging procedures.

- One person can place a patient in lateral recumbency (large breeds require two handlers):
  - Have the patient in a standing position
  - Place the hands over the patient's back and take hold of both forelimbs with one hand and both hindlimbs with the other
  - Carefully lift the patient and allow its body to slide gently and slowly against the handler's body into lateral recumbency
- Use the forearm restraining the front limbs to lie across the patient's neck to control the head
- The fingers should be positioned between the limbs to ensure a firm grip to prevent movement
- The limb to be bandaged is left free and supported independently.

Bandaging the thorax and abdomen

- Have the patient in a standing position
- Place an arm under the neck and gently turn the patient's head towards the handler.

Bandaging the head and ear

- Have the patient in a sitting position
- Place one hand over the back of the neck
- Use the other hand to support the muzzle.

Restraint for clinical examination

- Cardiorespiratory evaluation, taking of temperature, pulse and respiration – standing
- Ultrasonography, electrocardiography – lateral recumbency.

Cover the examination table with a fleece or similar. Patients are more likely to relax and tolerate the procedure if they are comfortable.

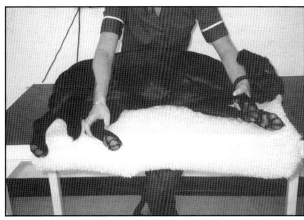

1.18 *Restraint in left lateral recumbency. Photo: Kate Wiggins.*

Aggressive patients
Some patients may require additional methods of restraint due to their aggressive behaviour.

Dogs

- Commercially available muzzles
- Tape muzzles, made from 5 or 7.5 cm white open weave bandage: a loop is placed over the dog's muzzle, crossed under the jaw and tied securely at the back of the neck.

Cats

- Commercial cat-calming muzzle (similar to the dog muzzle but it also covers the whole of the cat's face, including the eyes)
- Crush cage, useful for administering intramuscular injections
- Towel, rolled around the cat and covering the head, body and limbs (a limb can be excluded to access a vein)
- Commercial cat bag: the cat is placed in the bag for restraint (exclusion of a limb allows access to a vein).

Chemical restraint
In extreme cases, where manual restraint is impossible, it may be necessary to administer a sedative or general anaesthetic. These procedures must be under the direction of a veterinary surgeon.

Bandaging

Reasons for bandaging

- Protection
  - of wounds
  - of fractures
  - from self-mutilation
  - from the environment
- Support of fractures pre- and postoperatively
- Pressure
  - to control haemorrhage
  - to prevent and control swelling
- Immobilization
  - to provide comfort and pain relief
  - to restrict movement.

Bandage construction

The majority of bandaging procedures consist of the application of the following layers:

- Sterile wound dressing
- Padding layer
- Conforming layer
- Outer protective layer.

Sterile wound dressings

These dressings are applied directly to broken areas of skin. The type of dressing used depends upon the type of wound involved. Further information is given in Chapter 6.

- Clean wounds – post-surgical, use low-adherent dry sterile dressing
- Wounds with a small amount of exudate – use low/non-adherent sterile dressing
- Contaminated and exudating wounds may require wound dressings to assist with debridement and granulation, such as hydrocolloids.

Padding layer

This layer provides comfort, support and protection. The material used can be either a synthetic or a natural padding. With the exception of cotton wool, padding material is supplied in standard bandage sizes.

Conforming layer

Conforming bandage contours well to the area being bandaged. It compresses and holds the padding layer in place.

Outer protective layer

The final layer provides protection and support and assists with the overall position of the bandage. The types of bandage used are adhesive and cohesive; the latter is self-adhesive and has the advantage of not sticking to hair or skin.

Bandaging techniques

General important bandaging rules are outlined in Figure 1.19.

Robert Jones bandage

Uses

- First aid treatment for immobilizing a limb fracture
- To control swelling and oedema
- Postoperative support.

Materials

- Adhesive tape (2.5 cm)
- Cotton wool
- Conforming bandage
- Adhesive or cohesive bandage.

The bandage widths of the latter two will depend upon the size of the animal (Figure 1.20).

Procedure

Application of a Robert Jones bandage is illustrated in Figure 1.21.
Another method of applying a Robert Jones bandage is to alternate several thin layers of cotton wool and conforming bandage, but adequate and even compression may be more difficult to achieve this way.

1.19 General bandaging rules

Do:

- Prepare bandaging materials ready for application
- Use bandages of the same width and appropriate to patient size
- Have the patient suitably restrained, with assistance to support limb/area to be bandaged
- Clean wounds as necessary; clear away contaminated materials prior to bandage application
- Apply sterile dressings aseptically
- Clip patient's nails if including foot in bandage
- Apply stirrup tapes to distal limb, particularly if applying a Robert Jones dressing (see Figure 1.21)
- Pad between the toes with small amounts of padding
- Apply bandage from distal to proximal to prevent any compromise in circulation
- Apply evenly, overlapping each turn of the bandage by half a width
- Keep the roll of the bandage uppermost, with the flat of the bandage against the patient
- When bandaging limbs, include the foot or leave only the two central toes exposed
- Check the bandage for comfort and ensure that it fulfils the purpose for which it has been applied
- If applying a head bandage, check that the airway has not been obstructed
- Check that the bandage does not interfere with other areas of the patient (e.g. covering the eyes, occluding orifices)
- Check bandages regularly
- Provide the owners with written instructions regarding the care of their pet's bandage.

Do not:

- Use bandages of different widths
- Contaminate clean and sterile dressings
- Use large amounts of padding between the toes (moisture from the sweat glands will be absorbed, which can lead to pressure sores)
- Apply bandage material without a padding layer
- Apply adhesive bandages directly to the skin and hair
- Apply bandages too tightly, unless plenty of padding has been used first
- Apply bandage proximal to distal or start mid-limb
- Leave foot out of bandage – swelling can still occur even with a lightly applied bandage
- Leave pressure bandages on longer than 24 hours
- Use circular application of non-conforming adhesive tape to secure wound dressings prior to bandaging
- Use non-conforming adhesive tapes to hold splints in place without prior padding – be aware that circulation can still be compromised even with a padding layer
- Use safety pins or rubber bands to secure ends of bandages.

1.20 Bandage width and suitability

- 5 cm: cats and small dogs
- 7.5 cm: medium dogs
- 10–15 cm: large dogs.

1.21 Application of a Robert Jones bandage

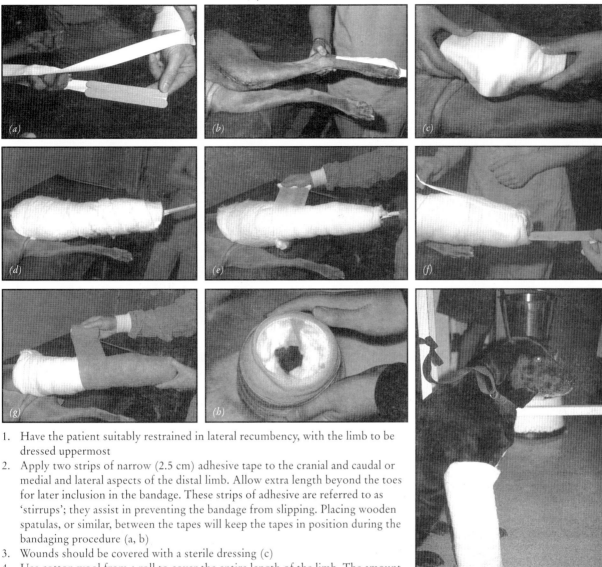

1. Have the patient suitably restrained in lateral recumbency, with the limb to be dressed uppermost
2. Apply two strips of narrow (2.5 cm) adhesive tape to the cranial and caudal or medial and lateral aspects of the distal limb. Allow extra length beyond the toes for later inclusion in the bandage. These strips of adhesive are referred to as 'stirrups'; they assist in preventing the bandage from slipping. Placing wooden spatulas, or similar, between the tapes will keep the tapes in position during the bandaging procedure (a, b)
3. Wounds should be covered with a sterile dressing (c)
4. Use cotton wool from a roll to cover the entire length of the limb. The amount to use depends upon the size of the animal – use at least three layers. Ensure an even thickness to prevent pressure points (d)
5. Compress the cotton wool with conforming bandage applied firmly from distal to proximal (e). Beginning at the toes and working up the limb will assist in preventing vascular constriction distally. The natural angles of the joints should be considered, especially at the elbow in the forelimb and the hock and stifle in the hindlimb. Retaining these angles will help to prevent the bandaged limb becoming effectively longer than the other limb
6. Reflect the stirrup tapes upwards and stick them to the conforming bandage (f)
7. Apply a final layer of adhesive or cohesive bandage, again from distal to proximal, overlapping evenly by half a width to complete the dressing (g). Some makes of adhesive bandage have a central line running through the bandage which assists with overlapping each turn evenly. Avoid applying adhesive bandages directly to the skin as this will be uncomfortable and irritating to the animal. Correctly applied stirrups and a well formed dressing will prevent slipping
8. Leaving the distal extremities of the two central toes exposed allows assessment of temperature and sensation (h). It also encourages the animal to use the limb, allowing some weightbearing on the bandaged structure (i)
9. The bandage should feel firm and solid. It should sound resonant when tapped.

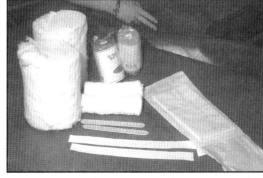

Materials for a Robert Jones bandage.

Photos: R.G. Whitelock.

Care of the dressing

- Check the dressing regularly – initially a few hours after application, to ensure that the toes are not swollen. If they are swollen, the distal end of the bandage may be loosened slightly
- The frequency of subsequent checks or dressing changes will depend upon the reason for the application. For example, any wounds under the bandage may require attention, but in some cases the bandage may be left on for up to 14 days
- Keep the dressing clean and dry. The cotton wool will act like a wick on contact with moisture. Covering the bottom of the bandage with a plastic bag will give some protection when the animal goes outside. The impervious cover should only be temporary and should be removed on return to a dry enviroment. Long-term maintenance of a plastic covering will result in skin complications.

Head and ear bandage

Uses

- As a first aid procedure to control haemorrhage from the pinna
- Postoperatively – to control haemorrhage and swelling following surgeries such as lateral wall resection, total ear canal ablation or drainage of an aural haematoma.

Materials

- Sterile wound dressing
- Cotton wool
- Synthetic padding bandage
- Conforming bandage
- Adhesive or cohesive bandage.

Procedure

Application of a head and ear bandage is described in Figure 1.22.

Care of the dressing

Check that the bandage has not been applied too tightly around the neck. This can be a particular problem in the anaesthetized animal. Observe carefully after extubation. A basic check is to be able to place the fingers easily under the completed dressing.

Ehmer sling

Uses

The Ehmer sling is used to support the hindlimb in abduction with internal rotation following the reduction of a hip luxation.

Materials

- Padding bandage
- Conforming bandage
- Cohesive bandage.

Procedure

Application of an Ehmer sling is illustrated in Figure 1.23.

Velpeau sling

Uses

The Velpeau sling is used to support the shoulder joint following luxation or surgery.

Materials

- Padding bandage
- Conforming bandage
- Cohesive bandage.

Procedure

Application of a Velpeau sling is illustrated in Figure 1.24.

1.22 Application of head and ear bandage

1. The animal must be suitably restrained if conscious, sitting with the head and muzzle supported
2. Wounds should be covered with sterile dressings
3. The ear to be dressed is reflected upwards
4. Place a pad of cotton wool on top of the head and fold the ear on to the pad. Apply another pad of cotton wool over the ear. This technique is particularly useful when controlling haemorrhage from the ear tip
5. Start at the top of the head and apply a padding bandage in a figure-of-eight pattern around the head, leaving the opposite ear out of the bandage
6. Use a conforming bandage to secure in place; again apply in a figure-of-eight pattern

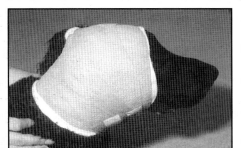
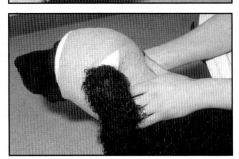
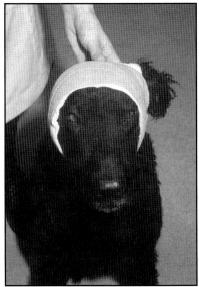

Photos: R.G. Whitelock.

7. A final outer layer of adhesive or cohesive bandage completes the dressing. This final layer is not always necessary, particularly if the dressing is only temporary to control bleeding in a first aid situation
8. Use a pen to indicate with an arrow the direction of the bandaged ear to prevent accidental damage when removing the dressing with scissors.

1.23 Application of an Ehmer sling

The correct application of an Ehmer sling immobilizes the hip joint. This is achieved by flexion and outward rotation of the hock joint, producing abduction and inward rotation of the hip. It is not an easy sling to apply, especially in the short-limbed animal.

1. Apply padding material to the metatarsal region (a). This will assist in preventing swelling but too much will allow the bandage to slip. A small amount of padding can be placed on the cranial aspect of the stifle
2. Apply a conforming bandage to the metatarsus and encircle several times from medial to lateral to secure the start of the bandage. Flex the whole limb, turning the foot inwards. This will turn the hock outwards and the stifle inwards (b)
3. Bring the conforming bandage upwards on the medial aspect of the stifle (c)
4. Return to the point of origin
5. Bring the bandage over the lateral thigh and medial hock (d)
6. Continue over the top of the stifle back to the metatarsus in a figure-of-eight pattern. The foot is rotated inwards and the hock outwards (e)
7. Repeat until full support of the hip is achieved. The bandage is secured with adhesive tape
8. In the short-legged dog and those with a lot of loose skin, the bandage can be taken over the back to encircle the abdomen to provide more stability. The use of a cohesive bandage is ideal in these situations. Conforming bandages tend to slip and the area is too large to be able to apply an adhesive bandage comfortably
9. The limb would generally be supported in an Ehmer sling for 4–5 days.

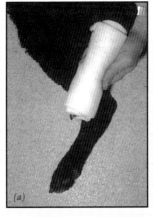
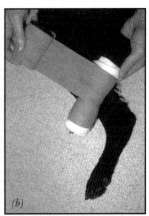
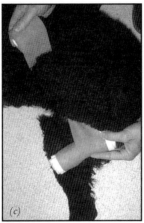
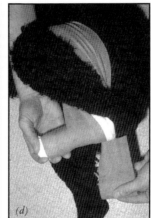
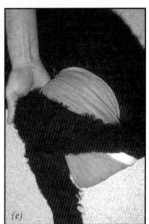
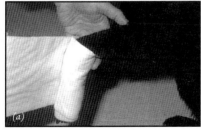

Photos: R.G. Whitelock.

1.24 Application of a Velpeau sling

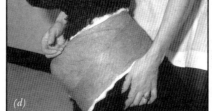
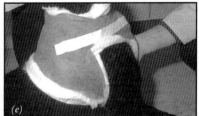

A Velpeau sling maintains the forelimb in flexion, preventing weight being borne by the shoulder joint. The flexed limb is bandaged close to the chest so that the foot is unable to slip out cranially and the elbow cannot move caudally.

1. Apply a layer of padding to the metacarpals and carpus. This will assist in preventing the conforming bandage from tightening excessively in this area. Apply a few turns of conforming bandage (a)
2. Take the bandage up over the shoulder and around the chest (b)
3. Take the bandage behind the elbow of the contralateral forelimb and continue again over the carpus of the flexed limb
4. To prevent the bandage from slipping caudally, it may be necessary to wrap the bandage in a figure-of-eight around the opposite elbow, under and over the chest. Care must be taken that this method does not compromise movement of the contralateral forelimb (c)
5. Continue around the chest, incorporating the flexed elbow and carpus in close proximity to the chest
6. A final complete covering of cohesive bandage will provide extra anchorage of the sling (d,e)
7. The limb would generally be supported in a Velpeau sling for 4–5 days.

Photos: R.G. Whitelock.

Thoracic bandage

Uses

- Trauma – as a first aid measure in the management of a flail chest or thoracic wound
- Postoperatively – to secure and cover a chest drain.

Materials

- Sterile dressing
- Padding bandage
- Conforming bandage
- Cohesive/adhesive bandage.

Use wide bandages (e.g. 10–15 cm width) for larger patients.

In some cases it may be necessary to stick the bandage slightly to the hair to prevent slipping, but be aware of the comfort factor when using adhesive bandages directly on to the patient's coat.

Cohesive bandage may be more practical, as it is easily removed – especially if frequent access to thoracic drains is required. Ensure that the bandage is comfortable and not too tight as this may compromise circulation and respiration.

Procedure

Figure 1.25 describes how to apply a thoracic bandage.

1.25 Application of a thoracic bandage

1. Apply sterile dressings to wounds. A chest drain requires sterile dressings around the insertion of the drain
2. Apply a padding layer in a figure-of-eight pattern around the forelimbs. It is usually easier to start this layer mid thorax, apply a few turns and then proceed from a dorsal to ventral direction, taking the bandage between the front legs
3. Apply another turn around the thorax, then proceed in a ventral to dorsal direction between the front legs to achieve a figure-of-eight. Repeat at least one more time to provide a reasonable padding layer
4. Conforming bandage is the next layer: this is applied in the same manner
5. Complete the bandage with cohesive/adhesive bandage, again in a figure-of-eight pattern.

Abdominal bandage

Uses

- As a first aid measure in the management of abdominal wounds
- Postoperatively – to hold dressings/drains in place
- As a pressure bandage to control haemorrhage.

Materials

As for thorax bandage.

Application

As for bandaging the thorax. If applying a pressure bandage, use a good quantity of padding as a primary layer. Cotton wool or an absorbent pad can be placed over the area of haemorrhage. Use a sterile dressing over open wounds first.

- It may be necessary to extend cranially over the thorax to prevent bunching up of the bandage
- A figure-of-eight pattern can be used around the hindlegs (Figure 1.26) but consider the anatomy of the male dog when applying an abdominal bandage – be careful not to cover the prepuce accidentally.

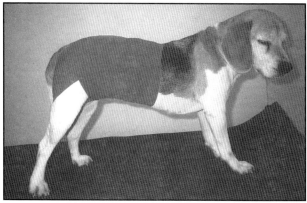

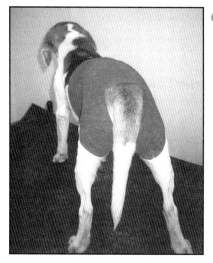

1.26 *Abdominal bandaging. Photos: K.A. Wiggins.*

Pressure bandages

Uses

- To control haemorrhage
- To control swelling.

Materials

- Sterile wound dressing
- Padding
- Conforming bandage, +/– adhesive/cohesive bandage.

Application

To control haemorrhage it is necessary to apply pressure. The easiest method is to apply a pressure bandage. It is possible to apply pressure bandages to most parts of the body but the common areas are the feet, particularly cut pads in a first aid situation. Figure 1.27 describes the application of a pressure bandage to the foot.

Care of the pressure bandage

- If bleeding is observed through the bandage, apply futher padding and conforming bandage
- Pressure bandages should be removed within 12 hours.

1.27 Application of a pressure bandage to the foot

1. Before applying a pressure bandage, check for obvious foreign bodies (see Chapter 3)
2. Surface debris can be gently removed by flushing with sterile saline. Deeper contaminants may require immediate surgical attention
3. Apply a sterile wound dressing to the haemorrhage site
4. It is often not practical to pad the toes
5. Apply three to four layers of cotton wool to cover the foot completely
6. Use a conforming bandage to cover the toes in a cranial-to-caudal and caudal-to-cranial pattern, then continue in a proximal direction, using the standard spiral procedure and covering the whole foot. Extend above the carpus/tarsus
7. It is essential to apply the conforming bandage tightly and firmly. The thick layer of cotton wool will prevent discomfort
8. An outer protective layer can be applied. If using an adhesive bandage, cut off two strips to cover the toe area before using the standard spiral bandage procedure. Cohesive bandage can be applied in the same way as the conforming layer.

Prevention of patient interference

In most cases animals do not interfere with well managed wounds. If patient interference occurs, wound healing is delayed and other complications may ensue. Methods for preventing patient interference are given in Figure 1.28. In some cases it is not apparent why the animal is irritated by the wound and in these situations the animal must be dissuaded from interfering. Surgical sites that are particularly prone to causing patient irritation and interference are:

- *Perineum* (e.g. perineal rupture repair, anal sacculectomy, perineal urethrostomy). This area is predisposed by the sensitive structures involved and the frequency of contamination of incisions. Elizabethan collars are required in many cases

- *Ears*. Surgery of the pinna and ear canal often provokes interference, probably because of the sensitivity of these structures and tendency for wound infection. Elizabethan collars or headbandages are often used
- *Tail*. The tail is a difficult site to protect but surgical wounds are often prone to damage, usually by impact with furniture and so on, rather than patient interference. The tail can be protected by a well constructed bandage
- *Scrotum*. Wounds involving the scrotum or close to it (such as castration) frequently provoke patient interference. This is often because of dermatitis of the scrotal skin initiated by rough surgical preparation. Some surgeons prefer to avoid clipping of this area for this reason. An Elizabethan collar is used if necessary, but in some cases surgery to excise the scrotum is necessary.

Casts and casting materials

Casts are custom-made forms of external coaption. They are used to provide support, particularly in fracture cases. They work by lying in close contact with the skin, conforming well to the area to be supported, to minimize movement at the fracture site and abrasion of the skin.

Uses

- As a temporary splint
- As sole method of management
- Postoperative support.

Casting materials

There are many casting materials available. An ideal casting material should be:

- Strong and relatively light in weight
- Easy to mould to the desired shape
- Simple to handle
- Waterproof but sufficiently porous to prevent maceration of the skin
- Rigid but not so brittle that it will splinter with normal use
- Radiolucent
- Easy to remove
- Cost effective.

1.28 Prevention of patient interference

Method	Application
Avoid iatrogenic problems: • Clipper rash • Topical skin irritants • Introduction of contamination or foreign material at surgery • Traumatic surgical technique • Irritating/tight skin sutures	All cases
Bandaging	All accessible sites (areas such as the perineum, groin and axilla are difficult to bandage without causing other difficulties)
Elizabethan collar	All sites except the neck, distal limb and tail
Devices to prevent body flexion (stiff collars, body brace)	Wounds of the trunk and proximal limbs
Tranquillizers	Used with caution and often ineffective alone Long-term use of questionable justification
Topical bitter substances	Sites prone to chewing rather than rubbing or scratching (e.g. not the head or perineum)

Types of casting materials

There are three main categories of materials in common use:

- Plaster of Paris
- Resin-impregnated
- Thermoplastic.

Cast application

Casts are normally applied to approximate a standing position. However, when protecting a tendon repair the limb is placed in a flexed position to relax the repaired tendon.

All limb casts, regardless of type, must include the whole foot or extend to the tips of the toes, leaving only the two central pads exposed for weightbearing. It is dangerous to end a cast above the foot, as circulation may be compromised distally.

Generally a cast should stabilize at least one joint proximal and one joint distal to the fracture. A cast for a fracture of the radius and ulna need not extend above the elbow joint, nor that for a fracture of the tibia above the stifle, as long as the cast is correctly applied and stabilizes the fracture site. However, fractures occurring close to the joints cannot be managed in this way.

Suitable fractures for external fixation by casting are transverse or short oblique fractures which are stable when reduced (see Chapter 6). If a fracture slips easily out of alignment, then it is not suitable for casting.

- General anaesthesia to facilitate muscle relaxation and abolish patient movement is essential for fracture reduction and cast application
- Great care should be taken to prevent a closed fracture becoming an open fracture
- Applying a good cast depends upon technique and efficiency
- It is important to have all materials prepared.

Materials and equipment

- Zinc oxide tape (2.5 cm)
- Padding bandage
- Casting material (number of rolls depends upon type of casting material and patient size)
- Adhesive/cohesive bandage
- Rubber gloves and plastic apron
- Bowl of water (temperature depends upon cast material used).

All types of casting material are activated by water immersion. The water temperature should be approximately 20°C – with the exception of the thermoplastic materials, which require hot water (generally 70°C). It is essential to check the manufacturer's recommendations.

Wear gloves and a protective apron when handling casting material.

Procedure

Figure 1.29 describes how to apply a cast.

Drying times

The length of time for the cast to dry depends upon the material used.

- Resins and thermoplastics feel hard and dry within minutes

1.29 Application of a cast

1. Pad between the toes – take care not to over-pad
2. Apply tape stirrups – cranial/caudal or lateral/medial aspect
3. Apply padding bandage as undercast padding – two evenly applied layers are usually sufficient. Over-padding could lead to loosening of the cast. To prevent soft tissue damage, the undercast padding should extend beyond the bottom and top of the cast material
4. Unwrap cast material. Resin materials harden with exposure to the atmosphere – only open when ready to use
5. Keep hold of free end of cast material roll (once wet, this end is often difficult to locate)
6. Immerse in bowl of water for 2–5 seconds; squeeze gently to encourage full saturation. Thermoplastics require longer (up to 5 minutes) and thicker rubber gloves are usually required, due to the higher water temperatures
7. Remove from water and squeeze gently to remove excess water
8. Apply to limb in a distal to proximal direction, overlapping the material by half a width to achieve an even covering. Do not pull, twist, apply pressure to or stretch the material, as this may result in circulation problems
9. The number of rolls depends upon the material being used. Resins and thermoplastics are very strong (one to two rolls are generally sufficient) whereas plaster of Paris materials are much softer and to achieve the same strength it may be necessary to apply three or more rolls. Patient size will also govern the amount of material required
10. Reflect the stirrups upwards, and apply a cohesive or adhesive bandage over the top of the cast. Do not allow this bandage to adhere to the skin or hair, as this would be uncomfortable and painful for the patient. This layer will assist in keeping the cast clean.

- Plaster of Paris materials can take several hours to become fully dry.

Cast removal

There are many implements for cast removal.

- Cast-cutting saw (electrical oscillating saw) – quick, accurate and easy to use, but very noisy: patients may require sedation. Operators should wear protective clothing, including a mask and goggles
- Plaster shears – good for plaster removal. Resin and thermoplastics are much harder constructions and therefore not easily removed with plaster shears
- Pre-placed embryotomy wire – threaded through a piece of drip tubing and placed between the padding layer and cast. To remove the cast, the wire is pulled at each end to cut through the cast material.

Bivalving

Bivalving is the cutting of the cast longitudinally along the medial and lateral aspects of the limb. This is best achieved with a cast-cutting saw and is more suited to the resin materials; it is not suitable for plaster of Paris. Before using the saw, draw pen guidelines on the cast.

Bivalving can be carried out during the initial cast application. Once the cast is dry, bivalve and then apply strips of 2.5 cm adhesive tape circularly around the cast; apply outer protective layer. The use of the saw is much easier in an anaesthetized patient.

Reasons for bivalving:

- Cost-effective – the cast can be removed and reapplied in situations of fracture assessment
- The split cast can be used to provide reduced support during the later stages of healing by using the caudal half to act as a splint.

Cast complications

Cast complications require immediate attention. Patients with casts should be checked by a veterinary surgeon or veterinary nurse at least every 7–10 days.

- Pressure sores – result from poor cast contouring and application or cast loosening
- Loosening can occur from:
    - Casting a swollen limb (a Robert Jones bandage should be applied initially before casting, until swelling has subsided)
    - Muscle atrophy due to long-term use of a cast
- Movement at the fracture site – can be caused by poor casting technique, resulting in delayed or no healing and skin abrasions
- Skin abrasions at the edges of the cast – due to insufficient undercast padding, causing the edges of the cast to rub the skin
- Ending a cast above the toes, compromising the circulation – causes pain, swelling and inflammation (if the toes are not included in the cast, only the two central toes should be visible)
- Patient interference – chewing cast edges and padding material (can be prevented by use of an Elizabethan collar)
    - May be due to an uncomfortable cast, particularly if the cast was initially well tolerated
    - Check for abnormal odour, swelling, areas of inflammation
    - Check the toes – they should feel warm to the touch

- Cast becoming wet – undercast padding will act as a wick when in contact with moisture; plaster casts soften when wet. Protect from moisture with a waterproof covering (old drip bags provide ideal coverings) but protective covers should only be used in the short term (e.g. when patient is taken outdoors to toilet).

Care of animal with limb cast

After care of an animal with a limb cast is vital to the success of the cast itself. Daily checks should be made and advice given to the owner on appropriate aftercare.

- Keep the cast as clean and dry as possible, waterproof protection is advisable
- Check the two exposed toes for warmth and lack of swelling
- Check for abnormal odours
- Watch for skin irritation at the top of the cast
- Watch for cast slipping
- Prevent patient interference
- Return to the veterinary surgery as soon as possible for a check up if:
    - the animal suddenly stops using the limb
    - the animal becomes lethargic or unwell
    - the animal shows discomfort with the limb

Further reading

Houlton JE and Taylor PM (1987) *Trauma Management in the Dog and Cat*. Wright, Bath

Lane DR and Cooper B (eds) (1999) *Veterinary Nursing, 2nd edn*. Butterworth-Heinemann, Oxford

McCurnin DM (1994) *Clinical Text for Veterinary Technicians*, WB Saunders

Pratt PW (1996) *Medical Nursing for Animal Health Technicians*. American Veterinary Publications, Goleta, California

Smith & Nephew Ltd, Bandaging Factsheets

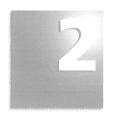

2 Pharmacology and pharmacy

Sally Anne Argyle

This chapter is designed to give information on:

- The different types of drugs used in veterinary practice
- Commonly used abbreviations associated with drug dosing, and their use in association with day-to-day nursing routines
- The different formulations and routes of administration of drugs
- Advantages and disadvantages of each formulation and route described
- Calculation of drug doses and infusion rates
- The different legal categories of drugs
- Safe handling, record keeping and storage of drugs, according to the existing legislation where applicable
- Labelling and dispensing of drugs where appropriate, in a safe and responsible manner and in compliance with the relevant legislation

Introduction

Pharmacology can be defined as the study of the way in which living organisms are affected by chemical agents. It encompasses pharmacodynamics and pharmacokinetics:

- *Pharmacodynamics* can be seen as the effect that the drug has on the body
- *Pharmacokinetics*, in contrast, can be seen as the way in which the body handles the drug. Pharmacokinetics therefore covers the absorption, distribution, metabolism and excretion of the drug.

Pharmacy focuses on the drugs themselves and encompasses the preparation, formulation and dispensing of drugs.
Figure 2.1 shows how drugs may be categorized by:

- Mode of action
- The body system on which they act.

Drugs categorized by mode of action

Chemotherapeutic agents

These are drugs used to treat either invading microorganisms or aberrant host tissue growth (neoplasia). Drugs in this category therefore include the *antimicrobial* and the *antineoplastic* agents. An important characteristic of these agents is that they should by some means be able, selectively, to affect the invasive agent or tissue without damaging healthy host tissue.

 Examples of how drugs may be categorized

Drugs categorized by mode of action	
Antimicrobial agents	Antineoplastic drugs
Anthelmintics	Corticosteroids
Analgesics	Sedatives/tranquillizers
Anaesthetic agents	Antiepileptic agents
Diuretics	Vaccines
Non-steroidal anti-inflammatory drugs	

Drugs categorized by the system on which they act	
Cardiovascular system	Respiratory system
Gastrointestinal tract	Urinary system
Endocrine system	Reproductive system
Nervous system	Immune system
The eye	The skin

Class	Examples	Bactericidal or bacteriostatic	Mode of action
Penicillins[a]	Ampicillin Amoxycillin	Bactericidal	Disrupt bacterial cell wall
Cephalosporins[a]	Cephalexin Cefoperazone	Bactericidal	Disrupt bacterial cell wall
Sulphonamides[b]	Sulphadimidine Sulfasalazine	Bacteriostatic	Block bacterial folate synthesis
Diaminopyrimidines[b]	Trimethoprim Baquiloprim	Bacteriostatic	Block bacterial folate synthesis
Aminoglycosides	Streptomycin Neomycin	Bactericidal	Inhibit bacterial protein synthesis
Tetracyclines	Oxytetracycline	Bacteriostatic	Inhibit bacterial protein synthesis
Macrolides	Erythromycin Tylosin	Bacteriostatic/bactericidal	Inhibit protein synthesis
Fluoroquinolones	Marbofloxacin Enrofloxacin	Bactericidal	Inhibit DNA gyrase – interferes with DNA processing and protein synthesis
Chloramphenicol	Chloramphenicol	Bacteriostatic	Inhibits protein synthesis
Nitroimidazoles	Metronidazole	Bactericidal	Prevent DNA synthesis
Lincosamides	Clindamycin	Bacteriostatic/bactericidal in some cases	Inhibit protein synthesis

a   *The penicillins and the cephalosporins are collectively known as the β-lactams.*
b   *The sulphonamides and the diaminopyrimidines are often combined; for example, trimethoprim and sulfadiazine may be combined in a single preparation. These combinations are known as potentiated sulphonamides.*

For example, the antibiotic benzylpenicillin prevents cross-linking of peptidoglycan, an important constituent of bacterial cell walls. This antibiotic will therefore disrupt the cell walls of susceptible bacteria, thereby killing the organism. Animal cells do not have cell walls and are therefore unaffected by the antibiotic.

Antimicrobial agents

Drugs within this group may be divided as follows:

* Antibacterial agents
* Antifungal agents
* Antiprotozoal agents
* Antiviral agents.

Antibacterial agents

By strict definition, *antibiotics* are the products of other microorgansims and are therefore naturally occurring agents, while *antibacterial drugs* include not only naturally occurring agents but also synthetic or semi-synthetic agents, such as the sulphonamides. However, the terms antibiotic and antibacterial are often used interchangeably, since many of the traditional antibiotics (e.g. those within the penicillin group) have been modified so that they too are synthetic or semi-synthetic and therefore the distinction is no longer relevant.

Antibacterials can be described as either bacteriostatic or bactericidal:

* *Bacteriostatic* implies that the drug slows down the growth of the bacteria, allowing the host's own defence system to overcome the infection
* *Bactericidal* agents kill the invading bacteria.

Figure 2.2 lists the main groups of antibacterial agents, together with examples and modes of action.

Antifungal agents

These are used to treat fungal infections and may be described as fungicidal or fungistatic:

* *Fungicidal* agents kill the fungus
* *Fungistatic* drugs slow or inhibit the growth of the fungal organism, thereby allowing the host's own defence system to overcome the infection.

They may be applied topically or given systemically.

Figure 2.3. summarizes the main antifungal agents used in small animal practice and gives examples of some of their uses.

2.3   **Examples of some of the antifungal agents used in companion animal practice**

Route of administration	Examples of drugs	Uses
Topical	Enilconazole Ketoconazole Miconazole	Treatment of *Malassezia pachydermatis* skin infection. Enilconazole may be used for irrigation of nasal *Aspergillus fumigatus* infection
Systemic	Griseofulvin Ketoconazole Itraconazole	Main use is in the treatment of ringworm

Antiprotozoal agents
These are discussed in the section on antiparasitic agents.

Antiviral agents
Treatment of viral infections generally involves supportive therapy and the use of agents, such as antibacterials, to control secondary infections. A number of antiviral drugs (such as acyclovir and zidovudine) are available but are not licensed for animal use. To date they have been used primarily for ocular manifestations of herpes virus infection in horses and cats. Antiviral agents are highly toxic, with a narrow safety margin, and should therefore be used with extreme care.

Antineoplastic and immunosuppressive agents
Drugs are frequently used in the treatment of neoplastic diseases of small animals. They are of particular importance in neoplastic diseases that are not amenable to surgical management (e.g. lymphosarcomas and leukaemias). They may also be used as an adjunct to surgery (e.g. to reduce tumour size prior to surgery). Drugs used to destroy tumour cells are termed *cytotoxic* drugs. Examples include vincristine, doxorubicin, cyclophosphamide and prednisolone.

 Many of these agents are highly toxic and safety precautions should be strictly adhered to in the handling, dispensing and administration of these drugs. Refer to the section on drug handling.

Many cytotoxic drugs are also immunosuppressants, and drugs such as prednisolone and cyclophosphamide are used in the treatment of conditions such as immune-mediated haemolytic anaemias and thrombocytopenias.

Antiparasitic agents
Antiparasitic agents encompass anthelmintics, ectoparasiticides and antiprotozoal agents.

- *Anthelmintics* are drugs that can be used to prevent or remove a parasitic worm infection from an animal. Most internal parasites (*endoparasites*) in dogs and cats are worms (helminths)

- Ectoparasites live on the surface of the animal and include fleas, ticks, mites and lice. Drugs used to kill ectoparasites are termed *ectoparasiticides*
- *Antiprotozoal agents* are used in the treatment of protozoal infections such as toxoplasmosis and giardiasis. Clindamycin may be used to reduce oocyst shedding in cats infected with *Toxoplasma gondii* as well as in the treatment of clinical signs due to this protozoan in both dogs and cats. A combination of a sulphonamide antibacterial and pyrimethamine has also been used in the treatment of toxoplasmosis. Metronidazole is effective in the treatment of giardiasis in cats; fenbendazole is used to treat giardiasis in dogs.

Anthelmintics
Figure 2.4. lists some of the anthelmintics commonly used to treat endoparasitic infections and provides information on their spectrum of activity. Many of the anthelmintics have a broad spectrum of activity, and drugs such as fenbendazole and mebendazole are effective against all stages of the parasitic life cycle. On the other hand, drugs such as piperazine have little effect on the larval stages of the parasite and therefore have a much shorter duration of effect.

The control of certain endoparasitic infections is of importance from a public health point of view. Parasites such as *Echinococcus* and *Toxocara* can cause zoonoses (disease in humans) and in order to prevent this type of infection, anthelmintics are often used routinely to prevent infection in pet animals and so reduce human exposure to these parasites. For example, the tapeworm *Echinococcus granulosus* inhabits the intestine of dogs, and the segments shed by the tapeworm, when passed by the dog, can be ingested by a number of intermediate hosts, including humans. The adult tapeworm in the dog does not cause disease, but the larval stage, on ingestion, migrates in the intermediate host, and results in the formation of hydatid cysts in tissues such as the liver and lung, which can result in serious illness.

Ectoparasiticides
Control of ectoparasitic infestations is also of importance in domestic animals. These parasites not only produce discomfort and skin disease in the host animal, but they may also be responsible for the transmission of other

2.4 Anthelmintics commonly used to treat endoparasites in the dog and cat

Anthelmintic	Tapeworms			Round worms					
	Echinococcus	*Taenia*	*Dipylidium*	*Toxocara*		*Uncinaria*		*Trichuris*	
				A	L	A	L	A	L
Fenbendazole		✓		✓	✓	✓	✓	✓	✓
Mebendazole	✓	✓		✓	✓	✓	✓	✓	✓
Pyrantel (not cats)				✓		✓			
Piperazine				✓		✓			
Praziquantal	✓	✓	✓						
Nitroscanate (not cats)		✓	✓	✓		✓			
Dichlorophen		✓	✓						

A = adult forms; L = larval stages.
Tapeworms have an indirect life cycle with only the adult inhabiting the intestine of the dog or cat. This means that part of the development (larval stages) occurs in an intermediate host. In the case of Dipylidium caninum, *the flea is the intermediate host. Therefore to control this parasite adequately, flea control should also be implemented.*

diseases or parasites. For example, fleas act as an intermediate host for the tapeworm *Dipylidium*, which infests dogs and cats; lice, fleas and ticks are involved in the transmission of *Haemobartonella felis*, a rickettsial organism which causes haemolytic anaemia in cats. Parasites may also infest and be responsible for skin lesions affecting in-contact humans.

There is now a vast array of veterinary ectoparasiticides. They can be broadly divided into those that act systemically and those that act topically. Figure 2.5 summarizes the main groups of drugs within these two categories. In the case of flea infestations, it is important not only to treat the animal, but also to treat the bedding and the environment. Some of the more novel preparations, such as fipronil and lufenuron, contribute towards environmental control of the parasite by affecting egg laying and larval development. In addition there are separate products specifically designed to treat the environment, e.g. methoprene combined with permethrin.

Anti-inflammatory agents

These are drugs that inhibit or reduce the formation of some of the mediators of inflammation and pain. The two main groups are:

- Corticosteroids
- Non-steroidal anti-inflammatory agents (NSAIDs).

Both groups of agents are anti-inflammatory, *analgesic* (reduce pain) and *antipyretic* (reduce fever).

Corticosteroids

Corticosteroids are frequently used for the management of inflammatory disease, such as arthritis or chronic bronchitis. An example is prednisolone. They also have an important role as antineoplastic and immunosupressive drugs, because in addition to reducing the formation of inflammatory mediators, they also reduce the cellular and (to a lesser extent) the antibody responses, which often play an important role in these diseases. A corticosteroid such as prednisolone is often used as part of a drug protocol for the medical management of neoplasia, or immune-mediated disease, such as autoimmune-mediated thrombocytopenia.

NSAIDs

NSAIDs are also used for the management of acute and chronic inflammatory conditions. Examples of NSAIDs include carprofen, flunixin, ketoprofen and phenylbutazone. Like the corticosteroids, these drugs reduce the formation of inflammatory mediators. The most common side effect involves gastrointestinal ulceration. Other side effects include renal toxicity, hepatotoxicity and blood dyscrasias.

 Cats are particularly susceptible to the toxic effects of paracetamol, due to a reduced ability to metabolize the drug. Its use should therefore be avoided in this species. Paracetamol may be used in dogs, although hepatotoxicity has been reported. Considering the number of alternative products available for use in dogs, paracetamol is probably best avoided.

Aspirin can also cause toxicity in cats, since the excretion of the drug is slow. Aspirin can still be used in cats provided that the dosing frequency is decreased.

It is usually administered only every second day in cats, as opposed to twice daily in the dog.

Antiepileptics

These drugs (Figure 2.6) are used to control epileptic seizures.

Key points relating to the use of antiepileptic drugs

- Start treatment if the seizures are more frequent than once every 6 weeks, or if they occur in clusters, or if status epilepticus occurs (i.e. repeated seizures with no conscious interval)
- Monitor for hepatotoxicity
- Sudden withdrawal of antiepileptic drugs can lead to seizures or status epilepticus
- Monitor plasma levels of the drug
- Avoid the administration of drugs that lower the threshold for seizures to occur. For example, the sedative acepromazine will have this effect and should be avoided in animals with epilepsy.

2.5 Ectoparasiticides commonly used in small animals

Group	Example	Route of administration	Target organisms
Systemic			
Organophosphates	Fenthion	Spot-on	Fleas
Benzoyl urea derivatives	Lufenuron	Oral	Fleas
Topical			
Amidines	Amitraz[a]	Topical	Mites
Carbamates	Carbaril Propoxur	Topical	Fleas
Organophosphates	Dichlorovos and fenitrothion combined	Topical	Fleas and ticks
Fipronil	Fipronil	Topical	Fleas and ticks
Imidacloprid	Imidacloprid	Topical	Fleas
Pyrethrins and synthetic pyrethroids	Permethrin	Topical	Fleas and ticks

a Amitraz is contraindicated in Chihuahuas.
Many of these products have age restrictions regarding use in young animals.
There will be certain species restrictions with different products. Always refer to the data sheet prior to administration.

2.6 Examples of drugs used in the control of epilepsy

Drugs used for seizure control	Comments
Phenobarbitone	Commonly used in canine epilepsy and can be used in cats
Primidone	Used in dogs, start at low doses and gradually increase
Phenytoin	Contraindicated in the cat and rapidly metabolized in the dog. Less commonly used
Potassium bromide	Can be used as an adjunct to therapy with phenobarbital where seizures are not controlled with phenobarbital alone. Very rapidly metabolized in the dog.
Sodium valproate	May help in refractory cases if used in conjunction with another agent

Drugs used to treat status epilepticus[a]	Comments
Diazepam	One of the drugs of choice if given intravenously
Pentobarbitone sodium	Intravenous administration

a Status epilepticus is life threatening and should be treated rapidly. Causes such as hypocalcaemia and hypoglycaemia should be ruled out concurrently.

2.7 Vaccines commonly used in small animals within the United Kingdom

Agents/disease	Species	Type of vaccine	Suggested regimen[a]
Canine distemper virus	Dog	Live	Initial dose at 12 weeks. Booster at 1 year and then every 1 to 2 years
Canine parvovirus	Dog	Live or inactivated	Initial dose depends on dose used. Boosters should be given annually
Infectious canine hepatitis	Dog	Live	Initial dose as early as 8 weeks but repeat at 12 weeks. Boosters every 1 to 2 years.
Kennel cough	Dog	*Bordetella bronchiseptica* live intranasal	From 2 weeks of age. Repeat every 6–10 months
		Parainfluenza virus live	Two doses 3–4 weeks apart, second at 12+ weeks. Annual booster
Leptospirosis	Dog	Inactivated	From 8 weeks, two doses 2–6 weeks apart. Annual booster
Rabies[b]	Dog and cat	Dead	
Chlamydia	Cat	Live	From 9 weeks, two doses 3–4 weeks apart. Annual booster
Feline panleucopenia	Cat	Live or inactivated	From 12 weeks single dose and a booster at 1 year. Immunity may last up to 4 years. Vaccinate every 1 to 2 years, depending on environmental challenge
Feline viral respiratory disease	Cat	Live or inactivated	From 9 weeks. Second dose 2–4 weeks later followed by annual vaccination
Feline leukaemia	Cat	Inactivated	From 9 weeks. Second dose 2–4 weeks later followed by annual vaccination
Myxomatosis	Rabbits	Live	From 6 weeks of age. Repeat every 6–12 months
Viral haemorrhagic disease	Rabbits	Inactivated	From 10–12 weeks of age and revaccinate every 12 months. If less than 10 weeks on first vaccination repeat in 1 month

a The regimens suggested here may vary depending on the particular vaccine used. Always refer to the data sheet.
b Used only with MAFF approval

Vaccines and immunological preparations

Immunity can be active or passive.

- *Passive immunity* can be either due to the transfer of maternal antibodies to offspring or due to the administration of antiserum containing antibodies. This type of immunity is short lived (1–3 months). Maternal immunity may interfere with vaccination and this is why vaccination programmes are not initiated until maternal immunity is considered to have waned (e.g. 12 weeks for canine distemper virus)
- *Active immunity* develops when the immune system is challenged either by a naturally occurring infection or by the administration of a vaccine. This stimulates the individual's own immune response. This type of immunity is in general much longer lasting than passive immunity
- *Vaccines* comprise antigenic material which is given to an animal in order to induce an immune response, usually against bacteria, viruses or parasites. The vaccine may contain *live organisms*, which are still capable of replication, or *inactivated organisms*, which will not replicate. Inactivated vaccines usually require two doses
- *Adjuvants* are agents that, when added to a vaccine, enhance the immune response. Examples are aluminium hydroxide and aluminium phosphate
- *Toxoids* are toxins, obtained from microorganisms, which have been modified so that they will still induce an immune response but are no longer harmful. Tetanus toxoid is the main example.

Figure 2.7 summarizes the vaccines routinely used in small animals in the United Kingdom.

Drugs categorized by the system on which they act

Drugs used in the management of cardiac disease

Cardiac disease is very common in dogs and cats. Figures 2.8 and 2.9 summarize the drugs used in the management of cardiac disease.

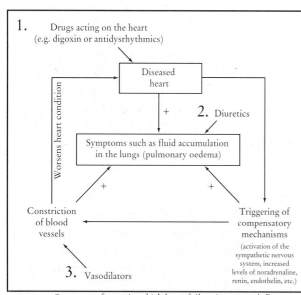

2.8 Summary of ways in which heart failure is managed. Drugs may (1) target the heart itself, (2) reduce the congestion caused by heart failure or (3) dilate the blood vessels.

Respiratory disease

Groups of drugs such as antibacterials, anti-inflammatories and antihistamines are used in the management of respiratory disease. In addition certain groups of drugs are used specifically for their effects on the respiratory system and three of these may require definition.

- In the presence of respiratory disease, the respiratory tract often becomes quite dry, with a reduction in volume and an increase in the viscosity of the secretions produced. This leads to a harsh dry non-productive cough. An *expectorant* increases the production of secretions, thus helping to alleviate the condition.
- A *mucolytic* is a drug that breaks down the secretions, making them less viscous
- An *antitussive* is a cough suppressant.

Figure 2.10 lists the main categories of drugs used in the management of respiratory disease. A couple of additional points are worth making.

- Antitussives should only be used when the coughing is such that it is causing discomfort and distress to the animal. These drugs should certainly be avoided in conditions such as bronchopneumonia, where inflammatory secretions are being produced.
- The main indication for respiratory stimulants is to stimulate respiration in newborn animals.

Gastrointestinal disease

Many of the drugs used in the management of gastrointestinal disease, such as antimicrobial agents and corticosteroids, may also be used for other conditions. Figure 2.11 lists a number of groups of therapeutic agents that are used more specifically for the management of gastrointestinal diseases.

Disease affecting the urinary system

Figure 2.12 summarizes some of the common conditions affecting the urinary bladder, together with examples of therapeutic strategies used to control or treat the conditions listed.

Chronic renal failure

Chronic renal failure is also frequently encountered. Treatment is largely palliative and is aimed at reducing the secondary changes associated with this disease. It includes:

- Fluid therapy
- Diet low in protein of high biological value
- Treatment such as aluminium hydroxide to lower blood phosphate
- Use of recombinant human erythropoietin to treat anaemia (note that this is not licensed in small animals and is not standard therapy at present).

Endocrine disease

Endocrine disorders are generally characterized by under- or overproduction of a variety of hormones. Figure 2.13 summarizes the more frequently encountered endocrine disorders of the dog and cat and also lists some of the drugs commonly used in the medical management of these conditions.

2.9 Summary of the main types of drugs used in the management of cardiac disease.

The categories are not absolute; e.g. venodilators will also help to reduce congestion and oedema formation

Drug type	Example	Effect
Drugs acting on the heart		
Cardiac glycoside	Digoxin	Increases the force of contraction and slows the heart rate
Antidysrhythmics	Lignocaine, procainamide	Reduce or abolish abnormal rhythms
Drugs to reduce congestion and oedema formation		
Diuretics	Frusemide, spironolactone	Increase water loss through the kidney
Drugs that dilate the blood vessels		
Arteriodilators	Hydralazine	Dilate the arteries
Venodilators	Glyceryl trinitrate	Dilate the veins
Mixed dilators	Enalapril, benazepril	Dilate both arteries and veins

2.10 Classification of drugs used in conditions affecting the respiratory system

Drug type	Examples	Action
Bronchodilators	Clenbuterol, etamiphylline camsylate	Dilate the airways
Expectorants	Ipecacuanha	Increase volume of secretions
Mucolytics	Bromohexine	Make secretions less viscous
Antitussives	Butorphanol, dextrometorphan	Suppress coughing
Stimulants	Doxapram hydrochloride	Act as central nervous system stimulants
Antibacterials	Tetracyclines, cephalosporins	Antibacterial
Nasal decongestants	Pseudoephedrine hydrochloride	Constrict the vessels in the nose and help to reduce congestion

2.11 Drugs used in the management of gastrointestinal disease

Drug category	Type	Example	Action
Emetics		Xylazine i.v. Washing soda orally Ipecacuanha	Induction of vomiting
Anti-emetics		Acepromazine, metoclopramide	Reduction of vomiting
Antidiarrhoeal agents	Adsorbents	Kaolin, charcoal	Adsorb toxins and coat the gut wall
	Agents that decrease gastrointestinal motility[a]	Loperamide	Reduce propulsive motility and increase segmental motility
Agents used in chronic diarrhoea	Anti-inflammatory	Prednisolone, sulfasalazine	Anti-inflammatory
	Antibacterials	Oxytetracycline, metronidazole	Used for bacterial overgrowth
Laxatives	Lubricant laxatives	Liquid paraffin	Soften and lubricate the faecal mass
	Bulk-forming laxatives	Bran, sterculia	Increase faecal bulk and promote peristalsis
	Osmotic laxatives	Lactulose, magnesium sulphate	Increase water in the bowel and induce peristalsis
	Stimulant laxatives	Bisacodyl	Promote colonic peristalsis
Antacids		Aluminium hydroxide	Neutralize gastric acid
Ulcer healing drugs	H_2 receptor antagonists	Cimetidine	Inhibit gastric acid secretion
	Sucralfates	Sucralfate	Protect the ulcer site
	Proton pump inhibitors	Omeprazole	Inhibit gastric acid secretion
	Prostaglandin E_1 analogues	Misoprostil	Inhibit gastric acid secretion

a   *Drugs that reduce motility are sometimes contraindicated in diarrhoea, since hypomotility rather than hypermotility may be a feature in some cases. Also, if invasive organisms are involved, reducing motility will only further decrease the rate of expulsion of the pathogens.*

Summary of some of the common conditions affecting the urinary bladder, together with examples of therapeutic strategies used in their treatment and control

Condition	Treatment
Cystitis	**Antibacterials**, e.g. amoxycillin, cephalexin **Acidifiers**[a], e.g. ammonium chloride **Alkalinizers**[a], e.g. sodium bicarbonate

Urinary retention due to:
  Paralysis of detrusor muscle
 	
  Excessive urethral sphincter tone
	
	Bethanecol – a parasympathomimetic drug that stimulates receptors in the detrusor muscle, causing it to contract
	Phenoxybenzamine – blocks receptors on the bladder neck and sphincter, allowing them to relax and allow urination

Urinary incontinence due to:
  Detrusor muscle instability (not common)
  Lack of urethral sphincter tone
	
	Propantheline – a parasympatholytic drug that blocks receptors in the detrusor muscle, reducing contraction
	Phenylpropanolamine – stimulates receptors of the sphincter, increasing tone and reducing urine leakage

a Acidification or alkalinization may improve the action of certain antibiotics. For example, penicillin is more efficacious in an acidic environment, while sulfadiazine is more efficacious in an alkaline environment.

Summary of the most frequently encountered endocrine disorders of the dog and cat, together with examples of drugs used in the medical management of these conditions

Gland	Endocrine disorder	Medical treatment/management

Thyroid	**Hypothyroidism**
	  Most common endocrine disorder in the dog
	  Due to underactivity of the thyroid gland
	Hyperthyroidism
	  Mainly in elderly cats
	  Due to overproduction of thyroid hormones
		
		Liothyronine sodium
		Levothyroxine sodium
		
		Carbimazole
		Radioactive iodine

Adrenal gland	**Cushing's disease**
	  Overproduction of adrenal glucocorticoids
	
	Addison's disease
	  Underproduction of mineralocorticoids and glucocorticoids
		
		Mitotane[a] is the preferred drug
		Ketoconazole
		
		Fludrocortisone acetate
		Prednisolone required initially

Pancreas	**Insulin-dependent diabetes mellitus** Reduced insulin production	 Insulin

Pituitary gland	**Diabetes insipidus**
	  Reduced production of ADH[b]
	  Can also be failure of the ADH to act on the kidney[c]
		
		Desmopressin for central form
		Hydrochlorothiazide for nephrogenic form

a Mitotane is a cytotoxic drug and should be handled with care. It is not generally available in the UK and a Special Treatment Authorization is required to obtain the drug. It should be administered with food to aid absorption.
b ADH is antidiuretic hormone. This hormone is normally produced by the pituitary gland and increases the reabsorption of water by the kidney. Central diabetes insipidus is due to an underproduction of ADH by the pituitary, while nephrogenic diabetes insipidus is where there is adequate production of ADH but the kidney is resistant to the effects of the hormone.
c Nephrogenic diabetes insipidus.

Reproductive system

Examples of drugs used to manipulate the reproductive system are listed in Figure 2.14.

Reasons for use in the female animal may include:

- Suppression of oestrus
- Prevention of pregnancy
- Abolition of pseudopregnancy.

In the male animal reasons for use may include:

- Management of aggressive behaviour
- Management of conditions such as prostatic hypertrophy.

 Care should be exercised at all times in the handling of hormonal substances. Some hormonal preparations should not be handled by pregnant women or asthmatics.

Categories of drugs that have an effect on the reproductive system

Drug	Classification or effect	Uses
Cabergoline	Stimulates dopamine receptors in the anterior pituitary, thus inhibiting the release of prolactin	Used to treat pseudopregnancy in the bitch. Prolactin controls milk production and also maintains pregnancy from day 35
Ethinyloestradiol and methyltestosterone combined	Oestrogen and testosterone	Used to treat pseudopregnancy in the bitch
Oestradiol benzoate	Oestrogens. Prevent implantation	Misalliance – used to prevent pregnancy in the bitch. Should be administered on the 3rd and 5th day following mating. A third injection may be given on the 7th day
Medroxyprogesterone acetate Megoestrol acetate Progesterone Proligestone	Progesterone-like activity	Used for prevention or suppression of oestrus in the bitch, the prevention of oestrus in the cat and (in the case of proligestone) the prevention of prolonged oestrus in the ferret
Methyltestosterone Testosterone esters	Androgens	Suppression of oestrus and pseudopregnancy in the bitch. Male dogs and cats for deficient libido. Hormonal alopecia in cats and dogs
Delmadinone acetate	Progesterone-like activity, acts as an anti-androgen	Used in male dogs in the management of prostatic hypertrophy and carcinoma and perianal gland tumours. Used in male cats and dogs for the management of male aggression and hypersexuality
Oxytocin	Normally secreted by the posterior pituitary; causes uterine contraction as well as stimulating milk letdown	Used in dogs and cats to promote milk letdown after parturition and also for the treatment of uterine inertia (lack of uterine contraction)
Vetrabutine hydrochloride	Inhibits oxytocin-induced contraction of the uterus	Used to inhibit uterine contraction in dogs. Used to delay parturition. Contraindicated in cats

Conditions affecting the eye

A wide range of conditions may affect the eye, either primarily or as part of a more generalized disease. Many of the drugs used to treat conditions affecting the eye are applied directly on to the surface of the eye itself in formulations designed specifically for this purpose. In addition, drugs may be injected into the subconjunctival region or administered systemically. Figure 2.15 lists some of the more frequently used ocular preparations together with their actions and some of the situations in which they may be employed.

Groups of drugs used for the treatment of conditions affecting the eye

Drug category	Examples	Uses
Antibacterial	Chloramphenicol Chlortetracycline	Bacterial infections
Anti-inflammatory	Corticosteroids[a] such as betamethasone	Inflammatory conditions such as uveitis[b]
Immune-modulating	Cyclosporin	Immune-mediated disease such as plasmacytic conjunctivitis of the third eyelid and keratoconjunctivitis sicca
Drugs that dilate the pupil (mydriatics) and reduce spasm of the ciliary muscle (cycloplegics)	Atropine sulphate	Anterior uveitis
Drugs that constrict the pupil (miotics)	Pilocarpine	Glaucoma[c]
Drugs that decrease the formation of aqueous humor	Acetazolamide Timolol	Glaucoma[c]
Tear replacement preparations	Hypromellose	Keratoconjunctivitis sicca[d]
Diagnostic stains	Fluorescein sodium	Diagnosis of corneal ulcers
Local anaesthetics	Tetracaine hydrochloride	Minor surgical procedures

a *Corticosteroids should not be used where there is corneal ulceration.*
b *Uveitis is inflammation of the uveal tract, which comprises the iris, the ciliary body and the choroid.*
c *Glaucoma is a condition associated with elevated intraocular pressure. Constricting the pupil may help to open the drainage angle, allowing the removal of excessive aqueous humor.*
d *Keratoconjunctivitis sicca is due to an underproduction of tears, associated with immune-mediated disease of the lacrimal gland.*

Conditions affecting the skin

Treatment may be achieved by either systemic or topical administration of drugs.

- Topical application allows the direct delivery of the drug to the affected site with minimal systemic effects. Topical treatment may be formulated as shampoos, sprays, powders, ointments, lotions, gels or creams. The formulation is important as it may aid in the penetration of the active ingredient to the skin
- A systemic approach may be more appropriate if the condition is affecting the deeper layers of the skin or if the disease is widespread.

Treatment should aim to:

- Alleviate symptoms
- Tackle the underlying cause.

While the symptomatic approach is quite straightforward, the aetiology of the skin disease may often be difficult to ascertain, or it may not be possible to prevent exposure of the animal even if the cause is identified. For example, many dogs suffer from allergic skin disease associated with allergens such as housedust mite and fleas. Flea control may be relatively straightforward to implement but exposure to housedust mite is unavoidable, although vacuuming may reduce levels of the mite.

Figure 2.16 summarizes the types of agent used in the treatment and control of skin disease.

Ears

A table summarizing the different types of drugs used in the treatment of otitis (inflammation of the ear) is included in Figure 2.16. Ear disease may occur as part of a generalized skin condition, or may be present in isolation. In addition to topical treatment of otitis, systemic administration of drugs such as corticosteroids and antibacterials may be necessary.

 Many of the agents used topically can penetrate the skin of the operator as well as the animal. In particular, care should be taken with the application of topical corticosteroids. Disposable gloves should always be worn when applying these agents. Gloves should be dispensed to owners, along with the drug.

2.16 Categories of drugs used for conditions of the skin and ear

Drugs used in the treatment and management of conditions affecting the skin

Classification	Route of administration	Examples	Uses
Corticosteroids	Topical Systemic	Betamethasone Prednisolone	Control of immune-mediated and inflammatory skin disease
Antihistamines	Systemic	Diphenhydramine	Allergic skin disease
Antibacterials	Topical Systemic	Neomycin Cephalexin	Pyoderma
Sunscreens	Topical	Titanium dioxide Butyl methoxydi-benzoylmethane	Prevention of sunburn and sun exposure, which can be associated with squamous cell carcinoma (white cat's ear tips)
Essential fatty acids	Systemic	Evening primrose oil	Coat condition and allergic skin disease
Antifungal agents	Systemic Topical	Griseofulvin Ketoconazole	Treatment of ringworm and *Malassezia pachydermatis* infections
Ectoparasiticides	Systemic Topical	Lufenuron Fipronil	Flea control
Keratolytic agents	Topical	Selenium sulphide Benzoyl peroxide	Promotion of loosening of the horny layer of the epidermis. Used in conditions such as pyoderma and seborrhoea

Examples of drugs used to treat otitis externa

Condition	Type of agent	Example
Otodectes (ear mites)	Ectoparasiticide[a]	Permethrin
Bacterial infection	Antibacterial	Neomycin
Fungal infection	Antifungal	Miconazole
Inflammation	Anti-inflammatory	Prednisolone

a *Some ear preparations contain no identified ectoparasiticide yet they are still effective against ear mites. Many ear preparations contain a combination of drugs (for example, they may contain an ectoparasiticide, an antibacterial, an antifungal and an anti-inflammatory drug).*

Administration and formulation of drugs

In order for a drug to have the desired effect, several criteria must be fulfilled.

- The drug must reach the site at which it is to act
- It must be present at the appropriate concentration
- The appropriate concentration must be present for a sufficient length of time.

In order to understand how this may be achieved, it is important to have some concept of the fate of a drug after it has been administered to the animal. Figure 2.17 illustrates the main steps involved in the disposition of drugs after administration.

- *Absorption* involves the movement of the drug from the site of administration into the plasma. By definition, drugs administered intravenously bypass the absorption stage. Local blood flow at the site of administration can have an important effect on the rate of absorption. Some drugs can be formulated as depot preparations. This means that there is a more prolonged release of drug from the site, decreasing the dosing interval required. A good example of this would be a depot preparation of penicillin that contains two salts of benzylpenicillin (penicillin G). One salt will give initial cover for 24 hours while the second less soluble, more slowly released salt will extend the antibiotic cover for up to 3 days
- *Distribution* is important as it determines whether the drug reaches the target tissue or not. Some drugs are widely distributed throughout the body and will enter most tissues, while others have a more limited pattern of distribution
- *Metabolism* involves alteration of the drug in some way. It is generally associated with inactivation of the drug but there are exceptions to this. The liver is the main organ involved in drug metabolism and liver dysfunction can reduce the body's ability to deal with certain drugs
- *Excretion* can occur through a variety of routes, such as the kidney, the gastrointestinal tract and the respiratory system. The presence of renal disease, for example, may reduce the ability of the body to excrete certain drugs.

As Figure 2.17 shows, two important factors that influence the fate of the drug within the body are:

- The site, or route of administration
- The formulation of the drug.

These two factors go hand in hand, in that in general drugs are formulated in a specific way in order to facilitate their administration by a particular route.

Routes of administration

Oral administration
This is a common route used in veterinary practice. Factors that can influence gastrointestinal absorption include gastrointestinal motility, splanchnic blood flow and particle size and formulation of the drug. There are several potential problems with the oral route:

- The drug may be inactivated by gastric acid or gastrointestinal enzymes. For example, penicillin G is unstable in the presence of gastric acid and therefore cannot be given orally
- The drug may not be absorbed from the gastrointestinal tract. In some instances this may be desirable. For example, some of the sulphonamide antibacterials are designed to remain in the gastrointestinal tract so that they have a local effect in the gut
- Drugs may be absorbed and undergo rapid metabolism and hence inactivation by the liver. This can preclude the oral administration of certain drugs. An example is glyceryl trinitrate, which is administered transdermally to avoid this effect
- The drug may interact with certain food components. For example, the tetracycline antibiotics bind to calcium-rich foods, hindering absorption
- Some drugs should be specifically be given with food (e.g. griseofulrin) or after fasting (e.g. ampicillin).

Formulation
Drugs for oral use are given as tablets, capsules or liquids (either solutions or suspensions).

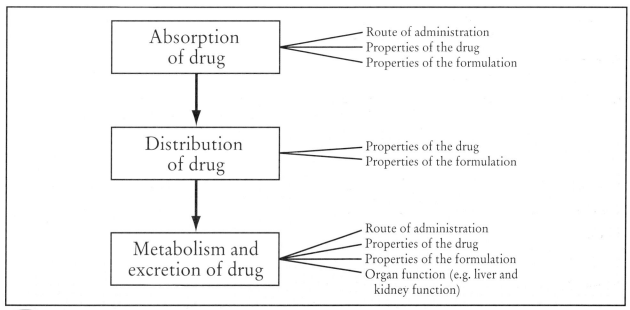

2.17 *The disposition of drugs within the body. On the left are the three main steps in drug disposition. On the right are some of the most important factors that influence drug disposition.*

Tablets may or may not be coated. Reasons for coating a tablet may include:

- Improving the palatability
- Protection from the atmosphere
- Protection from gastric acidity
- Reducing the rate of disintegration of the tablet in the gastrointestinal tract.

Capsules are made up of a hard gelatin case (generally two halves slotted together), containing the drug in granules or powder form. The capsule may contain a mixture of fast and slow release particles to produce a more sustained release of the drug and hence decrease the frequency of dosing required. Capsules should be given whole to the animal.

Liquids may contain the drug either in solution (the drug is dissolved in the liquid), or suspension (the drug particles are suspended in the liquid, and often settle to the bottom if left standing). Suspensions must always be well shaken prior to use, to resuspend the drug particles.

Parenteral administration

Parenteral administration implies injection of the drug. A number of different sites and routes may be used. Drugs may be injected rather than given orally for a number of reasons. For example:

- The drug may not be well absorbed by the oral route
- The drug may be inactivated by gastric secretions
- Injection of the drug may achieve more rapid and reliable therapeutic levels of the drug.

- All solutions, needles and syringes used for injection must be sterile and pyrogen free.
- Aseptic precautions should be observed at all times.
- Drugs should not be mixed in the same syringe as they may react with one another having a detrimental effect.

Drugs may be injected into the following sites:

- Intravenous (i.v.)
- Subcutaneous (s.c.)
- Intramuscular (i.m.)
- Intradermal
- Intrathecal
- Subconjunctival
- Intraperitoneal (i.p.).

Intravenous injection

This is the fastest route for drug administration, bypassing absorption. Intravenous administration requires the drug to be in solution, as particles in suspension may obstruct small vessels. Intravenous injection should be carried out slowly. Rapid injection of a drug bolus may cause adverse reactions, such as collapse. Drugs administered intravenously include some antimicrobials, diuretics and intravenous anaesthetics. The cephalic vein in the forelimb, the saphenous vein in the hindlimb and the jugular vein in the neck are examples of vessels used for intravenous injection of drugs.

Subcutaneous and intramuscular injection

The main determinant of absorption of drugs administered subcutaneously or intramuscularly is local blood flow.

Subcutaneous injections are administered in areas where the skin is loose (mainly the scruff of the neck in small animals). The plunger of the syringe should always be pulled back to ensure that the needle is not located within a blood vessel.

Intramuscular injections in general are more painful. The main site for intramuscular injection is the muscle mass of the hindlimb. Some drugs can cause marked local pain and inflammation at the injection site (e.g. the tetracycline antibiotics). Some drugs are so irritant that they may only be administered intravenously (e.g. the antitumour antibiotic doxorubicin and the intravenous anaesthetic thiopental). Extravascular injection of these substances can lead to severe tissue necrosis and sloughing of the skin overlying the site of injection.

Intradermal injection

This is used for intradermal skin testing: a panel of allergens is injected intradermally to determine the cause of allergic skin disease.

Intrathecal injection

This is injection of a drug into the subarachnoid space. It is rarely used in veterinary practice.

Intraperitoneal injection

This may be useful in very small animals (e.g. hamsters) for the administration of anaesthetic agents or fluids. The peritoneum provides a large surface area for the absorption of the drug.

Rectal administration

Rectal administration of drugs is not frequently used in veterinary practice.

Inhalation of drugs

This is the route of administration of volatile and gaseous anaesthetics such as halothane and nitrous oxide. Other drugs used in the treatment of respiratory conditions may also be administered by this route. For example, the antimicrobial gentamicin may be administered by nebulization to dogs with bronchopneumonia, in addition to the administration of systemic antimicrobials.

Transdermal administration

Drugs may be applied to the skin in order to produce a systemic effect. This can be useful to avoid first pass metabolism by the liver (seen with some drugs on oral administration). The vasodilator glyceryl trinitrite is administered this way, as is the ectoparasiticide fenthion.

Topical administration

In this case the drug is applied directly to the area where it is required. This is suitable for administration of drugs to a number of sites, such as the skin, the ear and the eye. Topical administration of a drug may avoid undesirable systemic effects, although in some cases drugs applied topically can be absorbed to give significant systemic levels. This tends to be the case with drugs that have good lipid solubility (fat solubility), which enables them to cross the barriers of the skin and conjunctiva (e.g. the topical administration of corticosteroids to the eye or ear). Figure 2.18 lists the different types of formulations used for topically administered drugs.

2.18 Different drug formulations used for topical administration

Formulation	Comments
Creams	Water-miscible, non-greasy and easily removed by washing and licking
Ointments	Greasy, insoluble in water and generally anhydrous More difficult to remove than creams
Dusting powders	Finely divided powders
Lotions	Aqueous solutions or suspensions Evaporate to leave a thin film of drug at the site
Gels	Aqueous solutions that are semi-solid Easy to apply and remove
Sprays	Disperse fine droplets
Shampoos	Convenient for skin treatment

Calculation of drug doses

 The ultimate responsibility for the calculation of doses lies with the veterinary surgeon. Nurses given the responsibility for calculation of doses should always check with the veterinary surgeon responsible for the case.

Most doses are described in terms of weight, and the recommended dose for an animal is generally expressed in terms of the weight of drug/kg body weight of the animal. Alternatively the dose may be expressed in terms of weight of drug per unit of body surface area (usually per square metre). This is the case for digoxin and some of the drugs used in the chemotherapy of malignant disease. Charts are available allowing the conversion of body weight into body surface area.

The main units of weight are: kilogram (kg); gram (g); milligram (mg); and microgram (can be abbreviated to mcg or µg but in handwriting may be difficult to distinguish mg and µg and it is therefore wiser not to abbreviate).

- 1 kg = 1000 g
- 1 g = 1000 mg
- 1 mg = 1000 micrograms.

- *Drugs in tablet and capsule form* state the weight of the active drug contained in each tablet or capsule. A particular drug may come in a variety of different strengths
- *Drugs in liquid form* contain the weight of drug per unit volume of liquid, e.g. the number of mg/ml, where 1 litre (1 l) = 1000 millilitres (1000 ml)
- The concentration of drugs in liquid form may also be expressed as percentage solutions. For example, a 1% solution means that there is 1 g of drug in 100 ml of the solution
- There are some exceptions to these formats. For example, insulin is expressed in international units/ml (IU/ml), and is administered in special 1 ml syringes that are graduated in international units rather than millilitres.

Example 1

A 25 kg collie requires treatment with ampicillin for 7 days. The recommended dose rate is 15 mg/kg twice daily. The capsules come in either 50 mg or 125 mg strengths. Calculate the daily dose of ampicillin for this dog.

15 (dose rate) x 25 (body weight of dog) = 375 mg twice daily.

Which strength capsule would you use?
The 125 mg size. The dog would require three tablets twice daily.

How many capsules should be dispensed to the owner?
Three tablets twice daily is six tablets per day x 7 days = 42 tablets required in total.

Example 2

A 30 kg dog requires treatment with oxytetracycline. The recommended dose for injection ranges from 2 to 10 mg/kg daily. There is a 10% solution of oxytetracycline for injection. Calculate a dose for this animal.

A 1% solution contains 1 g/100 ml. Therefore a 10% solution contains 10 g/100 ml, which is the same as 100 mg/ml.

Taking the top end of the dose range, the dose required by the dog will be 10 (dose rate) x 30 (body weight) = 300 mg dose.

The volume for injection will be the total calculated dose required divided by the concentration = 300 mg/100 mg = 3 ml of the 10% solution.

Example 3

A 10 kg dog has developed a heart rhythm abnormality after abdominal surgery. A bolus injection of lignocaine intravenously has abolished the rhythm but the dog now needs to be maintained on a constant rate infusion of the drug at a rate of 50 micrograms/kg/minute given in intravenous fluids. The fluids in a 1 litre bag are to be given at a rate of 10 ml/kg/h. How much lignocaine needs to be added to the bag to give the drug at a rate of 50 micrograms/kg/minute?

As both the rate of fluid administration and the rate of drug administration required are known, it is easier to express them both in the same units of time:

- Drug administration: 50 micrograms x 10 (weight of dog) = 500 micrograms/minute. This equals 500 x 60 = 30 000 micrograms/hour = 30 mg of lignocaine per hour
- Fluid administration: at a rate of 10 ml/kg/hour = 100 ml per hour for a 10 kg dog.

Therefore there needs to be 30 mg of lignocaine in every 100 ml of fluid.

In a 1 litre bag there is 10 x 100 ml, so it needs 10 x 30 mg of lignocaine. The 300 mg of lignocaine is added to the 1 litre bag of fluids which will give an infusion rate of 50 micrograms/kg/minute if the fluids are administered at a rate of 10 ml/kg/hour.

Legislation

In veterinary practice, legislation governs the handling, usage, storage and prescribing of veterinary medicines.

Veterinary surgeons and nurses working within veterinary practice must be aware of the legislation: it has been set in place to protect the animal, the practitioner, the nurse and the client.

The relevant legislation governing these areas includes the following:

- Medicines Act 1968
- Health and Safety at Work etc., Act 1974
- Control of Substances Hazardous to Health Regulations 1988 (enacted under the Health and Safety at Work etc., Act 1974)
- Misuse of Drugs Act 1971
- Medicines (Restrictions on the Administration of Veterinary Medicinal Products) Regulations 1994.

Classification of veterinary medicines

"A veterinary medicine is any medicinal product intended for animals and applies to veterinary medicinal products offered for sale *inter alia* (among others) in the form of proprietary medicinal products and readymade veterinary medicinal products" (Bishop, 1998).

Veterinary medicines may be classified as:

- General sales list (GSL)
- Pharmacy only (P)
- Pharmacy and merchants list (PML)
- Prescription only (POM)
- Controlled drugs (CD).

General sales list (GSL)

A veterinary surgeon may sell GSL medicines to anyone without restriction, whether they are a client or not. Examples include piperazine anthelmintic preparations.

Pharmacy only (P)

These medicines can be supplied by a veterinary surgeon for administration to an animal under their care or over the counter by a pharmacist. Very few veterinary medicines fall into this category.

Pharmacy and merchants list (PML)

PML medicines may be supplied by a pharmacist over the counter, or by veterinary surgeons for animals under their care. They may also be supplied by an agricultural merchant who is registered with either the Royal Pharmaceutical Society of Great Britain (RPSGB) or the Department of Agriculture in Northern Ireland (DANI). The merchant, however, may only supply to people who keep animals for the purpose of carrying on a business, although registered merchants and saddlers may also sell a small amount of anthelmintic to horse, dog and cat owners.

Prescription-only medicines (POM)

As with the P and PML medicines, POMs can be supplied by veterinary surgeons for administration to animals under their care. They may also be supplied by a pharmacist but only on a veterinary surgeon's prescription.

A veterinary surgeon may be prosecuted under the Medicines Act 1968 for supplying P, PML or POM drugs for the treatment of animals not deemed to be under his/her care. There is no legal definition of 'animals under his/her care' but the Royal Veterinary College requires that a number of criteria should be met for an animal to fall into this category:

- The veterinary surgeon should have been given responsibility for the animal's health by its owner
- The veterinary surgeon should have seen the animal for the purpose of diagnosis or prescription, or have visited the premises in which the animal is kept, sufficiently often and recently to have sufficient personal knowledge, enabling the veterinary surgeon to make a diagnosis and prescribe for the animal in question.

Controlled drugs (CD)

These are drugs that might be abused. Under the Misuse of Drugs Regulations 1985, controlled drugs are divided into five Schedules:

- *Schedule 1*. Veterinary surgeons have no reason or authority to possess or prescribe these drugs. This category includes LSD and cannabis
- *Schedule 2*. Examples in this group include fentanyl and morphine. There are special requirements concerning the prescribing, requisition, storage, record keeping and disposal of these drugs
- *Schedule 3*. This group includes buprenorphine, pentobarbitone and phenobarbitone. There are special requirements for the prescribing and requisition of these drugs, but they do not need to be entered on a drugs register
- *Schedule 4*. Benzodiazepines and anabolic substances are included. They do not require most of the restrictions required for drugs in Schedules 1–3
- *Schedule 5*. Preparations containing cocaine, codeine and morphine in less than specified amounts. They are exempt from the controlled drug requirements except that invoices must be kept for a period of 2 years.

Controlled Drugs Register: records are required for Schedule 2 drugs. This must be in a bound book with sections designated for each drug. An entry must be made within 24 hours of receipt of the drug and every time that it is used. Entries must be legible and indelible and must not be amended. The Register must be kept for 2 years from the last entry. Figure 2.19 shows the recommended layout of the Register.

Requisition of controlled drugs: a requisition in writing signed by the veterinary surgeon must be obtained by the supplier before delivery of Schedule 2 and 3 drugs. It must also state the name and address of the veterinary surgeon, the purpose for which the drug will be used and the amount of the drug required.

Prescribing and the 'cascade'

The numbered steps below summarize the legislation governing which medicines may be prescribed for a particular condition in a particular species. This system of prescribing comes under the Medicines (Restrictions on the Administration of Veterinary Medicinal Products) Regulations 1994.

Entries made on obtaining the drug:

Date supply received	Name and address of supplier	Amount obtained	Form in which the drug was obtained

Entries made when supplying the drug:

Date transaction occurred	Name and address of person supplied	Licence or authority of person supplied to be in possession[a]	Amount supplied	Form in which supplied

a In most cases the drug will have been directly administered to the animal by the veterinary surgeon and so direct administration would be entered here.

A veterinary medicine may only be administered to an animal if it has a product licence for the treatment of that particular condition in that particular species.

The exceptions to this are defined as the *cascade method of prescribing* and are numbered below.

If no drug is licensed for that condition in that species, then:

1. A veterinary medicine licensed in another species or for another condition in the same species may be used
2. If no product as in (1) exists, then a licensed human product may be used
3. If no product as in (2) exists, then a product can be prepared on a one-off basis by an authorized person in accordance with a veterinary prescription.

Prescriptions

Veterinary prescriptions are required to be written by a veterinary surgeon, to instruct a pharmacist to dispense either a prescription-only medicine (POM) or a controlled drug. There are legal requirements for prescriptions in both cases.

Requirements for a POM prescription

- Must be written in indelible ink
- Must state the name and address of the veterinary surgeon
- Must state the date
- Must state the name and address of the owner of the animal (it is good practice also to identify the animal to be treated)
- Must state the name and the strength of the drugs to be dispensed, using either the generic name or a proprietary (trade) name (it is not legally required to state the total amount and dose of the medicine to be supplied)
- Should state the directions that the prescriber wishes to appear on the label
- Should declare that the prescription is issued in respect of an animal under the veterinary surgeon's care
- Should be signed by the veterinary surgeon
- Should contain directions for repeat prescriptions
- May only be dispensed within 6 months of the prescription being issued.

Abbreviations

Abbreviations that may be used in prescription writing include:

- bd (*bis die*) – twice daily
- bid (*bis in die*) – twice daily
- od (*omni die*) – once daily
- qid (*quarter in die*) – four times daily
- sid (*semel in die*) – once daily
- tid (*ter in die*) – three times daily.

Additional requirements for prescriptions for Schedule 2 and Schedule 3 controlled drugs

- The prescription must be written in the veterinary surgeon's own handwriting (exceptions to this are phenobarbitone and phenobarbitone sodium)
- The form and strength of the drug to be dispensed must be included. The quantity to be dispensed must be written in both numbers and figures
- The drug may only be dispensed within 13 weeks of issue of the prescription
- Prescriptions for controlled drugs may not be repeated.

Special treatment authorization (STA)

If a product suitable for the treatment of a specific condition in an animal is not available in the United Kingdom, then a veterinary surgeon can apply to the Veterinary Medicines Directorate (VMD) for an STA allowing the importation of a suitable product which is available in another country.

Storage of veterinary medicines

Most of the requirements for the storage of veterinary medicines are based on common sense. The important points are:

- Store in accordance with the manufacturer's instructions
- Refrigeration must be available and maintained between 2°C and 8°C. Refrigerators should be fitted with a maximum/minimum thermometer to allow monitoring of the temperature. Insulin and vaccines are examples of products which must be kept refrigerated
- The designated storage area should not be accessible to the public

- Storage areas should be kept clean and should be well ventilated. Eating or drinking should be forbidden in this area
- Flammable products should be stored in appropriate cabinets
- Dates of delivery should be logged and marked on products and for multi-use products date of first use should be marked on the product
- Products returned by clients should not be reused as they may have been inappropriately stored
- An effective stock control system should be implemented allowing routine checking and detection of products requiring reordering or approaching their expiry date
- Controlled drugs in Schedule 2 and some in Schedule 3 should be stored in a locked cabinet. Keys for this cabinet should only be available to the veterinary surgeon and/or an authorized person designated by the veterinary surgeon. Other drugs such as ketamine, although not classed as controlled drugs, are liable to abuse and it is recommended that they also should be stored in a locked cabinet
- Drugs in consulting rooms and in vehicles should be kept to a minimum and should not include controlled drugs
- P, PML and GSL drugs may be displayed to the public but only 'dummy' packs may be used. POM drugs may not be displayed to the public although posters advertising them may be displayed within the veterinary practice since this is advertising only to clients and not the public.

Handling, labelling and dispensing of medicines

The important legislation involves:

- Health and Safety at Work etc., Act 1974
- Control of Substances Hazardous to Health Regulations 1988, enacted under the Health and Safety at Work etc., Act 1974 (COSHH).

In a practice situation a named person, who will be the veterinary surgeon, is responsible for ensuring that the requirements of the relevant legislation are fulfilled. A practice manual should be available which provides the staff with details of the practice policy, including handling and dispensing of medicines.

 Anyone involved in the handling or dispensing of veterinary medicines should be trained. Qualified veterinary nurses may supply POM products, provided they do so under the authority of the veterinary surgeon.

COSHH regulations

These regulations relate to work involving substances that are deemed to be hazardous to health — including certain veterinary medicines and animal products. It is the employer's responsibility to perform a risk assessment of each of these substances used. Manufacturers of veterinary products now provide a product safety data sheet to aid this risk assessment. The employer must aim to prevent or control exposure of employees to these substances by information, instruction and training.

Practical points for handling and dispensing of medicines

- Direct contact between the skin of the person dispensing the drug and the drug itself should be avoided. This can be achieved through wearing protective clothing, such as disposable gloves, or by using pill counters
- Notify the veterinary surgeon of skin abrasions and avoid dispensing drugs under these circumstances
- Particular care should be taken with drugs marked as teratogenic or carcinogenic
- The data sheet should always be consulted, especially if the dispenser is not familiar with the particular drug in question
- Drugs should be appropriately labelled and should be dispensed in an appropriate container (see separate section below)
- COSHH regulations extend to a responsibility to the client. The client should be given clear instructions with regard to the safe handling, storage and disposal of the medicine. For example, disposable gloves may need to be given to the client for the application of certain products for external application, or the client should be advised that some products should be kept refrigerated.

 Cytotoxic drugs, such as cyclophosphamide, require extreme care in handling and administration as many are highly toxic and irritant. Appropriate protective clothing should be worn and the drugs should be prepared in a designated area. Tablets must never be divided or crushed. These drugs should not be handled by pregnant women.

All drugs that are dispensed must be appropriately labelled. Figure 2.20 gives an example of a drug label showing the information that is legally required in addition to information that is recommended.

 2.20 Information required on the labels of dispensed medicines described under the Medicines Act 1968[a]

Legally required	For Animal Treatment Only Mr X's dog (name of dog) Address of owner Date
Recommended	Instructions for administration Instructions for storage Details of drug (i.e. name, strength and amount)
Legally required	Keep all medicines out of the reach of children
Legally required	Name and address of veterinary surgeon

This information should be written in an indelible manner on the container of the medicine or if this is not possible on the package of the medicine. The label should not obscure manufacturer's information. If the product is for topical application then **'For external use only'** should be included on the label. The omission of the recommended information could be considered professionally irresponsible and negligent if the product is used in an unsafe way.

[a] *Adapted from NOAH (1995)*

Containers

Many veterinary medicines may be dispensed from bulk containers and should therefore be packaged in suitable containers when dispensed to the public.

- Reclosable child-resistant containers made of light-resistant glass, rigid plastic or aluminium should be used. Elderly or infirm clients may require more easily opened containers and discretion may be operated in these circumstances
- Blister-packed medicines may be dispensed in paper board cartons or wallets
- Paper envelopes and plastic bags are not acceptable as sole containers of products
- Creams, dusting powders, ointments, powders and pessaries should be supplied in wide-mouthed jars made of glass or plastic
- Light-sensitive medicines should be in opaque or dark-coloured containers
- Certain liquids for external use, as specified under the Medicines (Fluted Bottles) Regulations 1978, should be dispensed in fluted bottles (vertical-ridged) so that they are discernible by touch. These bottles are no longer in production and so may be difficult to obtain at present. If possible these liquids should therefore be dispensed in the manufacturer's container.

Disposal of veterinary medicines

Tablets, capsules, creams, ointments, injections, etc. are classed as pharmaceutical waste and should not be included with clinical waste.

- Disposal is complex and local authorities can provide information on companies dealing with effective disposal
- Schedule 2 controlled drugs may only be destroyed in the presence of a person authorized by the Secretary of State, such as a police officer
- Once the product reaches the final user (i.e. the client) the legislation affecting disposal no longer applies, although advice should be given with regard to safe disposal of medicines.

Further reading

Bishop Y (1998) *The Veterinary Formulary*, 4th edn. Pharmaceutical Press, Wallingford

Bishop Y (1998) *British Veterinary Association Code of Practice on Medicines*. BVA Publications, London

Gorman NT (ed.) (1998) *Canine Medicine and Therapeutics*, 4th edn. Blackwell Science, Oxford

NOAH (1995) *Animal Medicines: A User's Guide*. National Office of Animal Health, Enfield, Middlesex

Tennant B (1999) *BSAVA Small Animal Formulary*, 3rd edn. BSAVA, Cheltenham

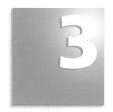

3 Nursing the emergency patient

Linda Oxley, Margaret Kane, Jane Pocklington and Kate Nichols

This chapter is designed to give information on:

- Evaluation of the emergency patient
- Application of ABC and ACRASHPLAN systems
- Emergency equipment
- Hydration status and fluid therapy
- Poisoning
- Monitoring the critically ill patient

Introduction

This chapter has been written to aid and support veterinary nurses in the care of the emergency patient, with the aim of preserving life, preventing suffering and preventing the situation from deteriorating. The importance of initial actions and the steps taken in further examination are shown within the framework of the mnemonics ABC and ACRASHPLAN. The principles of fluid therapy together with the clinical evaluation and treatment of shock are explained in more detail and there is a section devoted to poisoning. The chapter provides an easy reference guide for nurses confronted with an emergency situation. Much of the information is expanded in Chapter 4 of the *BSAVA Manual of Advanced Veterinary Nursing*.

 On all occasions when veterinary nurses are required to give first aid, they must inform the veterinary surgeon of the emergency as soon as possible.

Evaluation of the emergency patient

Animals may be examined at the site of an incident or at the clinic. The latter is often preferred as all the facilities for treatment are then at hand. Transport of injured animals is addressed in *BSAVA Manual of Veterinary Care*.

In the clinic, an area should be assigned for the assessment of emergency patients. It is preferable that the work station is close to the operating theatre and radiology areas so that emergency procedures can be performed if required. The area should be spacious and well lit. A well organized and fully stocked mobile emergency crash box should be available at all times. Figure 3.1 shows the items that should be included.

Assessment and examination

It is important to assess the patient quickly and to prioritize any potentially life-threatening problems. Note the general demeanour of the patient, e.g. bright, alert, responsive, nervous, disoriented, quiet, recumbent, ambulatory, comatose. If the patient is conscious, bright, alert and ambulatory, it may be referred to the veterinary surgeon. If the patient is collapsed, unconscious or cyanotic it needs immediate emergency measures.

 Remember your own safety
- If outside the clinic, check that there are no hazards in the area around the patient.
- Remember that even the friendliest of pets may become aggressive if frightened or in pain.
- Do not put your fingers into the mouth of a conscious patient without assistance, as it may bite.

When confronted with an emergency, the first questions to address are those raised by the mnemonic ABC:

- A – Airway
- B – Breathing
- C – Circulation

A supply of oxygen to the brain is necessary for life. Thus, the initial questions to be asked are:

- Is the airway clear?
- Is the patient breathing?
- Does the patient have a pulse?

Emergency equipment

Oxygen supply	Anaesthetic machine Anaesthetic curcuits and masks 'Ambu' bag	
Airway	Suction equipment: syringe with urinary catheter attached; hand-held suction; suction pump Range of cuffed endotracheal tubes with syringe attached for cuff inflation Stylet to facilitate difficult intubations Laryngoscope with range of blades Scalpel blades: no. 10, 15 Tracheostomy kit with range of sizes Curved haemostat Forrester forceps	
Drugs*	Lignocaine Atropine Adrenaline Methylprednisolone Calcium gluconate	Dobutamine Sterile water Doxapram Emergency drug chart (for quick reference by the veterinary surgeon)
Catheters	Various sizes of over-the-needle catheters Butterfly needles Central venous catheters Intraosseous needle Spinal needles Surgical scrub	Tape Heparin flush Scissors Three-way taps Giving sets
Fluids	Crystalloid Colloid Mannitol	
Electrocardiography	Electrocardiograph Electrode gel Defibrillator with external and internal paddles Wall-mounted chart for defibrillation guidance Clock	

* *Syringes to be preloaded and clearly labelled with content and date*

Once these questions have been addressed, a complete physical examination should be carried out, including the following:

1. Observe and define type of any haemorrhage
2. Record capillary refill time
3. Assess mucous membrane colour, noting any anaemia, jaundice or cyanosis
4. Observe and record any abnormalities, including pain, recumbency, respiratory distress
5. Record the peripheral pulse for strength, volume and rate
6. Determine hydration status
7. Examine for any skin wounds and fractures
8. Record rectal temperature.

These elements are incorporated into ACRASHPLAN (see Figure 3.3) for further examination and corrective action. During examination, it is important to limit the degree of movement of the head, neck and spine until fractures have been ruled out. Figure 3.2 shows normal values for vital signs.

Following any immediate action required, a detailed history should be obtained if possible. It is important to obtain relevant details of how the emergency arose, including any traumatic incidents or exposure to toxins.

Normal values for vital signs

Parameter	Dog	Cat
Temperature (°C)	38.3–38.7	38.0–38.5
Pulse (beats/min)	60–140	110–180
Respiration (breaths/min)	10–30	20–30
Capillary refill time (seconds)	1–2	1–2
Mucous membranes	Pink, moist	Pink, moist

ACRASHPLAN

The mnemonic ACRASHPLAN (Figure 3.3) outlines a logical approach to patient examination, resulting in a rapid and thorough patient assessment.

3.3 ACRASHPLAN

ACRASHPLAN shows the order of assessment, examination and treatment for an emergency case

A	=	Airway
C	=	Cardiovascular
R	=	Respiratory
A	=	Abdomen
S	=	Spine
H	=	Head
P	=	Pelvis
L	=	Limbs
A	=	Arteries
N	=	Nerves

Airway

Ensure the airway is patent by:

- Examining the mouth for obstructions, paying particular attention to the oropharynx
- Removing any fluids from the mouth or nose.

Observing respiratory rate and effort for visible signs of distress and monitoring any abnormal sounds will help to identify an impaired airway. If the airway is not clear, the steps in Figure 3.4 should be followed. When a clear airway is achieved, the patient may resume some voluntary respiratory effort.

3.4 How to maintain an airway

1. Insert a mouth gag – do not insert fingers
2. Extend the head and neck and pull the tongue forward
3. Clear the oropharynx using a swab wrapped around a pair of Allis forceps or a suction machine
4. Lower the head to prevent aspiration of foreign materials.

Airway obstructions

An object lodged in the trachea may obstruct the airway. It is often necessary to perform the Heimlich manoeuvre (Figure 3.5) to dislodge the object and aid elimination of the obstruction. The Heimlich manoeuvre should only be performed under the direction of a veterinary surgeon. It may be attempted up to four times before an emergency tracheotomy is considered.

Brachycephalic breeds of dog may have stenotic nares, an elongated soft palate, laryngeal malformation or a hypoplastic/stenotic trachea which predispose them to airway obstruction. The patient may present conscious, unconscious or in severe respiratory distress. Cooling, sedation and occasionally tracheal intubation may be necessary.

Cardiovascular

Cardiopulmonary arrest is usually defined as the sudden cessation of functional ventilation and effective circulation. The clinical signs are:

- Respiratory arrest, with or without cardiac arrest
- Sudden loss of consciousness
- Absence of pulse or weak, tachycardic pulse
- Agonal gasping
- Pupils fixed and dilated
- Absence of palpebral reflex
- Mucous membranes may be cyanotic, pale pink or grey.

3.5 The Heimlich manoeuvre for a dog or cat

1. Suspend the patient by its hind legs (either over a table or held up by another person). If the animal is too large for this, raise its hind quarters as high as possible and hang the head down before administering the blow
2. Administer sharp pressure to the abdominal wall just above the xiphisternum, angled down towards the diaphragm. This should cause the animal to cough and thereby dislodge the obstruction
3. If this is unsuccessful, place your hands on either side of the chest wall (with the animal still suspended) and deliver a sharp compression to the thorax.

Cardiopulmonary arrest is referred to as a 3-minute emergency, as brain damage may occur after this time due to hypoxia. There is a loss of consciousness, usually within 10–15 seconds of the event. There may be a short period of agonal gasping but, if there is a lack of circulation, tissues will not be oxygenated despite these respiratory movements. The pupils will become fixed and dilated within 30–45 seconds.

Capillary refill time (CRT) is not a reliable indicator of normal circulation, as it can appear normal even after cardiopulmonary arrest, usually due to venous flow back. Loss of blood pressure is a reliable sign that there is no cardiac output.

Cardiopulmonary resuscitation (CPR)

All staff within the clinic should be trained in CPR and be able to deal with the initial management of cardiopulmonary arrest. It is advisable that 'mock' CPR is practised for training purposes on a regular basis, as a successful resuscitation relies heavily on speed and teamwork. Within the CPR team there should be a group leader who will delegate to others, preventing confusion and time wastage. There should be an area within the workplace that is equipped for performing CPR. Artificial respiration must be maintained at the same time as cardiac massage is given; it is therefore best if at least two people work together to resuscitate the patient. The principles of performing CPR are shown in Figure 3.6.

3.6 Cardiopulmonary resuscitation

Artificial respiration

1. Check the animal for evidence of spontaneous respiration; proceed with artificial respiration if no spontaneous respiration
2. Place patient in right lateral recumbency (unless injury deems this inappropriate)
3. Extend the head and neck and pull tongue forward
4. Stretch the forelimbs cranially to allow the chest to expand
5. Attempt to pass an endotracheal tube and respirate, preferably using an anaesthetic machine and a resuscitation or Ambu bag. If you are not competent at this technique progress to 6
6. Place a flat hand or hands over the ribs, caudal to the scapula at the level of the costo-chondral junction
7. Compress the chest with a sharp downwards movement
8. Allow the chest to expand
9. Repeat compressions every 3–5 seconds
10. Check for spontaneous respiration every minute.

Figure 3.6 continues ▶

Cardiac massage

1. Follow steps 1–4 above
2. Commence artificial respiration, preferably using an Ambu bag
3. Auscultate or locate the apex beat of the heart to determine the requirement for cardiac massage
4. Place a sandbag or wedge under the sternum to aid cardiac filling. Alternatively a tight bandage can be applied to the abdomen to increase venous return
5. Commence cardiac compressions
   - In small dogs and cats pressure should be applied with the thumb and forefingers to the ventral third of the thorax between the 3rd and 6th ribs. Compressions should be at the rate of 120 per minute
   - In larger patients pressure should be applied using the flat of the hand against the thorax caudal to the triceps muscle of the forelimb and just below the costo-chondral junction. Compressions should be at the rate of 60 per minute
6. Check for spontaneous heart beat every minute.

Respiratory

Respiratory system examination includes:

- Assessing and recording respiratory rate, rhythm and effort
- Gentle palpation for fractured ribs and sternebrae
- Observation and recording of any penetrating foreign bodies. Do NOT attempt to remove them.

Presenting signs of a patient with respiratory distress may include any of the following:

- Dyspnoea
- Hypoxia
- Tachycardia
- Collapse/unconsciousness
- Hypovolaemia
- Cyanotic mucous membranes
- Increased respiratory effort
- Respiratory arrest.

Possible causes of respiratory emergencies are listed in Figure 3.7.

Resuscitation

The priority for patients in respiratory distress is to establish and maintain a patent airway (see Figure 3.4). Cardiopulmonary resuscitation is described in Figure 3.6. Where damage to the thoracic wall is suspected, mouth-to-nose resuscitation (Figure 3.8) may be employed.

 Always wear a face mask when performing mouth-to-nose resuscitation.

Oxygenation

Oxygen therapy is essential to prevent hypoxia in dyspnoeic patients. The method selected depends on the severity of the condition and what the animal will tolerate, as it is important not to stress these patients.

Airway obstruction
Brachycephalic respiratory obstruction
Bronchitis
Cardiopulmonary arrest
Diaphragmatic rupture
Emphysema
Haemothorax
Heart disease
Hydrothorax
Hyperthermia
Pain
Pneumonia
Pneumothorax
Thoracic penetrating foreign bodies

This technique can be used when intubation is not possible.

 Always wear a face mask!

1. Place the patient in sternal recumbency if possible, to allow inflation of both lungs
2. Pull the patient's tongue forward and close the jaws around it to ensure that the airway is unobstructed
3. Hold the patient's nose firmly in one hand, with your fingers holding the jaws together to create a tight seal with the lip folds. This is important because if the mouth is not sealed the air blown in will not reach the lungs but will escape through the mouth
4. Place your other hand under the lower jaw to support the weight of the animal's head
5. Take a deep breath. Place your mouth, covered by face mask, in front of the animal's nostrils and blow the air directly into the animal's nasal chamber in gentle puffs at 1-second intervals, expelling just enough air to allow the chest wall to lift slightly. Care must be taken not to over-inflate the lungs, as this can cause damage to the delicate lung tissue.

Emergency stabilization of a patient with severe respiratory distress should include increasing the inspired oxygen concentration. Ideally, the patient should be allowed to rest briefly in an oxygen-enriched environment before further diagnostic investigation and manipulation. This is particularly important for cats. An oxygen tank/tent can be created easily by covering the front of a cage/kennel with cling film, allowing the passage in of an oxygen pipe; a hole allows the expired air to escape. Further assessments can be carried out when the patient shows no exacerbated signs of respiratory distress.

If the animal is unconscious, the patient should be propped in sternal recumbency to allow expansion of both lung fields. In an unconscious or anaesthetized animal, oxygen can be administered via an endotracheal tube. When monitoring a patient with respiratory distress, the equipment necessary for intubation (Figure 3.9) should be placed on or beside the cage (Figure 3.10).

3.9 Equipment for endotracheal intubation

Light source/larygoscope
Laryngeal anaesthetic for cats
Syringe or cuff inflator
Range of suitable endotracheal cuffed tubes
Stylet to facilitate difficult intubation
Laryngoscope
Gauze for securing the endotracheal tube
Range of suitable canine and feline mouth gags

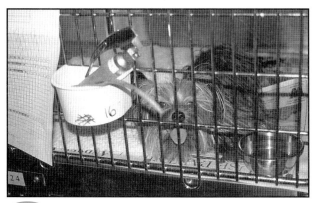

3.10 *Intubation equipment placed ready on a cage.*

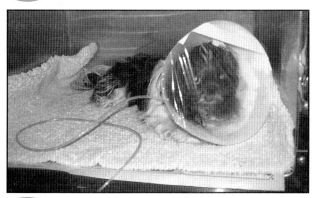

3.11 *Oxygenation via an Elizabethan collar.*

The most effective method of artificial ventilation is intermittent positive pressure ventilation (IPPV), which provides 100% oxygen from an oxygen machine.

Recommended rates for IPPV with 100% oxygen in dogs and cats:

- Two initial breaths of 1–1.5 seconds duration
- Then, one ventilation every 3–5 seconds between external chest compressions
- Or, two ventilations every 15 seconds if the resuscitation is being conducted by one person.

If using an anaesthetic machine, it is essential to flush it through first with 100% oxygen and ensure that all volatile anaesthetic agents are switched off. A self-inflating resuscitation bag ('Ambu bag') can be used but the concentration of oxygen provided is only 21% (the same as in normal room air). Mouth-to-tube resuscitation will only provide oxygen at 16-17%. If endotracheal intubation is not possible, a mask can be used around the patient's mouth and nose but a tight seal is required. Conscious animals with respiratory problems are often very distressed and may not tolerate oxygen therapy via a face mask. Alternatives are described in Figure 3.12. As patients may deteriorate rapidly, the simplest and quickest form of oxygenation should be chosen.

It is essential that long-term supplemental oxygen is humidified to prevent drying of the airway mucosa. Note that 100% oxygen should not be administered for longer than 24 hours as this may lead to oxygen toxicity. An attempt should be made to reduce the percentage of inspired oxygen to help wean the animal off oxygen therapy after this time. Management of long-term oxygen therapy is described in the *BSAVA Manual of Advanced Veterinary Nursing*, Chapter 4.

Pneumothorax

Pneumothorax is the presence of air in the pleural space. Presenting signs include:

- Mild tachypnoea to severe dyspnoea
- Cyanosis
- Fractures of the ribs
- Thoracic wounds

3.12 Methods of oxygen supplementation

Method	Advantages	Disadvantages
Oxygen mask	Increased oxygen supply	Mask may be too tight or too loose May cause rebreathing of carbon dioxide Poorly tolerated in distressed patients
Flow-by oxygen, provided by holding the oxygen supply pipe near the nostrils or mouth	Well tolerated	Difficult to monitor the exact oxygen intake
Oxygen tank/tent	Patient can rest without restraint during oxygenation	May increase patient warming and hyperthermia Makes monitoring and examination difficult Opening the cage door drops the oxygen concentration to room air almost immediately
Elizabethan collar (Figure 3.11)	Allows visibility	Poorly tolerated in distressed patients
Paediatric incubator	Good observation Useful for small dogs and cats	Expensive, unless obtained second hand from a human hospital
Nasal oxygen prongs (Figure 3.13)	Tolerated well in large breed dogs that are relatively immobile Useful for patients that are mouth breathing due to dyspnoea	Brachycephalic breeds are poor candidates for nasal oxygen supplementation (due to stenotic nares)

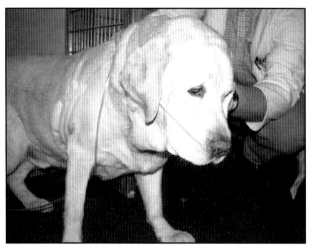

3.13 Oxygenation via a nasal cannula.

- Subcutaneous emphysema
- Dyspnoea
- Tachycardia
- Orthopnoea.

Pneumothorax is classified further as follows:

- Simple pneumothorax – Usually caused by non-penetrating trauma to the chest wall. Road traffic accidents are the most common cause
- Open pneumothorax – A penetrating wound in the thoracic wall, which results in collapse of the lung on the affected side. The usual causes are fights, penetrating stick injuries and fractured ribs
- Tension pneumothorax – A serious condition in which a large pulmonary leak acts as a ball valve, allowing air to enter the pleural cavity continuously but not to leave. This results in progressively increasing intrapleural pressure, leading to compression of the lungs and worsening respiratory compromise. This condition requires immediate attention by a veterinary surgeon (Figure 3.14), including emergency thoracocentesis.

Haemothorax

Haemothorax is an accumulation of blood in the pleural cavity. It prevents lung expansion and causes the lung to collapse. The severity of the haemothorax is dependent upon the volume of blood loss and rate, this may result in moist or noisy respiration.

3.14 Management guidelines for open pneumothorax

- Do NOT remove or cut any foreign bodies, as this may cause the situation to deteriorate. Removal of the foreign body may cause lung collapse due to air entering the thoracic cavity
- Provide supportive oxygen therapy
- Keep the patient warm and quiet. Sternal recumbency is the most comfortable position for these patients
- Monitor the vital signs
- A ring pad dressing may be applied and lightly bandaged around a penetrating foreign body
- Ensure all practice staff are aware of the presence and location of the foreign body underneath the dressing
- Keep stress and patient contact to the absolute minimum to avoid further distress.

Poisoning from inhalation
See section on Poisoning, below.

Abdomen
The abdomen should be examined externally for swelling, bruising or penetrating foreign bodies and for signs of abdominal distension.

> ⚠ To avoid damage do NOT palpate the abdomen. Do NOT attempt to remove any foreign bodies.

Diaphragmatic rupture
This is usually seen following a blunt blow to the thorax, often in cats that have been involved in road traffic accidents or in animals that have fallen from a height. A small tear in the diaphragm may go unnoticed, but problems arise when abdominal organs migrate through the tear into the thorax, preventing lung expansion. In the event of a possible diaphragmatic rupture, the patient should be encouraged to lie or stand with its head elevated to relieve pressure in the thorax. However, as these patients may show severe respiratory compromise and may not tolerate interference, it may be best to allow them to find a position that suits.

Spine
Record any obvious abnormalities, fractures or dislocations of the spinal column:

- Quadriplegia (paralysis of all four limbs)
- Hemiplegia (paralysis of one side of the body)
- Paraplegia (paralysis of any two limbs).

> ⚠ Do not move a patient with a suspected spinal injury unless instructed to do so by the veterinary surgeon.

Head
The head and face should be examined for:

- Facial/skull fractures, swelling or trauma
- Injuries to the head, neck, skull, nasal chamber, eyes or ears
- Epistaxis (nose bleed), swelling or haemorrhage
- Abnormalities of the head, such as head tilting.

Eyes

- Examination of the eyes should be conducted in a darkened/dimly lit room. Record any obvious ocular damage (e.g. exophthalmos)
- Note any discharges, fluid or blood from the eye and record the quantity
- Record palpebral reflex and colour of conjunctival mucosa for indication of anaemia, jaundice or cyanosis
- Examine for presence of wounds around the eyes or on the eyelids
- Note the position of the eyeball in the socket (in unconscious patients)
- Record any nystagmus (rapid involuntary movement of the eye) and if present the direction of the eye movement
- Record the size of the pupil in each eye, if abnormal, and monitor the response to a light stimulus.

Avoid touching the cornea, as this may cause ulceration and permanent damage. Do NOT attempt to remove any foreign body.
The tissues of the eye must be kept moist.

Clinical signs of ocular pain include:

- Affected animals may prefer to be in a darkened area due to photophobia (fear of bright light)
- Excessive tear production
- Inflamed sclera and conjunctiva of the eye ('red eye')
- Self-trauma, where the patient has rubbed an irritating eye on furniture or with its paw
- Severe oedema of the eyelid or conjunctiva.

Possible causes of injuries to the eye are listed in Figure 3.15.

The main priority before the veterinary surgeon arrives is to prevent the situation from deteriorating. An Elizabethan collar will minimize interference. Analgesia to minimize pain and discomfort should be administered at the discretion of the veterinary surgeon.

3.15 Causes of eye injuries

- Road traffic accidents
- Fighting
- Self-trauma – tissue around the eye may be red and swollen
- Foreign bodies e.g. grass seeds may become lodged under the eyelids or nictitating (third eyelid) membrane. The affected animal will be in severe pain and keep the eyelids tightly shut. The cornea may also be damaged if the foreign material is sharp. A purulent ocular discharge may be present if a foreign body has been in place for some time.
- Inflammatory reactions, due to insect stings: this type of reaction is often so severe that the oedematous conjunctiva swells over the eyelid margin, in some cases both upper and lower conjunctiva are affected which makes examination of the deeper structures very difficult.
- Lens luxation.

Prolapsed eyeball

When a patient presents with a prolapsed eyeball it is of paramount importance that the eyeball is replaced into the socket as soon as possible. Displacement of the eyeball can cause permanent damage to the eye very quickly. It is essential that a moist environment is maintained for the prolapsed eyeball. This can be achieved by dripping sterile saline or false tears over the eyeball itself or by covering the eyeball with a swab soaked in sterile saline until the veterinary surgeon is present.

Never attempt to replace the eyeball into the socket.

Lens luxation

This is where the lens moves from its normal position between the anterior and posterior chambers of the eye. It can be a primary condition, especially in certain terrier breeds. The lens can also luxate secondary to conditions such as glaucoma, uveitis, neoplasia or trauma. Clinical signs include:

- Abnormal iris movement
- A crescent shape around the lens edges
- Increased or decreased anterior chamber depth
- Pain.

Management:

- Inform the veterinary surgeon
- Keep the patient warm and quiet in a dimly lit room
- Prevent patient interference by fitting an Elizabethan collar.

Mouth

The following should be considered during the initial examination:

- Fractures of the mandible/maxilla or teeth
- Haemorrhage – record type and location
- Excessive salivation – may indicate poisoning; obtain relevant history
- Unusual breath smells – ketotic (sweet-smelling) breath may indicate ketoacidosis; creosote or phenol may be smelt in cases of toxicity
- Swellings, lacerations or haemorrhage on the tongue – record location and type
- Presence of foreign material or trauma in the roof of the mouth .

Poisoning is dealt with in detail later in this chapter.

Pelvis

The following should be considered during the initial examination:

- Abnormal gait
- Pain in the pelvic region
- Abnormalities involving the anal region, e.g. puncture wounds, discharging sinuses, blood/mucus from the anus, rectal prolapse.

If a fractured pelvis or dislocated hip is suspected, confine the patient (immobilize if possible). Do NOT attempt to move the patient unless instructed to so by the veterinary surgeon.

It is helpful to monitor and record urine output, as a fractured pelvis can cause damage to the bladder, or the bladder may have been ruptured by the trauma that fractured the pelvis. Faecal output and quality is also of interest.

Limbs

Any abnormalities of the limbs should be recorded, observing any signs of fracture, haemorrhage, swelling, pain, crepitus, or loss of feeling. Any fractures should be immobilized (see Chapter 6).

All limbs should be the same temperature; a cold limb may show that blood supply has been compromised.

Arteries

Cardiovascular circulation is considered early in the crash plan. Hypoxia (see above), haemorrhage and shock (see below) are the primary causes of death in the trauma case and require immediate attention.

Assessing the colour of the mucous membranes (Figure 3.16) and the capillary refill time may indicate a number of problems.

3.16 Mucous membrane colour

Description	Colour	Significance
Normal	Pale pink	Normal
Congested	Brick red	Toxins, septicaemia, heatstroke, smoke, cardiac disease
	Cherry red	Carbon monoxide
Pallor	Pale/white	Shock , haemorrhage
Cyanosed	Blue/purple	Lack of oxygen, severe dyspnoea, cardiac disease
Jaundiced	Yellow tinged	Acute hepatic failure, haemolysis

Haemorrhage

Figure 3.17 shows the types of haemorrhage and Figure 3.18 their presenting signs. Haemorrhage can be life-threatening. When haemorrhage is identified without evidence of trauma it is important to determine whether the bleeding is due to a systemic bleeding disorder or local factors. A detailed history is vital and should consider petechial haemorrhage, melaena or bleeding from the gingiva.

Patients with chronic blood loss generally do not become emergencies until they are severely anaemic.

The objectives of management are to:

• Arrest haemorrhage
• Treat shock (see below)
• Prevent sepsis.

Acute haemorrhage can be managed by arresting the bleeding and restoring the circulatory blood volume. Natural arrest of haemorrhage occurs in the body through retraction of cut ends of blood vessels, decreasing blood pressure, back

3.17 Types of haemorrhage

Primary	Occurs immediately following an injury
Reactionary	Occurs within 24–48 hours of injury May occur when blood pressure rises and dislodges a blood clot
Secondary	Can occur up to 10 days after injury May happen when a bacterial infection destroys the blood clot
Internal	Blood is lost into a body cavity, e.g. thorax or abdomen Presenting signs are often shock, dyspnoea or abdominal distension
External	Obvious bleeding from any open wound
Arterial	Bright red blood which spurts forcefully from the wound
Venous	Dark red blood
Capillary	Small volume of blood, oozes from damaged tissues with no definite bleeding point
Mixed	Blood from both arteries and veins, due to the close proximity of the vessels

3.18 Assessment of haemorrhage

Classification	Acute or chronic	Presenting signs
External		
Arterial, venous or capillary	Acute: ranges from minor problem to life-threatening emergency	Visible blood Evidence of hypovolaemic shock: pallor, tachycardia, rapid weak pulse, lowered rectal temperature, tachypnoea, depression, collapse, possible loss of consciousness
Internal		
Direct trauma to blood vessels, e.g. ruptured spleen, ruptured lung	Acute	Ballotment of thorax/abdomen may give a fluid wave, indicating free fluid Evidence of hypovolaemic shock: pallor, tachycardia, rapid weak pulse, lowered rectal temperature, tachypnoea, depression, collapse, possible loss of consciousness
Damage to walls of blood vessels, e.g. in immune-mediated disease, leptospirosis	Chronic, but may be seen as acute crisis	Chronic evidence: multiple petechial haemorrhage, melaena, haematuria, depression, exercise intolerance, tachycardia, tachypnoea, pallor May be presented for signs of other diseases or lethargy Acute crisis: collapse, with signs as for chronic condition
Defect in blood clotting mechanism		
– Primary, e.g. vasculitis thrombocytopenia	Chronic, but may be seen as acute crisis	Chronic evidence: multiple petechial haemorrhage, prolonged bleeding, e.g. after surgery
– Secondary, e.g. warfarin poisoning, haemophilia	Chronic, but may be seen as acute crisis	Chronic evidence: multiple petechial haemorrhage, melaena, haematuria, epistaxis

pressure and blood clotting. Methods of arresting haemorrhage are described in Figure 3.19. Blood transfusion is described later in the chapter in the section on Fluid therapy and in the *BSAVA Manual of Advanced Veterinary Nursing*.

Shock

Shock is a state of acute circulatory collapse, where the circulation is unable to transport sufficient oxygen and nutrients to vital organs such as the brain and heart. As shock progresses, changes to blood volume and arterial blood pressure are detected by the hypothalamus, which sends signals to the sympathetic nervous system. This results in a massive release of hormones, including cortisol, angiotensin, aldosterone and antidiuretic hormone. The effect of these is to retain salt and water, support blood pressure and supply energy. The sympathetic nervous system is responsible for increasing heart rate and constriction of peripheral arterial blood vessels in response to shock. This results in increased blood flow to vital organs. The heart receives adequate blood via the coronary artery, the brain via the carotid artery, and the lungs via the pulmonary artery. The kidneys receive blood only due to the special hormonal control of the renal artery via the renin–angiotensin mechanism. Initially these changes are beneficial to the patient, but later they may be harmful, leading to the worsening of shock.

Assessment

Animals presented as emergencies should be assessed for signs of shock:

- Collapse
- Decreased awareness
- Pale mucous membranes
- Prolonged capillary refill time of >2 seconds
- Tachycardia
- Weak peripheral pulses
- Hypothermia
- Oliguria.

Blood and urine samples should be obtained before starting treatment. As a minimum, the following diagnostic tests should be performed:

- Packed cell volume (PCV)
- Total protein (TP)
- Blood glucose
- Blood urea nitrogen (BUN) (plasma urea)
- Urine specific gravity
- Urine dipstick.

Figure 3.20 shows expected changes in blood and urine tests before and after treatment for shock.

3.19 Methods of arresting haemorrhage

Direct digital pressure	Use a sterile dressing/pad and apply pressure directly to the wound Take care to avoid any further contamination
Pressure pad	Adequate pressure over and around the bleeding vessel using absorbent pad and cohesive bandage
Pressure points	Only major arterial haemorrhage is controlled by this method Should only be used as a temporary measure as tissues supplied by the artery will be deprived of an arterial blood supply
Ring pad and pressure dressing	Preferred method when a foreign body or fracture of a long bone is suspected
Artery forceps	Very effective in controlling arterial or venous haemorrhage Care should be taken to avoid damage to nerves and other tissues
Tourniquet	No longer recommended, as the entire limb distal to the tourniquet is deprived of blood

3.20 Effects of shock on diagnostic test values

Packed cell volume (PCV)

Normal ranges: Dog 37–55%; Cat 24–45%
- May increase due to dehydration (after initial haemorrhage due to splenic contraction will increase circulating erythrocytes and PCV may be almost normal)
- Will decrease with chronic haemorrhage but may be unchanged during acute haemorrhage
- Treatment of shock with crystalloids or colloids causes a decrease in PCV due to haemodilution
- Administration of blood products increases PCV

Total blood protein

Normal ranges: Dog 5.5–7.0 g/dl; Cat 5.5–8.0 g/dl
- May increase due to dehydration
- Will decrease with chronic haemorrhage but may be unchanged during acute haemorrhage
- A further decrease will occur following treatment with crystalloid solutions, due to dilution
- If plasma or whole blood is administered, total protein levels will rise

Blood glucose

Normal ranges: Dog 3.5–6.0 mmol/l; Cat 3.5–5.8 mmol/l
- Corticosteroids released in shock cause elevated blood glucose levels
- Following treatment, blood glucose levels should return to normal

Figure 3.20 continues ▶

Blood urea nitrogen (BUN) (Plasma urea)

Normal ranges: Dog 2.0–8.0 mmol/l; Cat 4.0–11.0 mmol/l
- Increased by dehydration
- Increase by reduced renal blood flow in acute shock
- Levels return to normal once treatment for shock has been given and dehydration corrected

Urine specific gravity (SG)

Normal ranges: Dog 1.015–1.045; Cat 1.015–1.060
- Increased due to decreased circulation to the kidneys, resulting in a more concentrated urine and decreased urine production
- Once an adequate circulating volume and blood pressure are restored, urine production will increase and SG will decrease

Types of shock

Common causes include acute haemorrhage, trauma, gastric dilation volvulus and anaphylactic reactions.

Types of shock:

- Hypovolaemic – low circulating blood volume
- Haemorrhagic
- Traumatic – maldistribution of blood flow
- Anaphylactic – severe allergic reaction
- Cardiogenic – cardiac dysfunction
- Toxic – infection leading to a build up of toxins.

Treatment

Rapid treatment is essential if shock is to be reversed and the animal stabilized. The cause of shock should be identified if possible and specific treatment initiated, e.g. direct pressure to a site of external haemorrhage and administration of fresh whole blood if a large volume of blood has been lost.

In all cases the aim of therapy is to support the circulation, and intravenous fluid therapy should be started (see later in chapter for full details on fluid therapy). Hartmann's solution or 0.9% saline may be used in the emergency patient for the treatment of shock but dextrose saline should be avoided.

The fluid administration rate is determined by the animal's condition. Shocked or hypotensive animals will require a rapid infusion of crystalloids up to 90 ml/kg/h in dogs and 60 ml/kg/h in cats for the first hour only. Once the animal's condition improves, the infusion rate is normally reduced. The animal must be monitored carefully and the fluid rate adjusted accordingly. If there is no improvement following rapid administration of crystalloids, colloid administration should be considered. Care should be taken when administering intravenous fluids to animals with cardiac dysfunction to avoid development of pulmonary oedema. Monitoring of central venous pressure may be useful in these patients. A treatment plan is shown in Figure 3.21.

3.21 **Treatment plan for shock**

1. Provide intravenous access
   - Choose the largest gauge catheter possible, i.e. 18–14 G in dogs and 20–18 G in cats
   - The cephalic or saphenous vein should be aseptically prepared
   - More than one catheter may be necessary in larger patients (> 30 kg) to enable the desired fluid rate to be delivered
   - A jugular catheter may be useful to allow administration of drugs and intravenous fluids directly into the central circulation. The catheter should be fed into the jugular vein towards the heart and the tip should sit in the vena cava just cranial to the right atrium
   - If intravenous catheterization is not possible, the intraosseous route may be considered by the veterinary surgeon (see *BSAVA Manual of Advanced Veterinary Nursing*).

2. Intravenous fluid administration
   - Use crystalloids, colloids or whole blood (see text)

3. Maintain body temperature
   - Many animals in shock are hypothermic. Rectal temperature should be measured every 10 minutes until an improvement is seen, then every 30–60 minutes and the animal kept warm
   - Methods used to help prevent further heat loss include circulating warm water beds, heated pads, blankets, hot water bottles, warm intravenous fluids and a warm ambient temperature
   - Care should be taken so that heat is not directly applied to the patient, as this may cause thermal burns or peripheral vasodilation (can lead to pooling of blood in the periphery, so reducing blood flow to vital organs)
   - Limbs can be wrapped in aluminium foil and bubble wrap, though this is more useful in preventing heat loss rather than rewarming patients

4. Monitor urine output
   - Renal function is affected when arterial blood pressure falls below 60 mmHg, leading to poor renal perfusion. This leads to oliguria, a build up of toxins and development of acute renal failure
   - An indwelling urinary catheter should be aseptically placed when anuria or oliguria is suspected
   - Initially, urine output should be monitored every 30 minutes; every 4 hours may be sufficient later on
   - Normal urine output is estimated to be 1–2 ml/kg/h
   - The urinary catheter may be capped and periodically drained or a urine collection system can be attached. Closed urine collection bags are commercially available or an empty drip bag and giving set can be used. Urine collection bags must be placed lower than the patient, to allow urine to flow into the bag (Figure 3.22).

Figure 3.21 continues ▶

3.21 Treatment plan for shock *continued*

5. Frequent assessment of patient
    • Initially, the patient should be assessed every 10 minutes. Once it has begun to stabilize, assess every 30–60 minutes.
    • Monitor:
        – Demeanour
        – Rectal and peripheral temperature
        – Pulse rate and quality
        – Respiratory rate
        – Capillary refill time
        – Mucous membrane colour
        – Urine output.

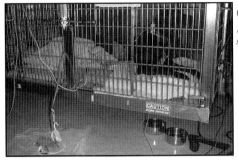

3.22
Urine collection system.

Nerves

Assessment:

• Note abnormal mentation
• Note any seizures
• Observe any head tilt
• Record posture – the ability to walk or stand, noting any ataxia
• Check limb posture – noting any flaccidity or rigidity
• Test the palpebral, menace and pupillary light reflexes.

3.23 Action plan for seizures

1. Ensure airway is clear
2. Place an intravenous catheter to provide access for administration of drugs
3. Obtain blood samples for haematology and biochemical analysis. Blood glucose, ammonia and ionized calcium should be measured as soon as possible, to assist in determining the cause of the seizure
4. Give therapy to control seizures if of prolonged duration (see Figure 3.24)
5. Measure the rectal temperature, as many seizuring animals become hyperthermic. If the rectal temperature is above 40°C cool the animal by wetting its coat with water or alcohol and placing a fan in front of the kennel
6. Seizure activity increases the oxygen requirements of the body, therefore oxygen administration may be necessary. If the animal is panting excessively or the mucous membranes appear cyanotic, oxygen therapy is indicated
7. Once the animal has been stabilized it should be placed in a quiet area away from stimuli. The animal must be closely observed.

3.24 Nursing considerations for animals having seizures

• Darken the room or place a towel over the front of the kennel
• Restrict access to the room – personnel should talk quietly and barking dogs should be moved away
• Pad the kennel with foam pads or bedding to decrease the risk of patient injury during seizures
• Only handle the animal when absolutely necessary. Care should be taken as the animal will be disoriented and may bite
• Maintain intravenous access by flushing the catheter with heparinized saline every 4 hours
• Observe for seizure activity and record
• Administer medications as directed by the veterinary surgeon
• Monitor respiratory and cardiovascular systems
• Ensure the patient does not become hyperthermic.

Seizures

There are many causes of seizure activity, including central nervous system disease, head trauma, hypoglycaemia, hypocalcaemia and encephalopathy. A detailed history is essential to try and establish the cause of the seizures so that appropriate therapy can be given. Most seizures are of short duration. They may be single or multiple. Where seizure activity continues for longer than 1 minute or cluster seizures are observed (lots of seizures of short duration), immediate action should be taken to control the seizures. An action plan is given in Figure 3.23. Nursing considerations are listed in Figure 3.24.

Poisoning

A huge number of substances are capable of causing poisoning; some are obvious and others require further investigation. Common clinical signs of poisoning are:

• Vomiting
• Diarrhoea
• Disorientation
• Abnormal behaviour
• Ataxia
• Shock
• Convulsions
• Profuse salivation
• Collapse
• Unconsciousness
• Death.

These clinical signs can also be associated with many other conditions, e.g. gastroenteritis and epilepsy. If poisoning is suspected, it is essential to obtain a comprehensive detailed history. The following questions should be asked:

- Have any medications (human or veterinary) been administered within the last 48 hours?
- Have toxic products been used recently by the owner in the house or garden?
- Has there been any accidental spillage in the house or garden?

Types of common poisons are listed in Figure 3.25.

3.25 Types of common poisons

Type	Example
Medicines	Sedatives, non-steroidal anti-inflammatory drugs, owner's medication
Herbicides	Weed killers
Insecticides	Flea spray
Rodenticides	Rat poison
Molluscicides	Slug bait
Household chemicals	Engine oil, antifreeze, disinfectant, bleach, wood preservative, petrol, lime scale removers, batteries (acid)
Theobromine	Chocolate
Plants	Foxglove, bluebell, acorns, deadly nightshade, ragwort, labernum
Venom	Snake bite
Insect stings	Wasp and bee stings (often presented as an anaphylactic reaction)

Poisoning through ingestion

The key aims in stabilization are:

- Prevent further absorption of the poison
- Identify the type of poison
- Treat the signs (under direction of the veterinary surgeon)
- Administer an antidote if a suitable preparation is available.

Management:

- Inform the veterinary surgeon
- Advise the owner to remove the source of the poison, if known, to reduce the risk of others becoming affected.

Induce vomiting (under the direction of the veterinary surgeon) by administering emetics such as apomorphine or xylazine, or by placing two crystals of washing soda on the back of the tongue. It is important to collect a sample of any vomit or faeces (label with date and time passed) for examination by the veterinary surgeon and for laboratory analysis. If the product was ingested more than 4 hours previously, there is little point in inducing vomiting as the poison will have emptied from the stomach into the small intestine.

- Do NOT induce vomiting where a corrosive or caustic substance is suspected, as the vomit can damage the gatrointestinal tract again when it is expelled.
- Do NOT induce vomiting in an unconscious patient as vomit may be inhaled into the lungs.

- Gastric lavage with warm saline may be performed (under veterinary direction) in an anaesthetized patient with an endotracheal tube secured in place
- Granules containing bismuth, calcium phosphate, charcoal and kaolin (1–3 tablespoons depending on size of patient mixed to slurry with water) or activated charcoal (made into a suspension using 1 g per kilogram body weight and mixing with water at 5 ml water per gram of charcoal) can be placed into the stomach via a stomach tube after gastric lavage, to aid adsorption
- Prepare fluid therapy infusion equipment for the veterinary surgeon to use if required
- Monitor vital signs and record regularly, especially capillary refill time, peripheral pulse, respiration, and rectal temperature
- Treat hypothermia or hyperthermia
- Keep the patient warm and quiet until the veterinary surgeon can treat the signs.

Poisoning through skin absorption

The appearance (e.g. paint, creosote) and odour (e.g. disinfectants, paint thinners, flea preparations) of the animal's coat are clear indications of a topical poisoning case.
Management:

- Inform the veterinary surgeon (there may be an antidote available)
- Fit the patient with an Elizabethan collar to prevent ingestion of a topical chemical through licking at the coat and grooming
- Keep the patient warm and quiet as it may be in shock
- Wearing gloves, remove the contamination from the patient's coat by clipping the area and/or washing the coat. Swarfega® applied directly to the patient's fur when dry will act as a binding agent and facilitate ease of washing, particularly of greasy or oily chemicals. Rinse with copious amounts of water.

Poisoning through inhalation

Signs of inhalation poisoning are:

- Dyspnoea
- Coughing
- Red mucous membranes.

Inhalation of carbon monoxide or smoke may require oxygen therapy with humidified oxygen. The oxygen is saturated with water vapour to prevent desiccation of the airways. This can be accomplished simply by bubbling the oxygen through a chamber of distilled water. If the animal is unconscious, intubation and intermittent positive pressure ventilation may be indicated.

Monitoring the emergency patient

Vital signs, including demeanour, temperature, pulse, respiration, capillary refill time and mucous membrane colour, should be monitored. These parameters should be assessed at least three times daily or as often as every 15 minutes, depending on the severity of the patient's condition. Whatever the frequency of observation, the details should be recorded so that abnormalities or trends can be easily identified and monitored.

Demeanour

The degree of awareness and response to the environment are useful in assessing patient status:

- Bright, alert and responsive (BAR)
- Quite alert and responsive (QAR)
- Depressed
- Comatose.

Patients in shock or severe pain, or those that are critically ill, may seem unaware of their environment. As their physical status improves, so does their level of awareness, and they will become more interested in their environment, and responsive to stimuli.

It is important to spend time with the patient so that you understand what the usual behaviour of that animal is and changes in behaviour can be easily identified. Regular contact with the patient will also be comforting, decreasing the stress associated with hospitalization. The well-being of the animal can be improved by ensuring that it is clean, dry and comfortable, that it has been given appropriate analgesia, and that it is stimulated to prevent or relieve boredom.

Temperature

Rectal temperature should be monitored for the development of pyrexia or hypothermia. If a pelvic fracture is suspected, an axillary temperature should be obtained. This may measure slightly lower than the rectal temperature but will provide some indication of patient status.

Palpation of ears or extremities may provide useful information about circulation. Where there is poor peripheral circulation, such as with cardiac disease or shock, the extremities will be cool. Return of warmth to the feet and ears may indicate an improvement in circulation.

Hypothermia is defined as a decrease in body temperature to below the normal range and is frequently seen in collapsed or shocked patients. Hypothermia leads to a decrease in metabolic rate, bradycardia and respiratory depression. As hypothermia worsens so does the severity of the clinical signs, and appropriate action must be taken to rewarm the patient:

- Warm intravenous fluids to 37°C
- Ensure the room is warm
- Use an insulating material such as 'bubble wrap' to cover the patient
- Ensure the patient's coat/skin is dry
- Use a heat lamp
- Use a hot water bottle, but do not place in direct contact with the patient.

The patient's body temperature should not be increased by more than 1°C per hour as this causes vasodilatation with transference of cool blood from the peripheral to the central circulation, and may cause ventricular fibrillation and death.

Hyperthermia (an increase in body temperature to above the normal range) can also be counteracted:

- Use a fan to blow cool air over the patient
- Pour alcohol over the pads and the body and allow to evaporate
- Pour cold water over the animal's body
- Soak towels in cold water and place them over the animal
- Cool any intravenous fluids before administration
- Place ice packs next to the animal, particularly in areas such as the axillary and inguinal regions.

Pulse

The pulse should be palpated to assess its rate, quality and rhythm. This provides information about cardiac output and blood pressure and is useful in detecting cardiac dysrhythmias.

Bradycardia

This is defined as an abnormally low heart rate. It may be caused by hypothermia, electrolyte imbalances or cardiac dysfunction. Bradycardia may lead to an inadequate cardiac output, so heart rates under 60 beats per minute should be investigated and treated. Treatment depends on the cause, e.g. warm up hypothermic patients, correct electrolyte imbalances. See the *BSAVA Manual of Advanced Veterinary Nursing* for further information.

Tachycardia

This is defined as an abnormally high heart rate. It may be seen in animals with shock, pain, sepsis or myocardial damage. Heart rates over 200 beats per minute may require treatment, and the animal should be attached to a continuous electrocardiograph. Tachycardia due to shock or hypovolaemia can be treated by rapid administration of fluids, either crystalloids or colloids (see below). Tachycardia associated with pain may be controlled by administration of appropriate analgesics, as directed by the veterinary surgeon. The myocardium is very sensitive to damage from hypoxia and trauma and this can lead to dysrhythmias such as ventricular tachycardia which may progress to ventricular fibrillation if left untreated. See the *BSAVA Manual of Advanced Veterinary Nursing* for further information.

Assessing cardiac rhythm

The cardiac rhythm can be assessed by auscultation of the heart and palpation of the pulse. The heart beat should be regular, although a phenomenon known as 'sinus arrhythmia' can occur in healthy animals and is normal. An irregular cardiac rhythm not associated with respiration is abnormal and the veterinary surgeon should be informed. An electrocardiogram (ECG) is necessary to identify the type of dysrhythmia present.

Assessing pulse rate

It is important to assess pulse rate together with heart rate to detect any pulse deficits. A pulse deficit occurs when cardiac output is not sufficient to pump blood around the body. A heartbeat will be heard but no pulse will be detected.

A peripheral pulse, such as the dorsal metatarsal or carpal pulse, should be palpated as these are more sensitive to changes in cardiac output and blood pressure than is the pulse.

When palpating the pulse, the strength should be assessed:

- Is the pulse weak or strong?
- Does the strength vary?

Weak pulses indicate poor peripheral perfusion and hypotension and may be seen in shock, hypovolaemia or cardiac dysfunction. Variation in pulse strength is related to cardiac output and is seen with cardiac dysrhythmias.

Respiration

Both respiratory rate and depth should be monitored:

- Tachypnoea – an increased respiratory rate – is seen in many critically ill animals. Causes include anaemia, pain, metabolic disorders and respiratory problems

- Bradypnoea – a decreased respiratory rate – is less common and is usually associated with central nervous system disorders or head trauma
- Hyperpnoea – an increase in respiratory rate and depth – is seen in acidotic animals as they try to eliminate carbon dioxide from the body.

Animals may exhibit respiratory effort on inspiration, expiration or both, and should be closely monitored. Breathing may be rapid and shallow with pneumothorax or pleural effusion. Dyspnoeic animals may stand with the forelimbs abducted and head extended in an attempt to increase oxygen intake. If an animal looks distressed and has increased respiratory effort, oxygen therapy should be considered (see above).

Pulse oximetry and arterial blood gas analysis provide further information about respiratory function (see *BSAVA Manual of Advanced Veterinary Nursing*).

Mucous membrane colour

Mucous membranes should be pink (see Figure 3.16). Pale membranes can be observed in states of poor peripheral perfusion such as in anaemic or shocked animals. Cyanotic membranes in conjunction with tachypnoea indicate hypoxia and oxygen should be administered. Icteric membranes may be observed with hepatic dysfunction or haemolytic disease.

Capillary refill time

Prolonged capillary refill time (CRT) above 2 seconds indicates poor peripheral perfusion and may be seen in cardiac dysfunction or shock. CRT is measured using the animal's gums. Pressing the gum causes it to blanche; the CRT is measured by estimating the length of time it takes for colour to return. Normal CRT in the dog and cat is 1–2 seconds.

Monitoring urine output

Urine may be collected in a bowl and measured. However, this can be difficult as you may be unable to catch every drop.

A kennel may be lined with incontinence sheets so that urine voided in the kennel will soak into the bedding. A 1g increase in the weight of bedding corresponds to approximately 1 ml of urine.

Alternatively, a soft urinary catheter can be aseptically placed to enable collection via a closed system. Indwelling urinary catheters are the most accurate way of measuring urine output and are useful for patients with acute renal failure or shock. Either routinely empty the bag or attach a giving set and drip bag or equivalent. Normal urine output from the dog or cat is 1–2 ml/kg/h. As there is a risk of ascending infection via the catheter, proper catheter care is essential:

- Place the urine bag on a sterile sheet and not directly on to the floor
- Wipe the outside of the urine collection system every 6 hours with alcohol
- Culture the urine and remove the catheter if infection is suspected.

Record keeping

When caring for critically ill animals, thorough and accurate record keeping is essential. A special hospital sheet should be used for this purpose.

- Vital parameters should be monitored (see above)
- Medications, fluid therapy and other nursing procedures should be written clearly on the record sheet and marked off once completed. This ensures that all treatments are administered and that all directions are strictly followed
- Observations such as vomiting, depression, nausea, etc. should be noted. This ensures that the veterinary surgeon is informed and that the frequency of any abnormalities can be easily assessed and any patterns identified
- Details about urination, including frequency and amount, should be monitored and recorded. Using the '+' system, where '+' indicates a small amount and '++++' indicates a large volume is the most basic method but is not accurate and should not be used in emergency or shock cases. Abnormalities such as straining or blood should also be noted.

Fluid balance and fluid therapy

Body water

Water makes up approximately 60% of an animal's body weight, the exact amount varying with age, gender and body fat content. Young animals tend to have a higher percentage, while obese animals have a lower percentage. Water is distributed throughout the body and can be categorized as intracellular and extracellular fluid (Figure 3.26). Intracellular fluid (ICF) is the

3.26 **Water distribution throughout the body**

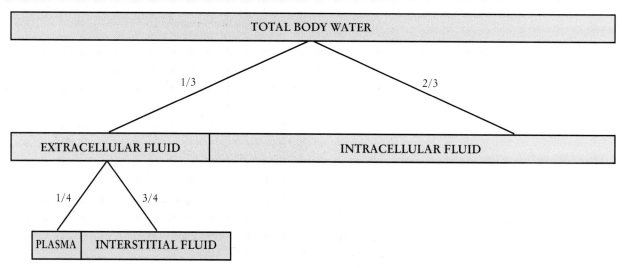

water contained within body cells and comprises two thirds of the body's water content. The remaining third is in extracellular fluid – that which is not contained within cells. Extracellular fluid (ECF) is further divided into interstitial fluid and plasma. Interstitial fluid is the fluid that exists between cells. Intracellular and extracellular fluid vary in composition: ICF contains higher concentrations of potassium and phosphate ions; ECF contains higher concentrations of sodium and chloride ions. Water can move between fluid compartments and its distribution is affected by osmolality, hydrostatic pressure (blood pressure), oncotic pressure (plasma protein levels) and electrolyte levels (mainly sodium and chloride ions).

Acid–base balance

The pH of blood is dependent upon the concentration of hydrogen ions [H^+]. The normal pH of blood is 7.35–7.45 and it must be maintained within this narrow range for normal cellular function to occur. Hydrogen ion concentration is controlled by bicarbonate ion and carbon dioxide levels. These, in turn, are regulated by the kidney and respiration, respectively.

The relation between carbon dioxide, bicarbonate ions and hydrogen ions is as follows:

$$CO_2 + H_2O \rightleftharpoons H_2CO_3 \rightleftharpoons H^+ + HCO_3^-$$

Carbon dioxide is carried in blood as carbonic acid (H_2CO_3). When a disease process causes a decrease or an increase in either hydrogen or bicarbonate levels it results in a change in blood pH.

3.27 Causes of acid–base imbalances

Type of imbalance	Causes
Respiratory acidosis	Hypoventilation, e.g. in anaesthetic depression, ruptured diaphragm, pneumothorax, pleural effusion, bronchitis
Respiratory alkalosis	Hyperventilation, e.g. in pain, stress, hyperthermia, excessive IPPV
Metabolic acidosis	e.g. Acute renal failure, ketoacidotic diabetes, vomiting and diarrhoea, shock
Metabolic alkalosis	e.g. Vomiting, pyloric obstruction, over-infusion of solutions containing bicarbonate

Acid–base imbalances

- Acidosis occurs when an animal has a blood pH below 7.35. This may be due to a loss of bicarbonate ions or a relative increase in hydrogen ions. The former is more common
- Alkalosis occurs when the blood pH is above 7.45. This may be due to an excess of bicarbonate ions or a loss of hydrogen ions.

Acid–base imbalances may have a respiratory or a metabolic cause (Figure 3.27). When ion levels increase or decrease to cause acidosis or alkalosis, equilibration occurs in an attempt to return the blood pH to the normal range. Therapy should be aimed at treating the underlying disease rather than the alkalosis or acidosis itself, since once the disease process concerned is addressed the blood pH should correct itself.

Fluid therapy (see below) should be administered to correct dehydration and to provide maintenance requirements and compensate for ongoing losses. In patients with acidosis an intravenous fluid such as Hartmann's solution (lactated Ringer's solution) should be considered. However, those fluids should be avoided in alkalotic patients because they contain bicarbonate; normal saline should be administered instead.

If acidosis is severe, i.e. if blood pH falls below 7.2 or the bicarbonate level below 12 mmol/l, the consequences may be life-threatening. Animals with severe acidosis exhibit deep rapid respirations in an attempt to dispose of carbon dioxide from the body. These animals require bicarbonate therapy. Sodium bicarbonate should be administered slowly by intravenous infusion over 30-60 minutes. See the *BSAVA Manual of Advanced Veterinary Nursing* for further information.

Electrolyte balance

Figure 3.28 lists normal ranges for electrolytes plus the clinical signs and causes of abnormalities.

Fluid requirements

Water intake must be sufficient to meet body needs and prevent dehydration. Fluid losses include sensible losses (in urine and faeces) and insensible losses (through panting, breathing, sweating). Sensible losses are those which can be controlled by the animal. Thus, when water availability is low, the animal is able to retain water through the kidneys and produce less urine. A certain level of urine production must be maintained, however, to allow elimination of waste products from the body. This is known as 'obligatory' urine production. Insensible losses are those over which the animal has no voluntary control and will continue independent of water availability e.g. respiratory losses.

3.28 Electrolytes: normal ranges and deficiencies

Electrolyte	Normal ranges in the dog (mmol/l)	Normal ranges in the cat (mmol/l)	Causes of deficiencies	Signs of deficiencies	Causes of increased levels	Signs of increased levels
Potassium	3.8–5.8	3.7–4.9	Anorexia, gastrointestinal disturbances, renal failure	Inappetence, weakness, cardiac abnormalities	Urinary tract obstruction, diabetic ketoacidosis, renal failure, Addison's disease	Bradycardia, cardiac arrest, collapse
Calcium (ionized)	1.0–1.5	1.0–1.5	Hyperparathyroidism, eclampsia	Twitching, seizures	Neoplasia (especially lymphosarcoma), Addison's disease	Polyuria/polydipsia, renal failure, vomiting lethargy
Bicarbonate	17–24	17–24	Ketoacidotic diabetic, acute renal failure	Rapid deep respiration	Iatrogenic	

Normal requirements

The daily water requirement for dogs and cats is 40–60 ml/kg per 24-hour period. Larger animals tend to require less water per kilogram and small animals to need more. This is because losses are greater with a higher body surface area. For convenience, an average of 50 ml/kg body weight is usually quoted for maintenance requirements for dogs and cats. In normal circumstances, this is provided by food and water.

Requirements for sick animals

In the veterinary clinic animals are often presented whose fluid requirements have not been met. They may have a facial injury which makes it difficult for them to take in fluid or may be losing fluid through vomiting, diarrhoea or disease. The outcome is an imbalance which may only involve the body water or may also involve other components of extracellular fluid.

3.29 Assessing the level of dehydration

Percentage dehydration	Clinical signs
<5%	No obvious signs Urine concentrated
5–8%	Slight tenting of skin Slightly prolonged capillary refill time Tacky mucous membranes Third eyelid visible
8–10%	Obvious tenting of skin Sunken eyes Prolonged capillary refill time
10–12%	Tented skin stands in place Oliguria May be signs of shock (tachycardia, cool extremities, weak pulse)
>12%	Progressive shock Coma Death

Assessing hydration status

When considering the hydration status of an animal, one should:

1. Assess how much fluid the animal has lost
2. Consider what type of fluid has been lost
3. Work out the daily maintenance requirement.

Figure 3.29 shows the clinical signs associated with differing degrees of dehydration. These changes occur over time and may not be detectable in an acutely ill animal. Where they are detectable, the percentage dehydration should be estimated.

Calculating fluid requirements

When calculating a rate for fluid supplementation, ongoing losses must be taken into account as well as the fluid deficit and maintenance requirement:

- Fluid deficit (litres) = body weight (kg) x dehydration level (expressed as a decimal)
- Ongoing losses – e.g. in vomit, diarrhoea, polyuria, pleural and peritoneal effusions
- Maintenance requirement = 40–60 ml/kg per 24 hours.

Where the animal is dehydrated but the cardiovascular system is otherwise stable, the fluid deficit should be replaced over 24 hours, along with maintenance fluid requirements (50 ml/kg/day) and ongoing losses. In more critical patients, where there is maldistribution of blood flow or hypovolaemia, rapid fluid administration is required with fluid deficits replaced over 4–6 hours. Figure 3.30 gives some examples of fluid requirement calculations.

Fluids for replacement therapy

Crystalloids

Once the fluid requirements for an animal have been calculated, a crystalloid solution may be selected (Figure 3.31). A replacement solution such as Hartmann's or 0.9% normal saline is usually selected. Dextrose saline is a maintenance solution and is only suitable for those animals that are fully hydrated.

A commercial intravenous fluid alone may not be sufficient to correct imbalances and stabilize the critical patient. Additional supplementation with potassium, dextrose,

3.30 Calculating fluid requirements

Example 1

Calculate the maintenance fluid requirement for a 5 kg cat. What drip rate would be required if a paediatric giving set (60 drops/ml) was used?

Maintenance fluid requirement	= 50 ml/kg per 24 h = 50 x 5 = 250 ml per 24 h
Requirement per hour	= 250/24 = 10 ml (approximately)
Requirement per minute	= 10/60 = 0.16 ml
The giving set delivers 60 drops/ml	= 60 x 0.16 = 10 drops/min required
Drip rate required	= 60 seconds/ 10 drops = 1 drop every 6 seconds

Example 2

Calculate the maintenance fluid requirements for a 20 kg dog. What drip rate would be required if a standard giving set (20 drops/ml) was used?

Maintenance fluid requirement	= 50 ml/kg per 24 h = 50 x 20 = 1000 ml per 24 h
Requirement per hour	= 1000/24 = 41 ml
Requirement per minute	= 41/60 = 0.69 ml
The giving set delivers 20 drops/ml	= 20 x 0.69 = 14 drops/min required
Drip rate required	= 60 seconds/ 14 drops = 1 drop every 4 seconds

Figure 3.30 continues ▶

Example 3

A 5 kg cat is 7% dehydrated. How much fluid does it need to receive over the next 24 hours to correct dehydration and provide maintenance requirements?

Fluid deficit	= body weight (kg) x dehydration (as a decimal)
	= 5 x 0.07 = 0.35 litres (350 ml)
Maintenance requirement	= 50 ml/kg per 24 h = 50 x 5 = 250 ml per 24 h
Total requirement over 24 hours	= 350 ml + 250 ml = 600 ml

Example 4

A 10 kg dog is 5% dehydrated. It vomits approximately 6 times a day and the volume is estimated at 4 ml/kg each time. What are the fluid requirements of this dog over the next 24 hours?

Fluid deficit	= body weight (kg) x dehydration (as a decimal)
	= 10 x 0.05 = 0.5 litres (500 ml)
Ongoing losses	= 4 ml/kg per vomit
	= 4 x 10 x 6 = 240 ml
Maintenance requirement	= 50 ml/kg per 24 h = 50 x 10 = 500 ml per 24 h
Total requirement over 24 hours	= 500 ml + 240 ml + 500 ml = 1240 ml

3.31 Crystalloid fluids: composition and indications

Name	Type	Composition (mmol/l)					Potential indications
		Na	Cl	K	Ca	Bicarbonate	
Hartmann's	Replacement solution	131	111	5	2	29	Metabolic disorders Endocrine disease Vomiting and diarrhoea Acidosis Dehydration
0.9% Sodium chloride (NaCl)	Replacement solution	150	150	–	–	–	Alkalosis Addisonian crisis Urinary obstruction Vomiting, pyloric obstruction Hepatic disease
0.18% NaCl & 4% Dextrose	Maintenance solution	30	30	–	–	–	Hypoglycaemia Hypernatraemia

calcium or bicarbonate may be required. Any syringe or fluid bag containing supplements must be clearly labelled. If the dose of the supplement or infusion rate is expected to change, a small volume of solution can be prepared by adding supplements to 100 ml fluid in a burette rather than a 500 ml bag of fluid.

Hypoglycaemia

Hypoglycaemic animals may require dextrose administration. Dextrose can be administered as a bolus (50% dextrose solution diluted 50:50 with saline) or as a continuous infusion (5% dextrose solution). A single bolus of dextrose is useful to control hypoglycaemic seizures, whereas a continuous infusion is needed to maintain blood glucose levels in the long term. An infusion of 5% dextrose is usually used for this purpose. Figure 3.32 shows how to prepare a 5% solution.

Hypocalcaemia

Either 40% calcium borogluconate (400 mg/ml) or 10% calcium gluconate (100 mg/ml) should be administered to control seizures associated with hypocalcaemia. They may be administered as a bolus or diluted and given as a continuous infusion.

 Many preparations are licensed for subcutaneous administration but care should be taken as these injections are painful and can be irritating to the skin

Colloids

Colloids may be administered when crystalloids alone are not sufficient to support the circulation. These solutions contain large molecules which remain in the circulation whereas

3.32 Preparation of a 5% (50 mg/ml) dextrose solution

	Volume of 50% dextrose solution added to a 500 ml bag of 0.9% NaCl	Volume of 50% dextrose solution added to a 1000 ml bag of 0.9% NaCl
5% dextrose solution	50 ml	100 ml

3.33 Commercially available colloid solutions

Type	Products	Duration of action	Fluid rate
Dextrans	Dextran 40 Dextran 70 (These fluids are hypertonic, not isotonic)	Up to 2 hours 6–24 hours	Up to 90 ml/kg/h (dog) Up to 60 ml/kg/h (cat) Maximum dose = 20 ml/kg
Gelatin solution	Haemaccel Gelofusine	Up to 6 hours	Up to 90 ml/kg/h (dog) Up to 60 ml/kg/h (cat) Maximum dose = 20 ml/kg
Starch	Hetastarch	24–36 hours	Up to 90 ml/kg/h (dog) Up to 60 ml/kg/h (cat) Maximum dose = 20 ml/kg

crystalloids are rapidly redistributed throughout the body. This results in plasma volume expansion, which may be useful in the treatment of shock, hypovolaemia or hypotension. Commercially available synthetic colloids are listed in Figure 3.33. Limiting factors include a maximum dose for dogs and cats of 20 ml/kg and also cost, as these solutions are relatively expensive. Disadvantages also include potential anaphylactic reactions and coagulopathies if administered in large doses. Some solutions may interfere with blood crossmatch results.

Blood

Collection of blood for transfusion is described in Chapter 4 of the *BSAVA Manual of Advanced Veterinary Nursing*. It should be noted that storage of blood and blood products is not approved by the RCVS. Further details of blood transfusion are also given in that chapter.

Blood administration sets are illustrated in Figure 3.38. Initially, blood should be administered slowly, at a rate of 1 ml/kg/h. The animal should be observed closely for signs of a transfusion reaction:

• Pyrexia
• Tachycardia
• Tachypnoea or panting
• Vomiting
• Depression
• Haemolysis
• Collapse.

Death can occur quickly if action is not taken.

Temperature, pulse and respiratory rates should be monitored frequently and recorded on a specially designed record sheet (Figure 3.34). The animal may be pre-treated with an antihistamine such as chlorampheniramine or with corticosteroids. The latter should be avoided in animals with surgical or traumatic wounds.

After 30 minutes and if no problems have been observed, the infusion rate should be increased to deliver the blood over the next 4 hours. Where severe blood loss has occurred it may be necessary to infuse the blood more rapidly to save the animal's life.

The animal should be monitored throughout the entire transfusion. If any signs of a reaction are noted, the transfusion should be stopped immediately and the veterinary surgeon notified. Other problems associated with blood transfusions include circulatory overload and a reaction to the citrate anticoagulant.

BLOOD TRANSFUSION
Monitoring Flow Chart

Type of blood component used: _____   PCV/TS of Donor: _____

Calculated amount of blood needed: _____

	Time	Flow Rate	Temp	Pulse	Resp	PCV/TS*
Pre-trans	—	—	—	—	—	—
15 min	—	—	—	—	—	—
30 min	—	—	—	—	—	—
60 min	—	—	—	—	—	—
Post-trans	—	—	—	—	—	—
6 hours PT	—					—

if serum is haemolysed STOP!

Transfusion Reactions: _____
_____
_____

3.34 *Record sheet for blood transfusion.*

Routes of fluid administration

The route chosen for administration will depend on the size of the patient, the reason for fluid therapy and the fluid to be administered (see also the *BSAVA Manual of Advanced Veterinary Nursing*). Routes include:

• Oral: does not need to be sterile. Inexpensive. Not appropriate for acute or emergency cases where rapid adjustment to the acid–base balance and circulatory volume is required. Cannot be given in gastrointestinal disease
• Intravenous: cephalic or saphenous veins. Used in severe dehydration and shock where rapid adjustment to the acid–base balance and circulatory volume is required. Only route for hypertonic solutions. Surgical preparation of the site is required. Catheters require changing every 48–72 hours
• Intraperitoneal: caudal to umbilicus. Useful in small mammals and possibly young animals. Not appropriate for acute or emergency cases where rapid adjustment to the acid–base balance and circulatory volume is required. Surgical preparation of the site is required
• Subcutaneous: multiple sites over the shoulders, back and hindquarters; possibly useful in small mammals and young animals. Not appropriate for acute or emergency cases where rapid adjustment to the acid–base balance and circulatory volume is required. Non-irritant and isotonic fluids only

- Intraosseous: Very useful in small mammals and young animals or animals in severe shock where venous access is difficult. Hypotonic fluids only.

Intravenous administration

The various types of intravenous catheters are illustrated in Figure 3.35.

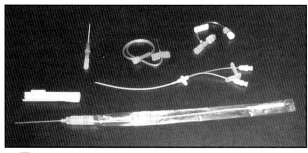

3.35 *Catheters.*

Over-the-needle catheters

These are short catheters, about 25–50 mm long. They have an inner stylet which is removed once the catheter has been placed into either the cephalic or saphenous vein. They can be left in place for up to 72 hours. They are made of Teflon™ or polyurethane, the latter being associated with less phlebitis.

Figure 3.36 shows how to place an over-the-needle catheter.

Butterfly catheters

These consist of a needle and plastic wings. The wings help to secure the catheter in place. Because the needle is rigid, there is an increased likelihood of dislodgement as the animal moves around. Other types of catheter are used more widely.

Through-the-needle catheters

These are generally longer than over-the-needle catheters and are most commonly used to catheterize the jugular vein, although certain types can also be placed in the medial saphenous vein. There are two types: some are provided as a closed system and others as a set. These must be placed in a sterile manner, using sterile gloves and drapes. Through-the-needle catheters may be left in place longer than over-the-needle catheters, for between 5 and 7 days. They can also be used to measure central venous pressure (see *BSAVA Manual of Advanced Veterinary Nursing*). Disadvantages include expense and being more difficult to place (Figure 3.37). If time allows, a topical anaesthetic cream may be applied to the skin 1 hour prior to placement to provide local analgesia at the site of catheter placement. A similar alternative catheter can be placed using the Seldinger technique (see Figure 3.37).

Methods of intravenous fluid administration

Various methods are available to enable intravenous fluid to be delivered at a set rate per minute or per hour. Methods include:

- Standard giving set – delivering 15 or 20 drops/ml
- Paediatric giving set – delivering 60 drops/ml
- Burettes
- Volumetric infusion pumps – delivering a set volume per hour
- Syringe drivers – delivering a set volume per hour.

Giving sets

Figure 3.38 illustrates the types of giving sets available.

Standard giving set

These are the basic type of fluid administration set.

3.36 How to place an over-the-needle catheter

Equipment

- Intravenous catheter
- T-connector or injection bung
- Clippers
- Heparinized saline (0.1 ml 1:1000 heparin in 100 ml 0.9% saline)
- Chlorhexidine surgical scrub
- Alcohol
- Swabs/cotton wool
- Adhesive tape for bandage
- Occlusive dressing
- Padding bandage
- Cohesive bandage

Method

1. Collect equipment and flush the T-connector or injection bung with heparinized saline
2. The patient should be restrained by an assistant
3. Clip a patch of hair from the leg over the vein to be catheterized
4. Clean the area with chlorhexidine
5. Wipe the area with alcohol
6. Ask the assistant to raise the vein
7. Identify the vein and push the catheter through the skin and into the vein. (Cut-down techniques should not be routinely performed but should only be used as a last resort in emergency cases when visualization of the vein is otherwise impossible due to low blood pressure)
8. Once blood returns into the catheter hub, hold the stylet still and advance the catheter into the vein
9. Ask the assistant to stop raising and press over the vein a few centimeters above the catheter entry site (this prevents contamination of the leg with blood when the stylet is removed). The stylet can then be removed and either a T-connector or injection bung attached
10. A piece of adhesive tape should be placed directly on to the animal's leg underneath the T-connector. The tape should be wrapped around the leg and then back over the top of the T-connector
11. Flush the catheter with heparinized saline to check placement
12. A further piece of sticking plaster tape may be required over the T-connector to ensure secure placement
13. The catheter site should be covered with an occlusive dressing. This provides a sterile covering and allows the catheter to be checked for dislodgement, phlebitis and infection. Alternatively, a plaster which has been impregnated with betidine ointment can be used
14. The catheter should be bandaged in place using a padding bandage and a cohesive bandage.

3.37 How to place a through-the-needle catheter

Equipment
- Jugular catheter
- T-connector or injection bung
- Clippers
- Heparinized saline (0.1 ml 1:1000 heparin in 100 ml 0.9 % saline)
- Chlorhexidine surgical scrub
- Alcohol
- Swabs/cotton wool
- Adhesive tape for bandage
- Occlusive dressing
- Fenestrated drape
- Surgical gloves
- Padding bandage
- Cohesive bandage
- Suture material

Method for placement of a closed system
1. Collect the equipment and flush the T-connector or injection bung with heparinized saline
2. Restrain the patient in lateral recumbency and place a sandbag underneath the neck. The head should be extended and the forelegs drawn backwards
3. Clip a patch of hair from the neck over the jugular vein
4. Clean the area with chlorhexidine surgical scrub
5. Wipe the area with alcohol
6. Ask the assistant to raise the jugular vein (this is done by gently pressing above the thoracic inlet)
7. Put on surgical gloves using the open method
8. Place the fenestrated drape
9. Remove the needle guard from the catheter. Tent the skin over the vein and push the needle through the skin. The needle is then pushed into the jugular vein (the needle should be directed caudally towards the heart)
10. When blood is seen to return along the catheter, thread the catheter through the needle into the vein. Once all the catheter has been threaded withdraw the needle and place the needle guard. Ensure all sections are connected tightly
11. Attach the pre-flushed T-connector. Take a 2 ml syringe containing heparinized saline, flush the catheter and then pull the plunger back to see if blood can be withdrawn easily. Then flush the catheter with fresh heparinized saline
12. Withdraw a small amount of catheter and form a loop (this helps to stop the catheter kinking)
13. Place the external part of the jugular catheter against the neck pointing dorsally
14. Place the transparent sterile dressing over the catheter site
15. Use strips of adhesive tape to secure the catheter or suture in place
16. Bandage with a layer of padding bandage followed by cohesive bandage.

Method for placement of a jugular catheter set (Seldinger technique)
Follow steps 1–8 above.
9. Tent the skin over the vein and push the needle through the skin
10. Push the needle into the jugular vein in a caudal direction (i.e. towards the heart)
11. Feed the guide wire through the needle into the vein. Now remove the needle leaving the guide wire in place
12. Feed the dilator over the guide wire and into the vein. Then remove the dilator
13. Feed the catheter over the guide wire. Once in place, remove the guide wire and attach a pre-flushed T-connector
14. Flush and withdraw as in step 11 of the previous catheter placement
15. Suture the catheter in place
16. Place transparent sterile dressing over the jugular catheter site
17. Bandage the catheter in place using padding bandage and cohesive bandage.

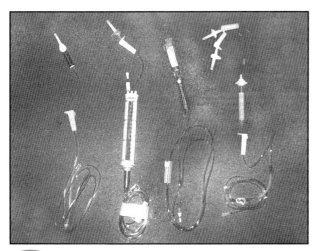

3.38 *Giving sets.*

- They consist of a length of tubing with a drip chamber and spike at one end and a luer lock connector at the other
- A flow regulator is positioned on the tubing below the drip chamber, allowing the fluid delivery rate to be controlled
- An injection port is incorporated into the drip tubing for administration of intravenous medications and to assist the removal of any air bubbles
- On average, standard giving sets deliver 20 drops/ml, but this can vary with the manufacturer, so the giving set packaging should be examined carefully.

Giving sets for use with volumetric infusion pumps
These are similar to the standard administration sets but have been adapted for use with fluid infusion pumps.

- A section of the tubing between the flow regulator and luer lock connector is designed to fit a particular fluid pump
- The drip is set up as normal and this section of the giving set is then fed through the pump

3.39 How to set up a drip

Equipment

- Intravenous catheter
- Giving set
- Extension set
- T-connector
- Heparinized saline (0.1 ml 1:1000 heparin in 100 ml 0.9 % saline)
- Intravenous fluids

Method

1. Collect equipment and flush the T-connector with heparinized saline
2. Ensure a catheter has been placed and is patent. Attach a T-connector to the catheter
3. Attach the extension set to the end of the giving set tubing
4. Remove the cap from the spike on the giving set and push into the port on the fluid bag
5. Squeeze the drip chamber to half fill it with fluid
6. Open the flow regulating clamp to allow fluid to flow through the giving set until both the giving set and extension set are full, this is known as priming. Check that there are no air bubbles left in the line. Fully close the flow regulator
7. Suspend fluid bag from a drip stand
8. Connect the end of the extension set to the T-connector. Open the clamp on the T-connector
9. Open the flow regulator to deliver the desired flow rate.

- The flow regulator is fully opened and the desired fluid rate per hour is programmed into the machine
- There are a wide range of infusion pumps available. The basic types are easy to use and have facilities to set a total volume, and record the volume infused as well as the fluid rate required
- These giving sets can also be used without pumps by counting the drops in the standard way.

Burettes

A burette is a graduated chamber. It is useful when either a small volume of fluid is required or when drugs need to be added to the infusion.

- The burette is incorporated into the administration system between the fluid bag and drip chamber, either as part of the giving set itself or as a separate piece of equipment added to a standard giving set
- The burette is filled by opening the flow regulator, situated between the fluid bag and the burette, and allowing the fluid to fill the burette to the desired level, up to a maximum of 150 ml. The gate clamp below the drip chamber should be left closed to prevent air entering the line
- Drugs may be added to the fluid in the burette via the injection bung in the top of the container
- Some of the combined burette and giving sets give 20 drops/ml, while others give 60 drops/ml (paediatric giving sets)
- Paediatric sets are usefull for small dogs and cats where a low fluid rate is required, as the rate can be more accurately controlled. These safeguards help to ensure that the appropriate amount of fluid therapy is given and prevent overinfusion which could cause pulmonary oedema and death.

Blood giving sets

Giving sets to be used with blood must contain a filter, to remove any blood clots or cellular aggregates and prevent them entering the circulation.

- Standard blood giving sets have a double drip chamber which contains a blood filter. When using these sets it is essential to ensure that the filter is completely covered with blood
- Blood giving sets providing 15 drops/ml and 20 drops/ml are available, so the information on the packet should be checked carefully
- Blood giving sets are also available for use with volumetric infusion pumps
- If only a small amount of blood is to be transfused, it can be administered using an extension set and syringe, but an in-line blood filter must be added.

T-connector

T-connectors are placed between the catheter and extension set. Features include an injection bung and white clamp. The catheter can be flushed with heparinized saline via the injection port when the clamp is across. Intravenous medications may also be administered via the injection port.

Extension set

An extension set is a length of tubing which can be attached between the T-connector and giving set. Its function is just to make the giving set longer and it is especially useful in medium and large dogs.

Setting up a drip with a T-connector and an extension set is described in Figure 3.39.

Further reading

King L and Hammond R (1999) *Manual of Canine and Feline Emergency and Critical Care*. BSAVA, Cheltenham

Mathews KA (1998) *Veterinary Emergency and Critical Care Manual*. Lifelearn, Guelph

Murtaugh RJ and Kaplan PM (1992) *Veterinary Emergency and Critical Care Medicine*. Mosby, St Loius

Welsh E (1999) Fluid therapy and shock. In *Vveterinary Nursing*, 2nd edn, ed. DR Lane and B Cooper, pp. 568–586. Butterworth-Heinmann, Oxford

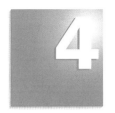

4 Medical conditions and medical nursing

James W. Simpson and Wendy Busby

This chapter is designed to give information on:

- Common infectious diseases of the dog and cat
- Diseases of the upper and lower respiratory system
- Diseases of the circulatory system
- Diseases of the alimentary tract
- Disorders of the kidney and lower urinary tract
- Neurological disorders in dogs and cats
- Diseases of the endocrine system
- Diseases of the musculoskeletal system
- Skin diseases
- The nursing role in medical diseases
- Nursing geriatric, recumbent or soiled patients
- Dealing with anorexic patients and providing assisted feeding
- Physiotherapy
- Administration of enemas
- Urinary catheterization

Introduction

The approach to every dog or cat presented with a medical condition should always start with the collection of a detailed history, followed by a thorough physical examination. This provides the necessary information required to determine if the animal has a systemic disease or a disease affecting only one body system, and in some cases allows a diagnosis to be reached. For example, a dog may present with chronic vomiting which, after careful clinical examination, reveals polydipsia, polyuria and pain over the kidneys – suggesting renal disease to be more likely than gastritis. This would be confirmed by carrying out a series of diagnostic tests.

The veterinary nurse's role may include assisting the veterinary surgeon in collecting the information required from the clinical examination and participating in the diagnostic procedures being carried out. This is only possible if the nurse has a clear understanding of the diseases being considered.

In addition, the veterinary nurse has a major role to play in administering treatment and monitoring the patient for signs of improvement or, more importantly, deterioration. Keeping the patient in a clean, warm and pleasant environment conducive to recovery has a major effect on the animal's desire to get better. These are extremely important and valuable responsibilities and

it is hoped that this chapter will provide the nurse with the information required to help to carry them out.

Canine infectious disease

Distemper
Causal organism: Morbillivirus related to measles and rinderpest.
Incubation period: 7–21 days.
Method of infection: Inhalation or ingestion following direct or indirect contact. Virus found in ocular and nasal discharge, urine and faeces.
Site of primary infection: Local lymphoid tissue, including submandibular lymph nodes and tonsils.
Target tissues: Epithelial cells of the respiratory and alimentary tract. Nervous system and other lymphoid tissue, including bone marrow.
Clinical signs: Anorexia, pyrexia, vomiting, diarrhoea, coughing, ocular and nasal discharge, tonsillitis, hyperkeratosis of pads and nose, nervous signs including chorea, muscle tremors, seizures.
Complications: Nervous signs developing years after initial infection; seizures, chorea, old dog encephalitis. Dental disease (Figure 4.1).

Diagnosis: Intracellular inclusion bodies, rising antibody titre, immunofluorescence for virus.

Treatment: Intravenous fluid therapy using Hartmann's solution, antibiotics, anti-convulsants, anti-emetics, anti-diarrhoeal agents.

Nursing care:
- Prevent spread of infection to other animals – isolation, barrier nursing
- Record episodes of vomiting and diarrhoea
- Maintain fluid lines
- Monitor vital signs
- Provide and maintain therapy prescribed by veterinary surgeon
- Bathe discharge from eyes and nose
- Clean and disinfect consulting areas.

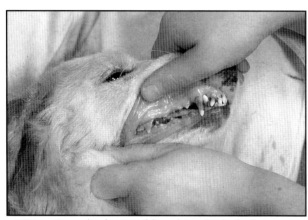

4.1 *Brown discoloration of the teeth in a dog that has had distemper prior to the eruption of its permanent dentition. The virus damages the enamel of the teeth before they erupt.*

Infectious canine hepatitis (ICH)

Causal organism: Canine adenovirus 1 (CAV-1).

Incubation period: 5–9 days.

Method of infection: Ingestion, following direct or indirect contact. Organisms found in saliva, vomit, faeces and urine.

Site of primary infection: Local lymph nodes, tonsils, submandibular lymph nodes and possibly mesenteric lymph nodes.

Target tissues: Hepatocytes, vascular endothelium, other lymphoid tissue and bone marrow.

Clinical signs: Sudden deaths in unweaned puppies. Acute vomiting, bloody diarrhoea, pyrexia, anorexia, abdominal pain, petechial haemorrhages on mucous membranes.

Complications: Corneal oedema or 'blue eye' and glomerular nephritis.

Diagnosis: Leucopenia, elevated liver enzymes, intranuclear hepatocyte inclusions, rising antibody titre and virus isolation.

Treatment: Intravenous fluid therapy using Hartmann's solution, whole blood where bleeding is extensive. Antibiotics, anti-emetics, intestinal protectants.

Nursing care:
- Record episodes of vomiting and diarrhoea
- Isolation procedures
- Monitor vital signs
- Provide and maintain therapy prescribed by veterinary surgeon
- Care of intravenous fluid lines
- Clean and disinfect consulting areas.

Leptospirosis

Causal organism: *Leptospira canicula* and *L. icterohaemorrhagiae*.

Incubation period: Approximately 7 days.

Method of infection: Penetration through skin, mucous membranes, cuts, transplacental and venereal. Urine a major source of infection. Direct and indirect spread possible.

Site of primary infection: Lymph nodes local to site of entry.

Target tissues: *L. canicola* – kidneys; *L. icterohaemorrhagiae* – liver; but each may target the other organ.

 Leptospirosis is a very important zoonosis. It is essential to consider personal safety when handling patients. Always wear protective clothing if this condition is suspected.

Clinical signs:
- *L. canicola* – acute vomiting, anorexia, polydipsia, initially oliguria, then polyuria, pain over kidneys, azotaemia
- *L. icterohaemorrhagiae* – sudden deaths in unweaned puppies; acute vomiting, anorexia, abdominal pain, jaundice, petechial haemorrhages on mucosa, collapse.

Complications: Excretion of organisms may persist for weeks following recovery.

Diagnosis:
- *L. canicola* – blood urea, creatinine, urinalysis and culture; rising antibody titre
- *L. icterohaemorrhagiae:* liver enzyme tests, bilirubin, urinalysis and culture; rising antibody titre.

Treatment: Intravenous fluid therapy, Hartmann's solution, possibly whole blood, antibiotics, anti-emetics.

Nursing care:
- Prevent spread of infection – isolation, barrier nursing
- Provide and maintain therapy prescribed by veterinary surgeon
- Maintain intravenous fluid lines
- Maintain a clean and stable environment
- Monitor vital signs
- Precautions required for zoonotic disease
- Clean and disinfect consulting areas.

Parvovirus

Causal organism: Canine parvovirus 2.

Incubation period: 3–5 days.

Method of infection: Ingestion following direct or indirect contact. Large amounts of virus found in faeces.

Site of primary infection: Replicates in local lymph nodes of gastrointestinal tract.

Target tissues: All rapidly dividing cells, including bone marrow, intestine and other lymphoid tissue. Myocardium in unprotected neonatal puppies.

Clinical signs: Sudden death from myocarditis rarely seen due to good level of maternal antibody. Gastroenteritis now most common form. Acute vomiting, diarrhoea, anorexia, abdominal pain, dehydration.

Complications: Malabsorption.

Diagnosis: Severe leucopenia, virus isolation from faeces.

Treatment: Intravenous fluid therapy using Hartmann's solution, antibiotics, anti-emetics.

Nursing care:
- Prevent spread of infection – isolation, barrier nursing
- Provide and maintain therapy prescribed by veterinary surgeon

- Record episodes of vomiting and diarrhoea
- Discuss with owner the need to protect in-contact animals.
- Clean and disinfect consulting areas.

Canine contagious respiratory disease (CCRD) (kennel cough)

Causal organism: *Bordetella bronchiseptica*, CAV-2, parainfluenza virus (CPIV), herpes virus (CHV), reovirus and secondary bacterial agents all implicated.

Incubation period: 5–7 days.

Method of infection: Aerosol spread and inhalation. Dogs in direct contact or within same air space.

Site of primary infection: Local lymph nodes such as tonsils and upper respiratory epithelium.

Target tissues: Upper respiratory epithelium.

Clinical signs: Dry 'hacking' cough, pyrexia, occasionally retching, mucopurulent nasal discharge. Possibly ocular discharge.

Complications: Chronic infection. Bronchopneumonia.

Diagnosis: Usually based on clinical signs. Pharyngeal swabs for culture.

Treatment: Antibiotics and cough suppressants.

Nursing care:
- Prevent spread of infection to other dogs – isolation, barrier nursing
- Provide and maintain therapy prescribed by veterinary surgeon
- Advise owners regarding in-contact dogs
- Clean and disinfect consulting areas.

Feline infectious disease

Feline panleucopenia (feline infectious enteritis)

Causal organism: Parvovirus.

Incubation period: 3–5 days.

Method of infection: Ingestion following direct or indirect contact. Virus found in saliva, vomit, faeces and urine. Transplacental.

Site of primary infection: Local lymph nodes of gastrointestinal tract.

Target tissues: All rapidly dividing cells, especially intestine, bone marrow and other lymphoid tissue.

Clinical signs: Acute vomiting, anorexia, abdominal pain, followed by fluid diarrhoea. Dehydration, weight loss. Fetal infection leads to cerebellar hypoplasia and ataxia after birth.

Diagnosis: Marked leucopenia, viral isolation from faeces.

Treatment: Intravenous fluid therapy using Hartmann's solution, antibiotics, anti-emetics and intestinal protectants.

Nursing care:
- Prevent spread of infection to other cats – isolation
- Clean and disinfect consulting areas
- Provide and maintain therapy prescribed by veterinary surgeon
- Advise owner regarding in-contact cats.

Feline upper respiratory disease (FURD) (cat 'flu)

Causal organism: Feline calici virus (FCV), feline herpes virus 1 (FHV1) and secondary bacterial infection.

Incubation period: 2–10 days.

Method of infection: Aerosol spread by direct or indirect contact. Viruses found in large numbers in ocular/nasal secretions and exhaled breath.

Site of primary infection: Local lymph nodes of respiratory tract.

Target tissues: Upper respiratory tract epithelium.

Clinical signs: Paroxysmal sneezing, serous ocular/nasal discharge changing to mucopurulent (Figure 4.2). Oral ulceration (Figure 4.3), blepharospasm, salivation, anorexia and pyrexia. Keratitis and corneal ulceration occasionally seen.

Diagnosis: Typical clinical picture and virus isolation from pharyngeal swabs.

Treatment: Correct dehydration if present; antibiotics, enteral feeding if anorexic.

Nursing care:
- Prevent spread of infection – isolation
- Clean and disinfect consulting areas
- Encourage patient to eat
- Provide and maintain therapy prescribed by veterinary surgeon
- Bathe ocular and nasal discharges to reduce complications.

Feline pneumonitis (chlamydiosis)

Causal organism: *Chlamydia psittaci*.

Incubation period: 4–10 days.

Method of infection: Direct contact via ocular discharge.

Site of primary infection: Ocular mucous membrane.

Target tissues: Ocular mucous membrane, nasal epithelium.

Clinical signs: Pyrexia, serous then mucopurulent ocular and nasal discharge, sneezing, blepharospasm and anorexia in some cases.

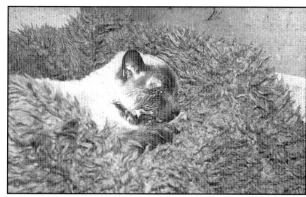

4.2 *Siamese cat with cat 'flu. Note the nasal discharge and closure of the eyelid due to the mucopurulent discharge.*

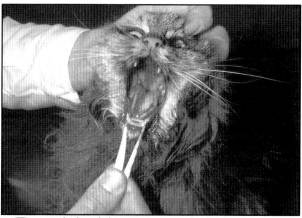

4.3 *Multiple oral ulceration in a cat with calicivirus infection. Courtesy of C.P. McKenzie*

Diagnosis: Conjunctival swabs. Rising antibody titre.

Treatment: Treat all cats in household with ocular tetracyclines and/or systemic tetracyclines.

Nursing care:
- Prevent spread of infection – isolation
- Advise owners regarding other cats in household
- Advise owners about vaccination
- Ensure treatment is carried out correctly.

Feline infectious anaemia (FIA)

Causal organism: *Haemobartonella felis.*

Incubation period: Not known, may have carrier states.

Method of infection: Cat bites, fleas, in utero, via milk.

Site of primary infection: Blood.

Target tissues: Red blood cells.

Clinical signs: Sudden onset of acute haemolytic anaemia, tachycardia, tachypnoea, pallor of mucous membranes, weakness, collapse.

Complications: Subclinical infection. Relapses common, especially following stress.

Diagnosis: Blood smears for extracellular parasite, using Giemsa stains. Confirmation of regenerative anaemia.

Treatment: Systemic tetracyclines. Possibly blood transfusion if severe. Clear flea infestations.

Nursing care:
- Provide and maintain therapy prescribed by veterinary surgeon
- Assist owner with flea eradication
- Observe vital signs while hospitalized
- Ensure stress-free environment.

Feline infectious peritonitis (FIP)

Causal organism: Coronavirus.

Incubation period: Variable.

Method of infection: Oronasal route.

Site of primary infection: Lymphoid tissue of gastrointestinal tract. Macrophages.

Target tissues: Vascular endothelium, peritoneum, pleura, eye, meninges, kidneys.

Clinical signs:
- Wet/effusive form (60%) – ascites, hydrothorax, pericardial effusion, anorexia, weight loss, diarrhoea
- Dry/non-effusive (40%) – no effusions, may affect abdomen, eye, central nervous system; liver, kidney or splenic dysfunction, retinitis, uveitis, ataxia, paresis, paralysis, convulsions.

Diagnosis: Serology debatable, biopsy of affected tissues, examination of ascitic fluid, high serum globulin (> 70 g/l).

Treatment: None.

Nursing care: Provide advice on prevention.

Feline leukaemia virus

Causal organism: Retrovirus (FeLV).

Incubation period: Variable, from weeks to months.

Method of infection: In utero, via milk, cat bites, mutual grooming (as saliva contains virus).

Site of primary infection: Local lymph nodes and circulation.

Target tissues: Bone marrow, intestines, salivary and lacrymal glands, urogenital tract.

Clinical signs: 40% of cats eliminate infection, in 30% the virus becomes dormant, and 30% of cats become infected. Leads to lymphosarcoma, non-regenerative anaemia, immunosuppression, glomerular nephritis, polyarthritis, polyneuritis, myeloproliferative disease, stillbirths, abortions, fetal resorption.

Complications: Generalized immunosuppression.

Diagnosis: ELISA test for viral antigen (P27). Virus isolation.

Treatment: None.

Nursing care:
- Advise owner regarding prevention – vaccination
- Prevent spread of disease – isolation, barrier nursing.

Feline immunodeficiency virus

Causal organism: Retrovirus (FIV).

Incubation period: Variable, from weeks to months.

Method of infection: Cat bites. High levels of virus in saliva.

Site of primary infection: Local lymphoid tissue.

Target tissues: Lymphoid tissue, bone marrow.

Clinical signs: Associated with immunosuppression. Chronic gingivitis, chronic upper respiratory tract disease, non-regenerative anaemias, development of FeLV, FIP, FIA, toxoplasmosis and other infections. Chronic weight loss.

Complications: Generalized immunosuppression.

Diagnosis: ELISA test for antibody.

Treatment: None. Treat secondary infections symptomatically.

Nursing care:
- Provide and maintain therapy prescribed by veterinary surgeon
- Advise owner regarding screening of other cats in household
- Isolation of infected and non-infected cats
- Advise owner regarding male cat aggression, roaming and fighting.

General infectious diseases

Rabies

Causal organism: Rhabdovirus.

Incubation period: 2 weeks to 4 months, with a mean of 3 weeks, depending on site and severity of bite wound and dose of virus.

Method of infection: Biting, but virus can cross mucous membranes.

Site of primary infection: Bite wound, multiplication in local tissue, usually muscle.

Target tissue: Neuromuscular junction and nervous system.

Clinical signs: Two forms recognized (furious rabies and dumb rabies) but signs of both types may be observed in any individual.
- Furious rabies – hyperexcitablity, aggression, depraved appetite, aimless walking for miles, with periods of normality in between; development of paresis and dysphagia, with facial asymmetry and finally seizures
- Dumb rabies – much more common, little observed until there is progressive paralysis involving limbs, facial asymmetry, salivation, dysphagia, coma and death.

 Great care is required when handling dogs with suspected rabies. Saliva contains large amounts of virus and this is a fatal zoonotic disease.

Diagnosis:
- Must inform Ministry of Agriculture, Fisheries and Food of suspected cases
- Keep animal in isolation until MAFF veterinary officer arrives to examine animal
- Examination of brain for negri bodies and fluorescent antibody test.

Treatment: None.

Nursing care:

- Where rabies is suspected, the nurse must ensure safety of personnel
- Do not allow animal to be handled unless essential
- Ensure animal is kept safely locked up
- Inform veterinary surgeon, or MAFF if unavailable.

Toxoplasmosis

Causal organism: *Toxoplasma gondii*.

Incubation period: 2–5 weeks.

Method of infection: Indirect, via ingestion of tissue cysts found in the intermediate host (rodent). Ingestion of oocysts in cat faeces less likely to induce infection.

Site of primary infection: Replicates in intestinal mucosa.

Target tissue: Muscle tissue and brain possible.

Clinical signs: Lethargy, depression, anorexia, pyrexia, weight loss, neurological signs, ocular disease and lymphadenopathy may occur.

Diagnosis: IgM titre useful to indicate active infection. IgG titre observed later in disease and in cases that have recovered.

Treatment: Antibiotics.

Nursing care:

- An important zoonosis so must discuss with owner.
- Especially important in immunosuppressed individuals; also in pregnant women, where abortion can occur – pregnant women should not handle cat litter
- Promote strict hygiene precautions
- Advice to owners:
  - Ensure all meat is thoroughly cooked
  - Wear rubber gloves when gardening
  - Prevent cats from hunting
  - Cover children's sandpits.

Salmonellosis

Causal organism: A bacterium called *Salmonella*, of which there are many serotypes.

Incubation period: 3–7 days.

Method of infection: Ingestion of contaminated food.

Site of primary infection: Gastrointestinal tract.

Target tissues: Gastrointestinal tract or circulation.

Clinical signs: Acute vomiting, diarrhoea, dehydration, weight loss, pyrexia, generalized lymphadenopathy. Abortion and arthritis are also possible.

Diagnosis: Blood and faecal culture.

Treatment: Only use antibiotics if systemic. Will naturally self-cure if enteric. Intravenous fluid therapy.

Nursing care:

- Potential zoonosis – isolation procedures
- Clean and disinfect consulting areas
- Advise owners regarding hygiene standards
- Provide and maintain therapy prescribed by veterinary surgeon.

Diseases of the respiratory system

Diagnostic procedures are described in detail in the *BSAVA Manual of Advanced Veterinary Nursing*.

Nasal discharge

Aetiology:

- Serous – early bacterial, viral and fungal infection or allergy

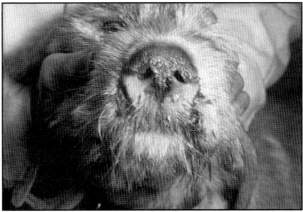

4.4 *Dog with a bilateral mucopurulent nasal discharge. This is associated with bacterial infection most frequently occurring secondary to viral infection.*

- Mucopurulent – established infections, foreign body, tumour and allergy (Figure 4.4)
- Epistaxis – trauma, tumour, clotting defect, severe bacterial or fungal infection.

Diagnosis:

- Radiographs – lateral, dorsoventral and rostrocaudal intraoral projections
- Bacteriology – culture and sensitivity of discharge
- Endoscopy – anterior and retrograde nasopharyngeal examinations
- Serology – rising titre to *Aspergillus* spp. and viral antigens.

Nursing care:

- Advise owners as to possible causes of nasal discharge
- Advise owners of diagnostic procedures that may be used
- Assist veterinary surgeon in carrying out procedures.

Coughing

Aetiology:

- Chronic bronchitis
- Cardiac failure
- Neoplasia
- Airway foreign bodies
- Tonsillitis, pharyngitis, tracheitis
- Tracheal collapse
- Pulmonary oedema
- Pulmonary haemorrhage
- Lungworm infection (*Oslerus osleri*, *Aelurostrongylus abstrusus*)
- Bronchopneumonia.

Treatment: Depends on the underlying cause (see above).

- Cardiac drug therapy
- Diuretics
- Antibiotics
- Anthelmintics
- Anti-tussants
- Corticosteroids
- Environmental improvements in air temperature and quality
- Bronchodilators.

Acute respiratory failure

Aetiology:

- Ruptured diaphragm
- Pneumothorax, haemothorax, pyothorax, chylothorax

- Airway obstruction: foreign body, laryngeal paralysis, tracheal collapse
- Neoplasia
- Infections: tetanus, botulism, bacterial and viral pneumonias
- Pulmonary embolism
- Paraquat poisoning
- Gastric torsion.

Clinical signs: May include some or all of the following, depending on underlying cause.
- Tachypnoea
- Dyspnoea
- Cyanosis
- Tachycardia
- Weak pulse
- Oral breathing
- Collapse.

Treatment: Procedures for treatment of airway obstruction are given in *BSAVA Manual of Advanced Veterinary Nursing*.

Diseases of the circulatory system

Normal heart rates and blood pressure measurements for dogs and cats are usually given as a range of values:

- Normal heart rates
  – Dogs: 60–140 beats per minute
  – Cats: 110–180 beats per minute
- Normal blood pressures
  – Dogs (oscillometric): average systolic 133 mmHg; average diastolic 75 mmHg; mean 98 mmHg
  – Cats (Doppler): systolic 118 mmHg; diastolic 83 mmHg.

Diagnostic procedures are described in detail in *BSAVA Manual of Advanced Veterinary Nursing*.

Congenital heart defects

There are many possible congenital heart defects which may occur in puppies and kittens. The commonest types are shown below.

Patent ductus arteriosus
- Fetal blood vessel between aorta and pulmonary artery remains patent
- Blood shunts from left to right
- Clinical signs depend on extent of shunting
- Clinical signs include: weakness, dyspnoea, exercise intolerance, cough, cyanosis
- Machinery murmur on auscultation.

Pulmonary stenosis
- Narrowing of blood vessel leaving right side of heart through pulmonary artery
- High pressure build-up on right side of heart
- May lead to right-sided heart failure (see congestive heart failure).

Aortic stenosis
- Narrowing of blood vessel leaving left side of heart through aorta (especially in Boxer dogs)
- High pressure build-up on left side of heart
- May lead to left-sided heart failure (see congestive heart failure).

Ventricular septal defects
- A hole exists between the right and left ventricle
- The size of the hole determines the clinical outcome
- Generally blood shunts from left to right
- Congestive heart failure is likely to occur.

Mitral and tricuspid dysplasia
- There is deformity of the atrioventricular valves
- Common cause of heart disease in young dogs, especially Golden Retrievers
- Regurgitation of blood between ventricles and atria
- Can lead to heart failure.

Tetralogy of Fallot
- A condition where several defects exist together
- Pulmonary stenosis, ventricular septal defect, dextraposed aorta, right ventricular wall hypertrophy
- Clinically causes cyanosis, exercise intolerance, systolic murmur and heart failure.

Persistent right aortic arch
- Right embryonic aortic arch persists instead of regressing
- Ligamentum arteriosus now lies across dorsal wall of oesophagus
- Oesophagus entrapped between ligamentum, aorta, pulmonary artery and base of heart
- Clinically causes oesophageal obstruction to passage of solid food
- Post-weaned puppies exhibit 'regurgitation' following eating. They may swallow liquids without difficulty.

Acute heart failure
Cardiac arrest is rare in dogs and cats.

Aetiology:
- Congenital defects
- Myocardial disease
- Dysrhythmias
- Hypoxia for any reason.

Clinical signs:
- Sudden onset, often during exercise
- Collapse
- Unconsciousness (flaccid collapse)
- Pallor or cyanosis of mucous membranes may be observed.
- Very weak or undetectable pulse
- Spontaneous recovery, which may be complete or include a period of lethargy.

Diagnosis: All or some of the following procedures may be used to reach a diagnosis.
- Auscultation
- Radiographs of thorax
- ECG measurements
- Blood gas analysis
- Blood pressure measurements
- Ultrasound.

Treatment:
- Establish and maintain patent airway
- Provide oxygen
- Cardiac massage at 60 compressions per minute
- Administration of drugs by veterinary surgeon
- Defibrillation
- Fluid therapy
- Monitor vital signs.

Nursing care:
- Assist veterinary surgeon with procedures listed above
- Monitor and record vital signs.

Congestive heart failure (CHF)

Aetiology: The heart is a muscular pump. When this muscle fails, cardiac output falls and clinical signs develop. The animal is said to have decompensated and developed CHF. Blood now pools in vascular beds, which may include the lungs or body tissues. This is called congestion. The location of congestion depends on whether pump failure is left or right sided.

There are many causes for pump failure, including:
- Myocardial disease – dilated or hypertrophic cardiomyopathy
- Arrhythmias
- Pulmonary or aortic stenosis
- Taurine deficiency in cats.

Clinical signs:
- General
  - Tachycardia
  - Weak pulse
  - Pallor of mucous membranes
  - Tachypnoea
  - Coughing
  - Exercise intolerance
  - Weight loss
- Right-sided heart failure
  - Poor venous return to heart
  - Congestion of liver, spleen and intestines
  - Hepatomegaly
  - Ascites
- Left-sided heart failure
  - Poor venous return from lungs
  - Pulmonary congestion and oedema
  - Tachypnoea and coughing.

Diagnosis:
- Auscultation
- Radiographs of thorax and abdomen
- ECG measurements
- Blood pressure measurements
- Blood gas measurements
- Ultrasound examination.

Treatment:
- Treat the underlying cause where known
- Cage rest
- Diuretics
- Angiotensin-converting enzyme inhibitors
- Cardiac drugs such as digoxin, propranalol
- Dietary management (salt restriction)
- Control of obesity.

Nursing care:
- Provide suitably quiet stress-free environment
- Provide and maintain therapy prescribed by veterinary surgeon
- Monitor vital signs
- Attend to dietary requirements.

Anaemia

Aetiology:
- Haemorrhagic
  - Acute blood loss – trauma, rupture to internal organs, clotting disorders
  - Chronic blood loss – haematuria, melaena, neoplasms, clotting disorder
- Haemolytic
  - Immune-mediated disease
  - *Haemobartonella felis* infection
  - Reactions to drugs, including sulphonamides, anti-convulsants
- Non-regenerative
  - Bone marrow hypoplasia
  - FeLV or FIV infection
  - Toxaemic states including pyometra and other septic conditions
  - Drugs, including chloramphenicol and oestrogens
  - Renal failure and erythropoietin deficiency
  - Neoplasia, including lymphosarcoma and leukaemias.

Clinical signs:
- Pallor of mucous membranes
- Jaundice
- Obvious signs of haemorrhage
- Weakness, collapse
- Tachycardia and weak pulse
- Tachypnoea
- Exercise intolerance and lethargy
- Signs of other system dysfunction, e.g. renal disease.

Diagnosis
- Physical examination
- Routine haematology, including reticulocyte count
- Check clotting factors: activated partial thromboplastin time (APTT) and prothrombin time (PT) and platelet count
- Coombs test
- ANA test
- Bone marrow biopsy.

Treatment:
- Control active haemorrhage by pressure bandaging followed by surgical correction
- Whole-blood transfusions in severe chronic cases when PCV < 0.15 l/l, and in all acute cases
- Correct underlying disease if present, e.g. renal disease
- Erythropoietin in cases of renal disease and in some other cases of marrow hypoplasia
- Stop any drugs known to affect haematology
- Immunosuppressive drugs for immune-mediated disease
- Vitamin K_1 for warfarin poisoning
- Provision of an adequate diet to ensure all haematinics are present
- Administration of tetracycline for *H. felis*.

Nursing care:
- Assist with administration of drug therapy
- Monitor vital signs
- General care of trauma patients
- Assist in carrying out diagnostic tests
- Advise owners where poisoning is suspected, to prevent further intake.

Diseases of the alimentary tract

Dysphagia
- Dysphagia is where the animal is unable to eat although maintaining the desire to do so
- Anorexia is where the animal has lost the desire to eat
- Dysphagia may be divided into:
  - Oral – fractured jaw, foreign body or neurological dysfunction
  - Pharyngeal – foreign body, tumour, neurological dysfunction
  - Oesophageal – megaoesophagus, stricture, vascular ring.

Clinical signs:
- Oral – inability to pick up food, food falls out of mouth; food held in cheeks
- Pharyngeal – retching, gagging, choking, food appears at nostrils
- Oesophageal – regurgitation, usually associated with eating; aspiration pneumonia.

Diagnosis:
- Observation of eating behaviour
- Radiographs of oral cavity, pharynx and oesophagus
- Barium swallow
- Endoscopy.

Treatment:
- Identify and correct underlying cause
- Nutritional management
- Antibiotics for aspiration pneumonia.

Nursing care:
- Carry out drug therapy as prescribed by veterinary surgeon
- Feeding procedures
- Ensure no excitement or exercise before and after feeding
- Observe for signs of complications (aspiration pneumonia).
- Assist with diagnostic procedures.

Vomiting

It is essential to make two important assessments in the patient presented with 'vomiting':

- Is the patient vomiting or regurgitating (dysphagia)?
- If vomiting: is this primary gastric disease or secondary to systemic disease?

Examples of conditions within these categories are:
- Primary vomiting
  - Acute and chronic gastritis
  - Gastric ulceration
  - Gastric neoplasia
  - Pyloric stenosis
  - Gastric foreign body
- Secondary vomiting
  - Azotaemia associated with renal disease
  - Ketoacidosis and diabetes mellitus
  - Pyometra
  - Addison's disease
  - Hepatitis, pancreatitis, colitis.

Diagnosis:
- History and physical examination of patient
- Radiographs of abdomen
- Barium studies
- Routine haematology and biochemistry
- Endoscopy.

Treatment: For treatment of secondary vomiting, see sections for appropriate systemic diseases elsewhere in this chapter.
Primary vomiting may be treated as follows:
- Identify and correct underlying cause (e.g. surgery to remove foreign body, correct pyloric stenosis or remove tumour)
- For gastritis:
  - Nil by mouth
  - Intravenous fluid therapy using Hartmann's solution
  - Anti-emetics
  - Gastric protectants such as sucralfate
  - Antacids such as cimetidine
  - Once vomiting stops, use low fat veterinary diets and return slowly to normal diet.

Nursing care:
- Provide and maintain therapy prescribed by veterinary surgeon
- Keep kennel and patient clean of vomitus
- Monitor vital signs
- Observe and record frequency of vomition and any deterioration in patient
- If infection is present – isolation, barrier nursing
- Inform owner of patient's progress.

Diarrhoea

It is essential to make two important assessments in the patient presented with a history of diarrhoea (Figure 4.5):

- Is the diarrhoea associated with primary intestinal disease or is it secondary to systemic disease?
- If the diarrhoea is primary: is it originating from the small or large intestine?

Examples of conditions within these categories are as follows:
- Primary diarrhoeas
  - Viral and bacterial infections
  - Hookworm and whipworm infections
- Giardiasis
- Inflammatory bowel disease (IBD)
- Tumours: lymphoma, adenocarcinoma
- Colitis
- Secondary diarrhoeas
  - Addison's disease
  - Azotaemia and renal failure
  - Liver disease
  - Pancreatic disease
  - Hyperthyroidism.

Inflammatory bowel disease (IBD) is a relatively new term used to describe chronic enteritis that results in malabsorption of nutrients from the small intestinal lumen into the enterocytes.

Patients with malabsorption or IBD must not be confused with patients with maldigestion (see exocrine pancreatic insufficiency). The clinical signs observed in malabsorption include:

- Marked weight loss
- Chronic diarrhoea
- Variable polyphagia.

4.5 Signs of small and large bowel disease

Sign	Small bowel	Large bowel
Weight loss	Present	Absent
Faecal volume	Increased	Reduced
Faecal frequency	Increased	Increased
Faecal fat (steatorrhoea)	May be present	Absent
Faecal starch	May be present	Absent
Faecal blood	May have melaena	May have fresh blood
Faecal mucus	Absent	May be present

Colitis is a common cause of chronic diarrhoea in dogs but not in cats. The aetiology of colitis is not frequently determined but may include:

- Bacterial infections, especially *Campylobacter* spp. and *Salmonella* spp.
- Parasitic infections with whipworms
- Food hypersensitivity reactions
- Secondary to colonic neoplasia.

Diagnosis: Diagnosis of both small and large intestinal diarrhoea (enteritis) may include some or all of the following procedures:

- Faecal analysis for
  - Undigested food components, especially fat and starch
  - Parasitic and protozoan examination
  - Bacteriology for pathogens, especially *Salmonella* spp. and *Campylobacter* spp.
- Serum folate and cobalamin estimations
- Endoscopic examination and biopsy collection.

Treatment: General treatments for small and large intestinal diarrhoeas (enteritis) without concurrent vomiting include:

- Nil by mouth for 24–48 hours
- Maintenance of oral fluids to prevent dehydration
- Anti-diarrhoeal drugs
- Low fat veterinary diets with slow return to normal diet
- Antibiotics should *only* be used where definite bacterial infection is confirmed.
  Treatment for IBD (malabsorption) and colitis differs from the general regimes:
- Feed exclusively hypoallergenic diets (single protein), which are gluten free
- Anti-inflammatory drugs
- Occasionally antibiotics for bacterial overgrowth.

Nursing care of diarrhoeic patients:

- If infection is suspected – isolation/barrier nursing
- Provide and maintain therapy prescribed by veterinary surgeon
- Ensure dietary management is carried out correctly
- Observe for signs of progression, especially dehydration and vomiting
- Provide a clean environment for the patient
- Record all episodes of diarrhoea or improvements in stool consistency
- Advise owner of patient's progress.

Constipation

Aetiology: The aetiology of constipation is long and varied and not necessarily directly associated with the alimentary tract.

- Dietary
  - Too high or low a level of fibre in the diet
  - Feeding of bones
- Colonic
  - Rectal strictures
  - Rectal foreign bodies (fur or hair balls)
  - Rectal tumours
  - Perineal rupture with rectal dilation
  - Megacolon
  - Anal sac disease or abscessation
- Orthopaedic
  - Pelvic fractures
  - Lumbar spinal lesions
  - Hindlimb instability

- Other
  - Neurological dysfunction
  - Prostatic hyperplasia.

Clinical signs:

- Failure to pass faeces
- Passage of small amounts of very hard faeces
- Vomiting
- Tenesmus
- Dyschezia
- Haematochezia/melaena.

Diagnosis: The diagnosis of constipation may be made using some or all of the following tests:

- Careful physical examination of the patient
- Rectal examination
- Neurological examination
- Radiographs of the abdomen, vertebrae and pelvis
- Endoscopic examination.

Treatment:

- Find and correct underlying cause, based on aetiology shown above
- Alteration of diet and ensuring that bones are not fed
- Stool softening agents
- Surgical correction of obstructions.

Gastrointestinal foreign body obstructions

Cats and (especially) dogs are prone to consuming foreign bodies. The most likely locations for foreign bodies to lodge in the alimentary tract are:

- Between the teeth and across the roof of the mouth
- Pharynx
- In the oesophagus between the base of the heart and the diaphragm
- Stomach, especially the pylorus
- Anywhere along the small intestine (Figure 4.6)
- Rectum.

The types of foreign body found within the alimentary tract are infinite but the commonest are:

- In dogs
  - Sticks wedged across roof of mouth
  - Balls, bone or hard pieces of food in pharynx
  - Chop bones or chicken bones in oesophagus
  - Balls, bones, stones or pieces of wood in stomach
  - Balls and stones within small intestine
  - Bone fragments and needles in rectum.

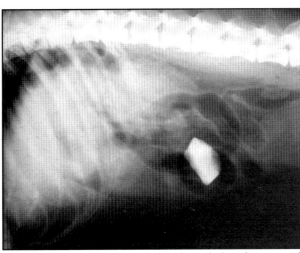

4.6 *Radiograph showing radiodense foreign body in the intestine of a dog.*

- In cats
  - Fish bones stuck between teeth
  - Loop of string round base of tongue and extending down alimentary tract ('linear foreign body')
  - Needles, fish hooks and chicken bones in pharynx, oesophagus and stomach
  - Fur balls in stomach.

Clinical signs: These depend on location of the foreign body and may be summarized as follows.
- Oral – salivation, pawing at mouth, dysphagia
- Pharynx – dysphagia, salivation, gagging, retching and difficulty in breathing
- Oesophagus – regurgitation
- Stomach – asymptomatic (unless in pylorus, when acute vomiting occurs)
- Proximal small intestine – acute vomiting
- Distal small intestine – chronic or intermittent vomiting
- Rectum – tenesmus, dyschezia, haematochezia and constipation.

Diagnosis: Diagnosis depends on the nature of the foreign body and its location. The following procedures may be used to detect foreign bodies:
- Oral examination
- Rectal examination
- Radiographs and contrast studies
- Endoscopy
- Exploratory laparotomy.

Treatment: Treatment depends on the location of the foreign body but usually involves some form of surgical intervention or endoscopic retrieval.

Hepatic disease

Hepatitis may be defined as inflammation of the liver. It is a general term used to describe most forms of hepatic disease. The causes of hepatitis are numerous and include:
- Primary hepatic disease
  - Infections such as infectious canine hepatitis (ICH) and leptospirosis
  - Toxic due to the ingestion of chemicals
  - Drug-induced due to anti-convulsants, azathioprine
  - Hereditary – copper accumulations
  - Portosystemic shunts
- Secondary hepatic disease
  - Metastatic malignant disease
  - Cushing's disease
  - Diabetes mellitus.

Clinical signs: Clinical signs of hepatic disease are frequently non-specific and could equally be associated with disease of another body system. There are other clinical signs that are considered more specific.
- Non-specific symptoms
  - Vomiting and diarrhoea
  - Weight loss
  - Polydipsia and polyuria
  - Anorexia
- Specific symptoms
  - Anterior abdominal pain
  - Jaundice
  - Ascites
  - Bleeding tendency
  - Hepatomegaly
  - Encephalopathy.

Jaundice is detected when the animal's mucous membranes and eventually skin are observed to be yellow in colour. There are many causes of jaundice and generally they are divided into three different categories:
- Pre-hepatic – associated with haemolysis of red blood cells
- Hepatic – due to various hepatic diseases
- Post-hepatic – associated with bile duct obstruction.

Diagnosis: Diagnostic procedures are described in detail in *BSAVA Manual of Advanced Veterinary Medicine*. They include:
- Clinical signs
- Elevation in liver enzymes
- Abnormal liver function tests.

Treatment:
- Hepatic support veterinary diets
- Antibiotics
- Anti-inflammatory drugs
- Intravenous fluid therapy
- Water-soluble bile acids.

Nursing care:
- Where infection is suspected – isolation, barrier nursing
- Provide and maintain therapy prescribed by veterinary surgeon
- Provide nutritional support
- Monitor all vital signs and report progress to veterinary surgeon
- Advise owner of animal's progress.

Pancreatic disease

The pancreas is composed of two types of tissue:
- Exocrine tissue (> 90%) – produces digestive enzymes
- Endocrine tissue (< 10%) – produces the hormones insulin and glucagon (see endocrine diseases, below).

Disease of the exocrine pancreas may be divided into:
- Pancreatitis – acute and chronic forms
- Exocrine pancreatic insufficiency (EPI)
- Exocrine tumours.

Pancreatitis (inflammation of the pancreas)

Acute pancreatitis is more common in dogs; chronic pancreatitis is more common in cats.

Aetiology: The aetiology of pancreatitis is extensive and includes:
- Obesity
- High fat diets
- Drug therapy
- Trauma
- Surgical manipulation
- Ascending infection, especially in cats
- Secondary to hepatic disease, especially in cats
- Bile duct obstruction, especially in cats.

Clinical signs:
- Sudden onset of anorexia and pyrexia
- Acute vomiting
- Anterior abdominal pain
- Dehydration, shock and collapse
- Later, diarrhoea may be observed.

Diagnosis: Diagnosis of pancreatitis is difficult and a variety of tests may be required in order to reach a definitive diagnosis. Diagnostic procedures are given in more detail in *BSAVA Manual of Advanced Veterinary Nursing* and include:

- Clinical findings
- Radiography to reveal dilated duodenum and local peritonitis in anterior abdomen
- Serum amylase, lipase and trypsin-like immunoreactivity (TLI) test
- Leucocytosis and shift to the left
- Ultrasonography of the pancreas.

Treatment:
- Nil by mouth for 3–5 days (includes fluids)
- Intravenous fluid therapy using Hartmann's solution
- Antibiotics
- Analgesics
- Low fat veterinary diet with replacement enzymes
- Restore body weight to normal
- Maintain long term on low fat diets.

Nursing care:
- Provide and maintain therapy prescribed by veterinary surgeon
- Monitor vital signs and report any progression
- Keep kennel clean of vomitus and provide a comfortable environment
- Provide and observe response to initiating feeding.

Exocrine pancreatic insufficiency (EPI)

This condition is rare in cats but relatively common in dogs. There is a total lack of digestive enzymes – hence the term maldigestion, which is often applied to this condition.

Aetiology:
- Hereditary deficiency in exocrine tissue, especially in German Shepherd Dogs
- Congenital condition in young dogs
- Following repeated episodes of pancreatitis with destruction of exocrine tissue.

Clinical signs:
- Ravenous appetite
- Coprophagia
- Marked weight loss
- Chronic large volume diarrhoea.

Diagnosis:
- Faecal analysis to detect undigested fat and starch (see Chapter 5)
- Serum trypsin-like immunoreactivity (TLI) test.

Treatment:
- Low fat veterinary diets
- Replacement enzyme supplement given with food
- Antibiotic for secondary bacterial overgrowth.

Nursing care:
- Advise owner on use of prescribed treatment
- Indicate how condition will improve
  - Faecal character will improve within 48 hours
  - Weight gain will occur slowly over several weeks
  - Ravenous appetite will be last to improve
- Offer encouragement to owner at repeat visits, as compliance is essential to success.

Renal disease

Various renal diseases occur dogs and cats, ranging from acute through to chronic disease.
- Acute renal failure
  - Mercury poisoning
  - Ethylene glycol poisoning (antifreeze)
  - Gentamicin administration
  - Sulphonamide administration
  - Leptospirosis
  - Hypovolaemia following haemorrhage
  - Addison's disease
  - Congestive heart failure
- Chronic renal failure
  - Progression from acute renal failure
  - Nephrotoxins
  - Congenital disease
  - Systemic lupus erythematosis (SLE)
  - Progression from glomerulonephritis
- Glomerulonephritis
  - Infectious diseases due to antibody/antigen complex
  - Immune-mediated disease, such as SLE
  - Endocrine disease, such as Cushing's disease and diabetes mellitus
- Nephrotic syndrome
  - End-stage kidney disease.

Acute renal failure

Clinical signs:
- Sudden onset anorexia, depression
- Anuria or oliguria followed by polydipsia and polyuria
- Vomiting
- Dehydration
- Halitosis.

Diagnosis:
- Elevated blood urea and creatinine
- Hyperkalaemia
- Metabolic acidosis
- Hyperphosphataemia
- Urinalysis may reveal isosthenuria, proteinuria, haematuria, casts and/or oxalate crystals.

Treatment:
- Identify and remove underlying cause (antifreeze or drugs)
- Intravenous fluid therapy using 0.9% saline or 5% dextrose saline
- Administer diuretics once dehydration is corrected
- Correct electrolyte disturbances
- Anti-emetics
- H_2 blockers
- Monitor urine production carefully – look for production > 2 ml/kg body weight per hour
- Antibiotics.

Chronic renal failure

Clinical signs:
- Anorexia
- Weight loss
- Lethargy
- Vomiting and diarrhoea
- Polydipsia and polyuria
- Non-regenerative anaemia
- Halitosis and oral ulceration.

Diagnosis:
- Elevated blood urea, creatinine and phosphorus
- Altered serum Ca:P ratio to > 1:4
- Urinalysis may reveal isosthenuria, casts, protein, blood (see Chapter 5).

Treatment:
- Intravenous fluid therapy
- Anti-emetics
- Antibiotics

- Dietary management using low phosphorus and protein diets
- Phosphate binders in food
- Anabolic steroids or erythropoietin to stimulate bone marrow.

Nephrotic syndrome

Clinical signs: Very similar to chronic renal failure, plus the following:
- May have signs of systemic disease
- Ascites, subcutaneous oedema and hydrothorax
- Severe weight loss.

Diagnosis: Similar to chronic renal failure, plus the following:
- Hypoproteinaemia associated with albumin loss
- Severe proteinuria.

Treatment:
- Plasma expanders (colloids)
- Diet using high biological value (BV) protein, low phosphorus, high levels of B vitamins and calories as fat and carbohydrate
- Anabolic steroids
- Diuretics for oedema, with care
- Antibiotics for secondary infection.

Nursing care for renal disease:
- Administer and maintain therapy as prescribed by veterinary surgeon
- Monitor urine production as described above
- Collect urine and blood samples for monitoring progress
- Provide stable and clean environment with regard to vomiting, diarrhoea and urine soiling
- Advise owner with regard to progress
- Advise owner if infections or poisons are implicated
- Assist in establishing nutritional management of patient
- Monitor oral water intake per 24 hours.

Lower urinary tract disease

Cystitis

Aetiology:
- Trauma
- Calculi (Figures 4.7 and 4.8)
- Ascending infections, especially in females
- Secondary to diabetes mellitus
- Secondary to Cushing's disease
- Secondary to neoplasia
- Secondary to immunosuppression (FIV, FeLV).

Clinical signs:
- Increased urinary frequency
- Urinary tenesmus
- Dysuria
- Incontinence
- Polydipsia.

Diagnosis:
- Urinalysis very important – catheterized or cystocentesis (see *BSAVA Manual of Advanced Veterinary Nursing*)
- Urine culture and sensitivity testing, ideally following cystocentesis
- Look for underlying cause.

Treatment:
- Antibiotic selection following sensitivity results
- Dietary management if calculi are present, to aid dissolution and recurrence

- Surgery to remove calculi or tumours
- Increase urine production by adding salt to diet.

Nursing care:
- Administer and maintain therapy prescribed by veterinary surgeon
- Collect samples for urinalysis
- Prevention of urine scalding (see 'Nursing the recumbent patient' below)
- Ensure dietary management is carried out.

Incontinence

Incontinence is an inability to control the passage of urine.

Aetiology:
- Sphincter mechanism incompetence
- Tumour – transitional cell carcinoma
- Prostatic disease
- Neurological defect
- Hypoplastic bladder
- Cystitis
- Behavioural.

Clinical signs:
- Passage of urine when lying down
- Passage of urine while walking about
- Wetness around perineum
- Urine scalding of perineum
- Signs of cystitis.

Treatment:
- Identify and treat underlying cause
- Use of barrier creams to prevent urine scalding
- Incontinence pads for bedding
- Offer frequent opportunities for passage of urine.

Nursing care:
- Administer and maintain therapy prescribed by veterinary surgeon

4.7 Urinary calculi

Type	Likely pH	Radiodensity	Location
Struvite	Alkaline	Radiodense	Bladder/urethra
Oxalate	Acid/alkaline	Variable	Urethra
Urates	Acid/alkaline	Radiolucent	Bladder
Cystine	Acid	Radiolucent	Bladder

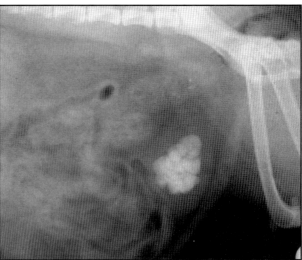

4.8 *Radiograph revealing multiple radiodense calculi in the urinary bladder of a dog. These were subsequently found to be struvite calculi.*

- Prevent urine scalding as described above
- Clip and clean perineal region
- Offer advice to owner.

Feline lower urinary tract disease

Previously known as feline urological syndrome (FUS), this disease includes a group of conditions that affect the lower urinary tract.

Aetiology:
- Nutritional factors
- Infectious disease
- Trauma
- Neurogenic causes
- Neoplastic disease
- Congenital abnormalities
- Iatrogenic causes.

Clinical signs:
- Signs of cystitis (see above)
- Dysuria
- Anuria and secondary azotaemia
- Haematuria
- Azotaemia
- Tenesmus
- Distended bladder.

Diagnosis:
- Radiographs of abdomen
- Catheterization of urethra, or inability to do so (see 'Urinary catheterization', below)
- Urinalysis
- Blood urea and creatinine where post-renal uraemia is present.

Treatment:
- Identify and treat the underlying cause where possible
- Antibiotics
- Urinary acidifiers
- Dietary management; low magnesium, phosphorus in particular.

Nursing care:
- Administer and maintain therapy prescribed by veterinary surgeon
- Monitor urine production
- Monitor for signs of dysuria and uraemia
- Collect samples for assessing progress of case.

Diseases of the nervous system

Seizures

Several terms are used to describe seizures, including fits and convulsions. Epilepsy is the term used to describe a central nervous disorder in which an irritable focus leads to disordered brain activity. Continuous seizures are called status epilepticus.

Seizures may be caused by primary nervous system disorders or occur secondary to systemic diseases:
- Primary
  - Infections, both viral and bacterial
  - Trauma with increased intracranial pressure
  - Congenital conditions such as hydrocephalus
  - Epilespy
  - Brain tumours
- Secondary
  - Hypoglycaemia
  - Portosystemic shunts
  - Hypocalcaemia
  - Hypokalaemia
  - Uraemia
  - Poisons such as metaldehyde.

Clinical signs: The clinical signs exhibited by animals having a seizure usually take the form of three phases:
- Preictal – just before the fit the animal will usually be asleep or resting and awaken suddenly, appearing restless and anxious
- Ictal – the actual fit: collapse, tonic and clonic activity, salivation, jaw champing, vocalization, voiding of urine and faeces are all possible
- Postictal – following the fit the animal may appear exhausted, dazed and anxious again. This will last for variable periods of time.

 When a pet dog or cat is having a seizure, the owner will be greatly distressed. The veterinary nurse should take command, calm the owner and give advice on what action the owner should take:
- Do not handle or restrain the animal
- Do not drive the animal to the surgery during its fit
- Remove children and others from the vicinity of the animal
- Provide a quiet dimly lit room
- Remove any objects that may injure the animal during the fit
- Stay with the animal but only observe
- Once the fit has finished, *then* bring the animal to the surgery.

Treatment:
- Identify and correct underlying cause
- Where epilepsy is diagnosed, start anti-convulsant treatment.

Opinion varies as to when anti-convulsants should be started. Usually if the animal has epilepsy and has a fit more frequently than every 3 months, then anti-convulsants should be prescribed.

Nursing care:
- The nurse should advise the owner on how to deal with an animal having a seizure (see above)
- Administer drugs as prescribed by veterinary surgeon
- Advise owner on:
  - Safe handling and storage of anti-convulsants
  - Recording episodes of fits
  - Looking out for recurrence of fits which may manifest as minor episodes, initially called petit mal, rather than typical fits
- Advise owners that fits are often progressive with time and may therefore require more treatment.

Loss of consciousness

This is sometimes called syncope or fainting. Unlike the seizure, syncope is a flaccid collapsing episode, with none of the activity observed with seizures. It should not be confused with seizures – there is no tonic or clonic muscle activity.

Aetiology:
- Cerebral anoxia
- CNS trauma
- Cardiopulmonary disease
- Barbiturate poisoning
- Heat stroke
- Airway obstruction

- Hypocalcaemia
- Narcolepsy
- Addison's disease.

Clinical signs:
- Sudden onset, with no preictal phase (see above)
- Flaccid collapse for variable periods of time
- Occasionally associated with exercise
- Cyanosis or pallor of mucous membranes
- Other signs if systemic disease
- Spontaneous recovery.

Diagnosis:
- Check for patent airway and mucous membrane colour
- Assessment of cardiopulmonary function: ECG, radiography, ultrasonography, blood gases
- Biochemistry profile for metabolic disease
- Neurological examination if primary CNS.

Nursing treatment of the unconscious patient:
- Send for veterinary surgeon
- Monitor vital signs
- Establish patent airway
- Supply oxygen and artificial respiration
- Assist veterinary surgeon in collecting blood samples
- Assist veterinary surgeon with additional therapy as required.

Paresis and paralysis

When the spinal cord is injured it may result in paresis (weakness) or paralysis of the fore and/or hindlimbs. Spinal cord injury is most likely following:
- Trauma such as road traffic accidents
- Intravertebral disc protrusion
- Neoplastic lesions.

Clinical signs:
- Paresis or weakness of one of more limb
- Paralysis of one or more limbs
- Paraplegia (hindlimbs paralysed)
- Tetraplegia (all limbs paralysed)
- Hemiplegia (limbs down one side paralysed)
- Urinary and/or faecal incontinence
- Lack of skin sensation (panniculus reflex)
- Loss of tail function.

Diagnosis:
- Physical examination of the patient
- Radiographic examination of the vertebral column
- Neurological examination, including
  - Withdrawal reflex: noxious stimuli to foot results in withdrawal and awareness

- Anal reflex: observe if anal sphincter contracts when inserting thermometer
- Panniculus reflex: pin prick on skin along flank results in skin twitching
- Patellar reflex: hold hindlimb partially extended and tap patellar ligament – limb should extend, but not excessively
- Tail function: pin prick for sensation – no tail wagging with motor loss
- Conscious proprioception: knuckle each paw – animal should immediately correct so pads touch floor
- Assess muscle tone in limbs
- Assess ability to urinate and defecate.

Nursing care:
- Help veterinary surgeon to carry out neurological examination
- Monitor vital signs
- Assist with radiographic procedures
- Prevent pressure sores by frequent turning and suitable bedding (see 'Nursing the recumbent patient', below)
- Avoid excess movement which may damage spine
- Assist in emptying bladder and rectum
- Prevent urine and faecal soiling
- Apply physiotherapy as directed by veterinary surgeon (see 'Physiotherapy' section, below)
- Ensure adequate nutrition is provided.

Endocrine diseases

Figure 4.9 describes components of the endocrine system.

Diabetes mellitus

Aetiology:
- Relapsing pancreatitis
- Influence of progesterone – oestrus
- Progestagens
- Obesity
- Cushing's disease and use of corticosteroids
- Acromegaly, growth hormone
- Immune-mediated disease.

Pathophysiology of ketoacidosis:
- Absolute or relative lack of insulin
- Leads to hyperglycaemia
- Failure of cells to take up glucose as energy source

4.9 Main components of the endocrine system

Organ	Location	Hormones produced	Disease
Pituitary gland	Base of brain	ACTH, TSH, FSH, oxytocin, ADH, LH	Irregularities in these hormones have their action through their target endocrine gland (see below)
Thyroid gland	Behind larynx	Thyroxine Calcitonin	Hypothyroidism/hyperthyroidism
Parathyroid gland	Next to thyroids	Parathormone	Hypo-/hyper- parathyroidism
Pancreas	Contiguous with stomach/duodenum	Insulin Glucagon	Diabetes mellitus Insulinoma
Adrenal glands	Cranial to kidneys	Cortisol Aldosterone	Cushing's disease Addison's disease
Ovaries	Abdomen	Progesterone Oestragen	Reproductive problems
Testes	Scrotum	Testosterone	Reproductive problems

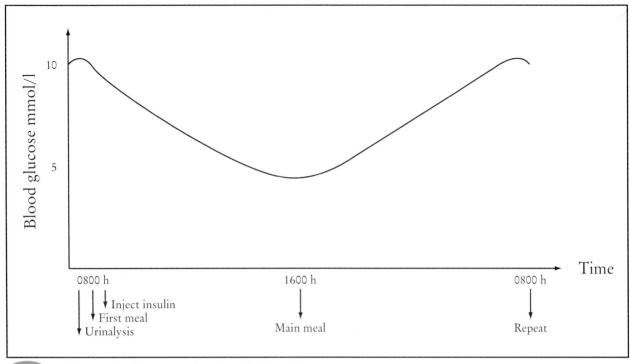

4.10 *Daily routine for administration of insulin and food to a diabetic patient.*

- Mobilization of fat as alternative energy source
- Incomplete degradation of fat, leading to formation of ketone by-products
- Excess mobilization of fatty acids results in metabolic acidosis.

Clinical signs: These change as the disease progresses:
- Initial
  - Polyphagia
  - Polydipsia
  - Polyuria
  - Bright alert animal
- Ketoacidosis
  - Anorexia
  - Vomiting
  - Dehydration
  - Ketotic breath
  - Polydipsia and polyuria.

Diagnosis:
- Clinical findings
- Glucosuria
- Ketonuria
- Hyperglycaemia
- Elevated fructosamines.

Treatment:
- Ketoacidosis
  - Nil by mouth
  - Intravenous fluids as Hartmann's solution, then 0.9% saline
  - Soluble insulin
  - Monitor blood sugar, sodium, potassium
- Routine management (started once ketoacidosis is resolved and animal is eating) (Figure 4.10)
  - Measure urine glucose in early morning
  - Calculate insulin dose (Figure 4.11)
  - Feed one quarter of daily ration
  - Administer depot insulin subcutaneously
  - Feed remainder of diet 8 hours later
  - Repeat each day.

Insulin
Calculation of insulin dose is explained in Figure 4.11.

There are two types of veterinary insulin licensed for dogs and cats:
- 100 IU/ml bovine insulin
  - Use 1 ml insulin syringe marked in *black*
  - Available in soluble form and depot insulins lente and protamine zinc
- 40 IU/ml porcine insulin
  - Use 1 ml insulin syringe marked in *red*
  - Available as a mixed insulin.

- Soluble or neutral insulin is a clear solution that can be given intravenously, intramuscularly or subcutaneously
- Depot insulins are all-white suspensions and must *only* be used subcutaneously
- All insulins should be kept at 4°C
- Gently mix insulin before loading syringe. *Do not shake bottle.*

Feline diabetes mellitus
It is usually impossible to obtain regular urine samples from cats. For indoor cats, special litter is available that will not affect the urine glucose estimation.

Most cats are stabilized using blood glucose levels. The aim is to get blood glucose levels between 5 and 12 mmol/l in each 24 hour period.

4.11 **Calculating insulin dose**

Urine glucose	Insulin dose
> 2%	Previous day's + 2 IU
1%	Previous day's + 1 IU
0.1%	Previous day's
0%	Previous day's – 2 IU

Fructosamine assays should be used to assess glycaemic control:
- High fructosamine levels mean poor glycaemic control over previous 3 weeks
- Low fructosamine levels suggest excessive glycaemic control over last 3 weeks
- Normal values suggest good glycaemic control over previous 3 weeks.

Dietary management
A high fibre diet should be used:
- Helps to treat obesity
- Helps to slow down glucose absorption from intestine and so glucose surges postprandially
- Diet should contain adequate protein of high BV, fat and carbohydrate for calories
- Carbohydrate must be complex and *not* simple sugars; therefore semi-moist foods should not be used
- Titbits should not be fed
- The same diet at the same amounts should be fed at the same times each day.

Exercise
- Moderate exercise (similar from day to day) should be provided
- Exercise should be increased gradually as the animal's weight falls to normal
- There should be no major changes in exercise from day to day.

Insulin overdose
Causes:
- Usually owner error in calculation or administration
- Animal refusing to eat after being given correct insulin dose
- Insulin peaking before main meal in afternoon.

Clinical signs:
- Muscle tremors
- Ataxia and incoordination
- Weakness
- Collapse
- Unconsciousness
- Death.

Treatment: Treatment depends on the clinical condition of the animal.
- If conscious, give a high sugar solution or food
- If unconscious, seek immediate veterinary assistance for intravenous glucose infusion.
- May need to change time of main meal if insulin is peaking early.

Complications
- Chronic renal failure
- Cataracts
- Insulin resistance.

Diabetes insipidus
Often called 'water diabetes', this endocrine disorder has two possible causes:
- Central form – associated with a deficiency in ADH production from pituitary
- Nephrogenic form – associated with failure of collecting ducts to respond to ADH.

Clinical signs:
- Polyuria, due to inability to concentrate urine
- Compensatory and marked polydipsia, often exceeding 150 ml/kg body weight per day
- Animal may vomit after ingesting large amounts of water
- Weight loss, due to failure to eat.

Diagnosis:
- Routine haematology and biochemistry are normal
- Urinalysis reveals no abnormality except very low specific gravity (< 1.009)
- Water deprivation test (WDT) normally carried out as modified WDT
  - Deprive animal of water at 10% per day for several days, under observation
  - Empty urinary bladder and measure specific gravity (SG)
  - Weigh animal and determine 5% of body weight
  - Keep in kennel without food or water
  - Empty urinary bladder every hour, weigh animal and measure SG
  - Once 5% body weight has been lost, stop test; *or* at anytime if animal becomes distressed
  - If SG > 1.025 after this test, animal is normal
  - If SG < 1.020, suspect diabetes insipidus.
- ADH test
  - Once rehydrated, repeat test as above *but* give ADH injection
  - If urine SG increases, then animal has central diabetes insipidus
  - If SG does not rise, then animal has nephrogenic diabetes insipidus.

Treatment:
- Central diabetes insipidus – ADH as intranasal drops daily
- Nephrogenic diabetes insipidus – chlorothiazides.

Nursing care:
- Assist veterinary surgeon in carrying out tests described above
- Assist in collection of samples, as required
- Administer therapy as prescribed by veterinary surgeon
- Advise owner on condition and treatment regimes
- Measure water intake on daily basis.

Hyperadrenocorticism (Cushing's disease)
In this condition the adrenal cortex secretes excessive amounts of cortisol. It may occur due to one of two causes:
- Pituitary tumour – producing excess ACTH, which stimulates the adrenal glands
- Adrenal tumour – producing cortisol autonomously.

Clinical signs:
- Polyphagia, polydipsia, polyuria
- Bilateral flank alopecia, becoming generalized
- Change in coat colour
- Pot-bellied appearance, due to liver enlargement and loss of muscle tone
- Muscle weakness and exercise intolerance.

Diagnosis: Diagnostic techniques are explained in more detail in *BSAVA Manual of Advanced Veterinary Nursing*.
- Elevations in alkaline phosphatase, leucocytosis, neutrophilia
- ACTH test – excessive response
- Dexamethasone suppression tests – failure to suppress
- Ultrasonography of adrenal glands.

Treatment:

- Surgery to remove adrenal tumours
- Mitotane for pituitary-mediated disease
- Alternatively ketoconazole may be used.

Hypothyroidism

This condition is most frequently seen in dogs and only rarely in cats. There is a failure to produce adequate levels of thyroxine, which in turn results in a reduction in metabolic rate. This leads to the classic signs of the condition:

- Anorexia
- Weight gain
- Marked lethargy
- Muscle weakness
- Bilateral alopecia
- 'Tragic' expression
- Bradycardia.

Diagnosis: Diagnostic techniques are explained in more detail in *BSAVA Manual of Advanced Veterinary Nursing*.

- Measure T4 levels in serum (usually very low)
- TSH test to assess thyroid function (poor response).

Treatment:

- Thyroid replacement therapy
- Monitor T4 levels and cardiac function.

Hyperthyroidism

This condition is observed most frequently in cats (but rarely in cats less than 6 years old) and is only very infrequently seen in dogs. There is an excessive production of thyroxine, which results in a marked increase in metabolic rate and the following clinical signs:

- Polyphagia
- Polydipsia and polyuria
- Weight loss
- Aggression, hyperexcitability, restlessness
- Occasionally chronic vomiting and diarrhoea
- Hypertrophic cardiomyopathy
- Palpable mass at neck

Diagnosis:

- Based on clinical features
- Measurement of high T4 levels.

Treatment:

- Carbimazole given daily, which stops T4 production
- Propranolol to assist cardiac function
- Surgical intervention to remove neoplastic thyroid gland(s).

Nursing care:

- Assist veterinary surgeon with diagnostic tests
- Monitor patient's vital signs and water intake
- Administer and maintain therapy prescribed by veterinary surgeon
- Assist with surgical procedures where appropriate.

Diseases of the musculoskeletal system

Ninety per cent of the calcium and phosphorus in the body is found in bone. In addition, calcium is required for blood clotting and for nerve and muscle function. Phosphorus is used in enzyme systems throughout the body.

The relationship between plasma calcium and phosphorus is important and is expressed as a ratio. Normally this is in the region of 1.5:1 (Ca:P).

Vitamin D, which is activated by the kidney, is required to:

- Assist in the absorption of calcium and phosphorus from the small intestine
- Reduce loss of calcium and phosphorus from the kidney
- Increase mineralization of bone.

Bone disease may be metabolic or non-metabolic. For example:

- Metabolic bone disease
  - Secondary nutritional hyperparathyroidism
  - Metaphyseal osteopathy
  - Rickets
- Non-metabolic bone disease
  - Pulmonary osteopathy
  - Osteomyelitis
  - Bone tumours
  - Arthritis.

Secondary nutritional hyperparathyroidism

- Caused by deficiency of calcium or excess of phosphorus in the diet
- Most commonly associated with feeding 'all meat' diets
- Often associated with young growing puppies of the giant breeds
- Results in secretion of parathormone from parathyroid glands to release calcium from bone in order to maintain blood calcium level
- Renal excretion of phosphorus is increased to restore Ca:P ratio.

Clinical signs:

- Depression
- Lameness
- Pain on locomotion
- Compression fractures and pathological fractures occur following minor trauma
- Demineralization may lead to 'rubber jaw' and loosening of teeth.

Treatment:

- Most effective treatment is dietary correction
- Use a suitable commercial puppy food
- *Do not* supplement a bad diet with calcium.

Metaphyseal osteopathy

This is also known as Moller-Barlow's disease, juvenile scurvy and hypertrophic osteodystrophy. The true cause is not known but it is thought to be associated with a deficiency in vitamin C.

The disease affects the metaphysis, where a necrotic band develops next to the growth plate, followed by deposition of a band of osseous tissue in the metaphysis and periosteal reaction.

Clinical signs:

- Always young growing dogs (clinical signs will disappear as dog matures), often large breeds
- Often severe lameness and pain on movement
- Some dogs are totally unable to walk
- Swollen and very painful growth plate regions of all four limbs
- Pyrexia often > 40.5°C.

Treatment:

- Powerful analgesics are required
- Correct the diet to a commercial puppy growth diet
- Ensure adequate fluid intake
- Nursing care to turn animal regularly
- Ensure urination and defecation are possible.

Rickets

Rickets is the term used for this condition in young animals; in adult animals it is termed osteomalacia. In this condition there is failure of mineralization around growth plates. The cause is not fully understood but it is thought to be due to a deficiency in vitamin D. Calcium and phosphorus deficiencies may also be involved.

Clinical signs:

- Most frequently observed in young growing dogs
- Marked enlargement of growth plates
- Bowing of limbs
- Enlargement of costochondral junctions ('rickety rosary')
- Lameness, less severe than metaphyseal osteopathy
- Spontaneous fractures may occur.

Treatment:

- Correct the diet to an appropriate puppy growth diet
- Give analgesics initially to control pain.

Pulmonary osteopathy

Often known as Marie's disease, this is a condition of the bones of the lower limbs, especially forelimbs, associated with a thoracic mass. Marked periosteal proliferation occurs in the carpal and metacarpal bones and digits. There is no joint involvement. The reason for these changes is not known.

Clinical signs:

- Bilateral painful soft tissue swelling of lower forelimbs
- Lameness
- These changes are often observed *before* thoracic signs develop.

Treatment:

- None – usually by the time limb changes occur the mass in the thorax is inoperable
- Euthanasia.

Osteomyelitis

This inflammation of the bone usually involves both cortex and medulla. The condition is classified as follows:

- Infectious causes
  - Bacterial infections
  - Fungal infections
- Non-infectious causes
  - Trauma to the bone
  - Sequelae following fractures
  - Foreign bodies and implants.

Clinical signs:

- Pyrexia
- Bone pain
- Lameness
- Loss of function.

Diagnosis:

- Radiographs reveal lytic areas in bone together with other areas of proliferation
- Failure of fractures to heal
- Obvious bone fragments may be seen.

Treatment:

- Identify and correct underlying cause
- Remove bone fragments and foreign bodies surgically
- Antibiotics where infection is present.

Bone tumours

Several bone tumours may be observed in dogs and cats. The two most important are osteoma and osteosarcoma:

- Osteoma
  - Benign slow-growing tumour
  - May cause mechanical interference with function if near a joint
  - May be found anywhere on axial and appendicular skeleton
- Osteosarcoma
  - Primary malignant and aggressive tumour
  - Initially spreads to local lymph node, then lung
  - More common in giant breeds (St Bernard, Great Dane, Dobermann)
  - More common in dogs older than 7 years
  - Most often involves proximal humerus, distal radius/ulna, distal femur and distal tibia
- Chondrosarcoma – slow-growing tumour of flat bones
- Fibrosarcoma – rare tumour affecting growth plates and periosteum
- Osteochondroma
  - Most frequently observed during bone growth
  - Affects limb bones and vertebrae
- Chondroma – affects the skull and spreads locally to brain.

Arthritis

By definition, this refers to inflammation of the joint. Several forms of arthritis are classified in Figure 4.12.

Clinical signs:

- Variable degrees of lameness
- Degenerative types slow onset, improve with exercise, crepitus on movement
- Pyrexia and joint pain associated with infection
- Immune-mediated cases have multiple joint involvement, other signs of systemic disease
- Recent history of drug administration or vaccination.

4.12 Classification of arthritis

Degenerative	Primary	Aetiology unknown
	Secondary	Hip dysplasia
		Cruciate ligament rupture
Inflammatory	Infective	Bacterial, viral, fungal and mycoplasmal
	Non-infective	Crystal formation (gout)
Immune-mediated	Erosive	Rheumatoid
		Polyarthritis
	Non-erosive	Systemic lupus erythematosus (SLE)
		Polyarthritis nodosa
		Drug-induced
		Vaccination reactions

Diagnosis: Diagnostic procedures are explained in more detail in *BSAVA Manual of Advanced Veterinary Nursing.*

- Radiographic changes to joint and periosteal regions around joint
- Check for systemic disease
  - Routine blood tests
  - Coombs test
  - ANA test
  - Rheumatoid factor
  - Cytology of joint fluid.

Treatment:

- Identify and treat underlying cause
- Antibiotics where infective
- Immunosuppressive drugs in immune-mediated disease
- Non-steroidal anti-inflammatory drugs for degenerative disease
- Surgery to correct joint instability.

Nursing care:

- Assist veterinary surgeon in taking of radiographs
- Assist veterinary surgeon in collection of blood samples, joint fluid and other tests
- Administer and maintain therapy prescribed by veterinary surgeon
- Assist animal with locomotion in order to allow defecation and urination
- If recumbent, turn frequently to prevent bed sores
- Physiotherapy where appropriate
- Maintain comfortable environment
- Advise owner.

Muscle disease

Myositis disease refers to inflammation of the muscle. This may involve one muscle group or be associated with multiple muscle groups (polymyositis). There are many causes of myositis, including infections and immune-mediated disease.

Myopathy or muscle weakness and loss of function may also occur with metabolic diseases such as Cushing's disease and hypothyroidism (see section on endocrine disease).

Diagnosis:

- Check routine bloods for systemic disease
- Collection of muscle biopsy
- Electromyography (EMG) assists in detecting disease of muscle fibres and associated nerves.

Treatment: Treatment depends on the underlying cause but may include antibiotics, immunosuppressive drugs and treatment for metabolic disease.

Cutaneous disease

Parasitic skin disease

- *Cheyletiella* spp.
  - Surface-dwelling mite
  - Can live off host
  - Affects dogs, cats, rabbits and humans
  - Life cycle 5 weeks
  - Marked pruritus over whole body
  - Often referred to as walking dandruff
- *Sarcoptes scabiei*
  - Burrowing mite
  - May live off host
  - Mainly affects dogs

- Can affect owner
  - Life cycle 3–4 weeks
  - Intense pruritus often starts around head and legs but often generalized
- *Demodex*
  - Lives in hair follicles
  - Cannot live off host
  - Specific to dog and cat
  - Life cycle very variable
  - Initially pruritus and alopecia around eyes and feet but can be generalized
- Fleas
  - Surface-dwelling
  - Can live off host
  - Not host specific – may affect humans
  - Life cycle 3 weeks to 2 years
  - Miliary dermatitis, allergic reactions, pruritus
- Lice
  - Surface-dwelling
  - Must live on host
  - Host specific
  - Life cycle 3 weeks
  - Pruritus often around ears and neck initially; can be generalized
  - May be able to see 'nits' or eggs attached to hairs
- *Neotrombicula* spp.
  - Surface-dwelling mite
  - May live off host
  - Not host specific and may affect humans
  - Life cycle up to 70 days
  - Intense pruritus, especially around paws but may be generalized
  - Seasonal occurrence
- *Notoedres* spp.
  - Burrowing mite
  - Must live on host
  - Primarily in cats
  - Life cycle not known
  - Initially pruritus around ears, then face, and extends to neck
- *Otodectes* spp.
  - Surface-dwelling mite
  - Can live off host
  - Affects only dogs and cats
  - Life cycle 3 weeks
  - Pruritus of external ear canal – head tilt, head shaking, pawing at ears
- Ticks
  - Surface-dwelling
  - Can live off host
  - Not host specific, may affect humans
  - Life cycle 2 months to 2 years
  - Local reaction and pruritus where tick attaches to host. May spread infections such as Lyme's disease.

Diagnosis:

- Surface mites – adhesive tape preparations, superficial skin scrapings and brushings (see Chapter 5)
- Burrowing mites – deep skin scrapings
- *Trombicula* spp. – look between digits for clusters of red mites
- Lice – look on pinna initially for adults and eggs
- Fleas – look for flea dirt on skin, as well as adults (which are more difficult to find)
- Demodectic mange – squeeze pustules, which are loaded with mites; or skin scraping if non-pustular form.

Treatment:
- Sarcoptic and demodectic mange
  - Clip out coat if longhaired breed
  - Wash in amitraz solutions
- *Cheyletiella* spp., lice, *Neotrombicula* spp.
  - Shampoo using pyrethrin-based products
  - Needs to be repeated at least twice
  - Fipronil spray may also be used
- Ear mites – ear ointments containing monosulfiram
- Fleas and ticks
  - Dichlorvos and fenitrothion sprays
  - Fipronil spray or spot-on (kills fleas on contact)
  - Lufenuron tablets for dogs and injection for cats (chitin inhibitor only kills larvae – no action on adults)
  - Permethrin and methoprene sprays for environmental control of fleas.

Ringworm

Also known as dermatophytosis, this is a fungal infection of the skin, hair and nailbed areas of dogs and cats. It is more common to see clinical disease in cats than dogs.

Infection is obtained by direct contact and indirect contact (fomites). It is an important zoonosis.

There are two main types of organism involved:
- *Microsporum canis*
  - Accounts for around 95% of feline disease
  - Accounts for around 40–80% of canine disease
- *Trichophyton* spp.
  - Accounts for around 4% of feline disease
  - Accounts for between 12 and 60% of canine disease.

Clinical signs:
- Dogs
  - Initial circular rings of alopecia with grey crusting coloration
  - Most often seen around head and forelimbs
  - May become generalized
- Cats
  - May initially appear as circular areas of alopecia, grey and crusting
  - May also appear as miliary dermatitis
  - May remain asymptomatic.

Diagnosis: Diagnostic procedures are explained in more detail in Chapter 5.
- Pluck out hairs for culture using Sabouraud's medium
- Ultraviolet light fluorescence
- Skin scrapings to observe spores.

Treatment:
- Oral griseofulvin tablets given with food
- Clip hair from lesions in longhaired breeds
- Apply local enilconazole solutions to lesion
- For cats, use chlorhexidine solutions on lesions
- Burn bedding where possible
- Disinfect with sodium hypochlorite, formalin or enilconazole solutions.

Nursing care:
- Assist veterinary surgeon in carrying out diagnostic tests
- Administer and maintain therapy prescribed by veterinary surgeon
- Help to prevent self-damage by animal
- Advise owners where zoonotic disease exists
- Advise owners on precautions that may be taken
- Advise owners on importance of cleaning environment.

Hormonal alopecia

The conditions in this group are usually associated with one of the following.
- Hypothyroidism
- Hyperadrenocorticism (Cushing's disease)
- Sertoli cell tumour (hyperoestrogenism)
- Canine ovarian imbalances (hyper- and hypo-oestrogenism)
- Feline hormonal alopecia.

Clinical signs:
- The majority of cases have bilateral alopecia, usually starting on the flanks
- There is rarely pruritus. The skin is unreactive
- There are frequently other signs of systemic disease.

Diagnosis:
- Find and correct the underlying cause
- Blood tests
- Hormonal assays.

Treatment: Treatment depends on identifying and correcting the underlying cause.

Pyoderma

Pyoderma is more common in the dog than in the cat. There is frequently an underlying cause for its development, such as *Demodex* infection or immunosuppression.

Pyodermas are usually classified as follows:
- Surface dermatitis
  - Acute moist dermatitis and skin fold dermatitis
  - Frequently involves the side of the face, or hindquarters
  - Associated with ear infections and anal sac disorders
  - Significant self-trauma involved in aetiology
  - Skin fold dermatitis due to anatomical problem with folding of skin preventing proper ventilation
  - Seen mostly in Sharpei, Pug, Pekingese
- Superficial dermatitis
  - Impetigo, puppy dermatitis or juvenile dermatitis
  - Often seen on ventral abdomen of puppies
  - Multiple yellow pustules
  - Also occurs as folliculitis where the hair follicle is involved
  - Ring formations develop, giving moth-eaten appearance
  - Formations spread out radially
- Deep pyoderma
  - Pododermatitis (i.e. affecting feet)
  - Paws become swollen and painful and exude pus
  - Fistulas and sinus tracts may be seen
  - Furunculosis associated with ringworm and *Demodex* infection
  - Very serious deep-seated infection which may be generalized
- Feline pyoderma
  - Associated with cats biting each other
  - Oral bacteria 'injected' under skin, leading to cellulitis
  - Usually involves a limb with swelling, pain and pyrexia

Treatment:
- Involves identifying and correcting the underlying cause
- Culture and sensitivity of purulent material
- Long-term antibiotic use.

Allergic skin disease

Various forms of allergic skin disease are seen in dogs and cats.

Urticaria
- Induced by drugs, vaccines, insect bites/stings
- Sudden development of multiple oedematous-like swellings over skin surface, with erection of hairs at each site
- Diagnosis based on presentation and known cause
- Treat by removing cause and giving anti-inflammatory drugs.

Atopic dermatitis
- Large number of known antigens, including housedust mites, fungi, pollens and danders
- Usually affects dogs 1–3 years old
- Intense pruritus, especially around eyes, feet, axilla and ventral abdomen
- May get otitis externa and ocular discharge
- Miliary lesions may develop, especially along the back
- Diagnosis with intradermal skin test
- Treatment is lifelong using antihistamines, anti-inflammatory drugs, shampoos, desensitization.

Food hypersensitivity
- May occur due to consumption of food proteins such as beef, pork, milk, eggs, etc.
- Pruritic skin disease and/or chronic vomiting and diarrhoea may occur
- Diagnosis on clinical presentation, use of elimination diets
- Treatment requires avoidance of initiating agents.

Contact dermatitis
- May be induced by soaps, detergents, chemicals of any kind
- Develops about 5 weeks after initial exposure
- Pruritus and erythema involving feet, ventral abdomen, face
- Diagnosis requires patch testing with suspect agents
- Treatment involves avoiding contact with known agents.

Nursing the geriatric patient

As pets become older they require special consideration from the veterinary practice, the veterinary surgeon and the veterinary nurse. In general giant breeds of dog tend to age more rapidly than smaller breeds and cats tend to age less rapidly than dogs.

'Geriatric' or 'senior' animals are:

- Large-breed dogs aged 6 years and older
- Smaller-breed dogs aged 8–9 years and older
- Cats aged 9 years and older.

As an animal enters old age it has a decreased ability to adjust to change, there is a reduction in body cells (as those worn out are not readily replaced) and the surviving cells do not work as efficiently as before. Two main factors are responsible for these changes:

- Ageing – physical and behavioural changes (Figure 4.13)
- Accumulated injury.

Accumulated injury
Injuries sustained during a lifetime plus an age-related loss of functional reserve mean that maximum organ function is reduced with age. This becomes apparent when the animal is stressed due to:

- Severe exercise
- Changes in routine – hospitalization/boarding kennels
- Changes in environmental temperature
- Acute illness
- Anaesthesia
- Inadequate nutrition
- Dehydration.

A number of diseases associated with decreased cell and organ function are commonly seen in geriatric animals (Figure 4.14). Common problems associated with ageing in the main body systems are listed in Figure 4.15. All these factors must be taken into consideration when nursing a geriatric patient.

4.13 Common physical and behavioural age-related changes

Physical factors that are reduced in geriatric animals
- Stamina
- Agility
- Metabolic rate – an average 20% decrease which often leads to obesity exacerbating many other geriatric disease processes
- Regenerative powers
- Protein levels
- Muscle mass – less efficient cells, and decreased replacement leads to atrophy
- Bone mass
- Immune responses – therefore increased susceptibility to disease including neoplasia
- Sense of smell/taste/sight and hearing
- Hair – becomes sparse, dull and listless, and white hairs appear on muzzle
- Elasticity of the skin, some thickening of the skin, callus formation
- Ability for producing melanin – nose may become pinker

Behavioural changes seen in geriatric animals
- Forgetting basic obedience and house training
- Irritable when disturbed
- Slower reactions to stimuli
- Developing sleep disorders
- Less adaptable to change
- Disorientation
- Inappetence

4.14 Common diseases seen in geriatric animals due to decreased cell function

Neoplasia (e.g. oral, skin, mammary, prostate, testis)
Chronic renal disease
Chronic heart disease
Diabetes mellitus
Osteoarthritis
Bone fractures
Periodontal disease
Ear/eye problems
Constipation
Urinary and faecal incontinence
Obesity
Weight loss

Common problems associated with ageing in the main body systems

Digestive system	
Oral cavity	Increased dental calculus Periodontal disease leading to atrophy and retraction of the gums, with increased tooth loss Infected teeth can lead to absorption of bacterial toxins/periodontal bacteraemia Ulcerative lesions – bacterial/uraemia/decreased saliva production Tumours
Oesophagus	Loss of muscle tone
Stomach	Reduced hydrochloric acid secretion in the stomach, resulting in vomiting/flatulence and intermittent diarrhoea
Liver	Decreased hepatocyte numbers leading to reduced liver function, biliary and intestinal secretions
Intestine	Impaired intestinal motility Decreased rate of intestinal epithelial renewal leading to decreased lipid absorption Decreased villous height and width thus decreased areas for nutrient absorption
Anal glands	Impaction due to increased thickness of fluid, irregular defecation, decreased bulk of faeces

Cardiorespiratory system	
Heart	Cardiac output decreased by 30% in last third of animal's life span Fibrous thickening of the valves (endocardiosis) Red cell counts and haemoglobin levels decrease Reduced peripheral circulation
Lungs	Atrophy of secretory structures may cause obstructive lung disease Chronic bronchitis Increased susceptibility to infection Reduced ability to expel air Alveolar capillary membrane has reduced diffusing capacity Atrophy and weakening of respiratory muscles Loss of elastic tissue Increased pulmonary fibrosis, eventually leading to increased intrapleural pressure, decreased cardiac output and ultimate right-sided cardiac failure

Urinary system	
Kidneys	Reduced function Scarring of medulla and cortex Decreased glomerular filtration rate as a result of interstitial pressure, reduced renal perfusion and altered permeability of glomerular membrane
Bladder	Incontinence due to reduced bladder sphincter tone particularly in spayed bitches Chronic cystitis from incomplete bladder emptying

Endocrine system	
	Decreased secretion of hormones by thyroid glands, testes and ovaries Geriatric hormonal activity may affect skin and coat condition, and encourage weight gain Lethargy

Reproductive system	
	Mammary gland tumours Pyometra in unspayed bitches and queens Testicular atrophy Testicular tumours Pendulous prepuce due to oestrogen secretion from sertoli cells or androgen deficit Prostatic hyperplasia Prostatic disease – enlarged due to hypertrophy, infection, cysts and neoplasia Perineal rupture

Musculoskeletal system	
	Loss of muscle mass Deterioration of neuromuscular function Loss of bone mass Thinner cortices of long bones Split and fragmented cartilage Thickened synovial fluid and joint capsules Osteophyte formation Arthritis – wear and tear of joints.

Figure 4.15 continues ▶

Nervous system and special sense organs

General	Chronic hypoxia of the brain
	Sleep disorders
	Neuromuscular disorders
	Depression
	Reduced reaction to stimuli
	Reduced response to pain
Eye	Impaired sight
	Retinal atrophy
	Iris atrophy
	Cataracts
	Increased density of the lens (nuclear sclerosis)
	Increased tear viscosity
	Increased susceptibility to infection
	Warts
Ear	Chronic otitis
	Wax accumulation
	Impaired hearing
Nose	Decreased sense of smell

Hair and skin

	Prolonged healing time of skin
	Reduced general condition
	Thinned coat
	Greasy skin
	Calluses and pressure sores
	Increased frequency of sebaceous gland adenomas, cysts, lipomas, skin tumours
	Hyperkeratinized footpads
	Nails, including dew claws, often become overgrown and sometimes malformed, due to reduced exercise and cell dysfunction

Feeding

Dietary needs

The gastrointestinal tract of a geriatric animal may have reductions in muscle tone, ability to absorb nutrients and provision of gastric juices. The diet must be adjusted accordingly, and should be fed in divided meals two to four times daily. The animal may also need encouragement to eat.

Dietary factors to consider include:

- Increased palatability
- Increased digestibility
- Protein of high biological value
- Fibre (aids digestive tract function and used to control obesity, but may reduce the palatability of the diet)
- Carbohydrate levels to maintain normal body weight
- Sufficient vitamins, minerals and essential fatty acids (EFA)
- Freely available fresh water.

Further adjustments should be made for a patient with concurrent disease:

- Obesity – reduce fat
- Cardiac disease – reduce sodium
- Renal disease – reduce phosphorus
- Liver disease – increase vitamins B, C, D and K.

Monitoring water intake

Water intake may be slightly increased in older animals because of reduced organ efficiency. Water should always be freely available to the patient (see Figure 4.16).

If an animal drinks more than the average requirement, enough extra water should be provided each day to meet its daily need. If the water intake is significantly elevated or decreased, the veterinary surgeon must be notified. Polydipsia is usually defined as a water intake in excess of 100 ml/kg/24 h.

4.16 **Calculating an animal's water intake**

1. Calculate the average daily water requirement for the patient (40–60 ml/kg body weight per 24 h)
2. Measure out the water required, rounded up to the nearest half litre, and give to the animal
3. Replenish with fresh measured water if required
4. Measure any water left after 24 h to calculate the animal's actual daily water intake.

A 10 kg dog is given 1 l water in the morning. Within 8 h the water has been consumed, and is replenished immediately with a further 1 l water. When measured the following morning there is 700 ml water left in the bowl.

This dog has consumed 1.3 l water over 24 h, which is equal to 130 ml/kg/day (calculated by dividing the total consumed by the weight of the animal). A minimum of 1.5 l must be given to the patient for the next 24 h period. This animal is polydipsic and the veterinary surgeon must be notified.

It should be noted that the amount of moisture contained within the food provided (i.e. canned versus dry) will influence the animal's daily water intake.

Owners can be taught how to monitor fluid intake at home and instructed to contact the surgery if there are any marked changes.

Exercise

A change in exercise regime may be required in the geriatric pet due to reduced stamina or concurrent disease. Short and frequent exercise is beneficial as it helps to maintain joint movement and muscle tone, reduce adhesions and stiffness, and will also help control obesity.

When walking:

- Allow frequent opportunity for urination and defecation
- Observe frequency of urination and defecation
- Note any respiratory change or coughing
- Look for lameness or stiffness of gait
- Avoid sudden changes in routine.

In lethargic or hospitalized patients, passive physiotherapy of the limb joints may help to maintain joint mobility and muscle tone.

Mental stimulation

Geriatric pets may need more attention than younger adult animals, which can be time consuming for both owners and nurses. Although older animals tend to sleep more often, they benefit from extra stimulation and care.

Ways of stimulating geriatric pets include:

- Exercise
- Daily grooming
- New and interesting toys
- Television/radio/music, especially if the animal is left alone
- Socialization with other animals and people
- Fish in a tank (closed!) for older cats.

Grooming

Regular grooming is essential for the geriatric patient, who is often less able or less willing to self-groom. It enables the handler to observe what is 'normal' for that animal, and therefore detect and report any changes to the veterinary surgeon more promptly. Geriatric patients must be handled confidently and gently while grooming, with particular consideration given to an arthritic patient.

Grooming prevents matting, stimulates skin and sebaceous glands and maintains the coat in good order. It provides regular mental stimulation for the patient and improves the bond between the handler and the animal.

It also provides the opportunity to check for:

- Discharges (regular cleaning of eyes, ears, prepuce and vulva)
- Nail health (nails, including dew claws, often become overgrown and sometimes malformed)
- Skin lesions or growths
- Parasites.

Any abnormalities detected should be recorded and brought to the attention of the veterinary surgeon.

Bedding

Consider the special needs of a geriatric patient in relation to bedding:

- Increased need for sleep
- Increased need for warmth
- Peripheral circulation is not as efficient in the geriatric and calluses or bedsores may occur
- Incontinence.

Adaptations

- Raise the bed and place in a draught-free area
- Provide warm and insulative bedding
- To give support, provide cushioned/thick bedding (e.g. PVC-covered foam, synthetic fleece, blankets)
- For patients with normal bladder control, provide beanbags
- For incontinent patients, provide bed with urine-proof base containing washable bedding.

Hospitalization of the geriatric patient

Hospitalization periods should be kept to a minimum, as geriatric patients are less adaptable to change and become stressed when taken out of their normal environment. They may also be susceptible to nosocomial infection.

Before admitting the patient:

- Gather information from the owner regarding routine, care, feeding, medication, apparent disabilities, commands, etc.
- Assist veterinary surgeon to carry out a general health check
- Assist veterinary surgeon to carry out any tests required to investigate abnormalities.

With geriatric in-patients:

- Observe closely for signs of chronic disease
- Monitor vital signs on a regular basis – body temperature may be at the lower end of the normal range; pulse and respiration rates may be at the higher end of the normal range
- Consider their special needs – bedding, nutrition, exercise, grooming, mental stimulation
- Physiotherapy can be used as a supportive therapy (see later)
- Reduce stress.

 Blind patients should be spoken to before being approached, so that they are aware of your presence.
If the patient is deaf, approach through its line of sight.

Anaesthesia

Special consideration must be given to the geriatric patient admitted for an operation or investigation requiring a general anaesthetic. The geriatric patient may have:

- Reduced ability to distribute, metabolize and excrete drugs
- Reduced distribution and clearance rates
- Reduced renal reserves
- Compromised cardiac function
- Increased susceptibility to stress.

Preoperatively

- Water should only be withdrawn 30 min prior to operation
- Pre-anaesthetic health check including blood profiles may be undertaken.

Premedication and induction of general anaesthesia

The anaesthetic regime should be carefully selected for the geriatric patient (see Chapter 8).

Postoperatively

Geriatric patients may have a longer recovery time due to the possibility of hepatic or cardiovascular insufficiency. Precautions must be taken:

- Provide external warmth
- Observe regularly and monitor temperature, pulse, respiration, capillary refill time and colour of mucous membranes
- Consider other predisposing factors to apparent prolonged recovery, e.g. osteoarthritis.

Advice to the owner

Advice concerning a geriatric pet may be complicated. After discussing care and treatment with the owner, advice should be backed up with leaflets and written instructions.

Factors to discuss with the owner (some of which have already been detailed) include:

- Exercise
- Urination and defecation
- Eyesight and hearing
- Feeding and water intake
- Mental stimulation
- Bedding
- Grooming
- Veterinary care.

Veterinary care

The importance of annual vaccinations should be emphasized to the owner. The older pet may have increased susceptibility to disease due to decreased immune resistance.

A regular 6-monthly check as part of a geriatric healthcare programme can be undertaken. These checks may detect problems early, before advanced disease disabilities become apparent (which are then often more complex to control).

The check by the veterinary surgeon may include:

- Weight
- Feeding (dietary advice and provision of clinical diets)
- Teeth, gums and eyes
- Gait and mobility
- Heart and lungs
- Organ function (a blood sample may be taken)
- Urine (urinalysis may be performed to look for signs of renal disease).

Nursing the recumbent patient

A recumbent patient is one that is unwilling or unable to rise. Problems occur because of this inability and the fact that the patient is in the same position for prolonged periods of time.

Causes of recumbency include:

- Anaesthesia (particularly in the geriatric patient)
- Spinal surgery
- Fractured pelvis
- Surgery for multiple fracture injuries

- Paraplegia
- Shock
- Head injuries
- Neurological disorders (e.g. coma)
- Debilitating medical disease (e.g. cardiac disease).

Problems associated with recumbent patients are more easily prevented than cured. In addition to general nursing care, other factors must be considered when nursing recumbent patients:

- Hypostatic pneumonia
- Bed sores (decubitus ulcers)
- Soiling
- Problems associated with urination and defecation
- Temperature control
- Musculoskeletal problems
- Inappetence/inability to eat or drink
- Coat/skin problems
- Depression.

Hypostatic pneumonia

When a patient is recumbent for long periods, blood pools in the lower lung. The alveoli tend to collapse, causing oxygen deficiency and static blood supply. This in turn is an ideal medium for growth of microorganisms causing pneumonia.

Prevention
- Turn the laterally recumbent patient every 2–4 h, 24 h per day
- Alternate lateral recumbency with supported sternal recumbency for 30 min periods. Patients can be supported using sandbags, rolled-up blankets and towels, or beanbags
- Encourage active assisted or supported exercise
- Give respiratory physiotherapy – positioning, postural drainage, coupage and vibrations
- Record all treatments, including time in each position.

Supported exercise and respiratory physiotherapy are discussed in the physiotherapy section.

Clinical signs of hypostatic pneumonia
- Increased rate and depth of respiration
- Increased effort of respiration
- Abdominal breathing
- Increased lung sounds, gurgling – moist breathing
- Depression.

Treatment
If hypostatic pneumonia develops, the veterinary surgeon must be informed so that treatment may be given promptly. Nursing techniques used to treat hypostatic pneumonia are as those listed in 'Prevention' above.

Bedsores

Bedsores, or decubitus ulcers, occur on areas of little subcutaneous fat and over bony prominences. Pressure on these areas in the recumbent patient is almost continuous, resulting in a decreased local blood supply and anoxia of tissues.

Areas that may develop decubitus ulcers are:

- Facial prominences, including point of jaw
- Point of shoulder
- Elbow
- Wings of ilium

- Ischial tuberosity
- Greater trochanter of femur
- Hock
- Tarsus.

Prevention
- Turn or reposition patient every 2–4 h
- Supportive and comfortable bedding, e.g. PVC-covered foam mattresses, synthetic fleece or bubble-wrap (multiple layers of bedding are sufficient if PVC foam beds are not available)
- Physiotherapy (orthopaedic and neurological, massage – see later)
- Pad and bandage potential problem areas
- Close attention to hygiene
- Check problem areas twice daily.

Clinical signs
- Redness
- Inflammation
- Ulceration.

Treatment
If decubitus ulcers develop, the veterinary surgeon must be informed. Nursing techniques are as those listed in 'Prevention' above. In addition the area should be clipped, cleaned with a mild antiseptic, dried thoroughly and a soothing barrier or therapeutic cream applied.

Problems associated with urination and defecation
Constipation, diarrhoea, urine retention, urinary incontinence and patient soiling are some of the problems encountered with the recumbent patient. Nursing patients with soiling problems from urinary incontinence and diarrhoea are dealt with under the section on the soiled patient, below.

Constipation
Due to decreased circulation, decreased activity and decreased intake of food and water, constipation may occur.
Factors to consider:

- A patient should pass faeces at least once every 48 h. If this does not occur, inform the veterinary surgeon
- Diet may need to be adjusted to try to reduce the occurrence of constipation
- Treatment may be prescribed by the veterinary surgeon (e.g. oral liquid paraffin, or an enema).

Diarrhoea
Faecal incontinence, diarrhoea or a rectal enema may cause problems.
Factors to consider:

- Treatment of the cause
- Adjusting the diet
- Nursing of the soiled patient (see later).

Urinary incontinence
Urinary incontinence may occur in a patient with neurological disease, nerve damage due to trauma, or debility.
Factors to consider:

- Nursing of the soiled patient (see later)
- Catheterization.

Because a debilitated patient is unable to rise, urine is retained for long periods. When it is eventually released, the patient may appear 'incontinent'. A bladder sphincter weakness can develop. Regular supported exercise and encouragement to urinate may be all that is required to keep the patient clean and comfortable.

Urine scalding
If urine scalding occurs, dermatitis (inflammation of the skin) will be evident. Care and treatment for urine scalding are outlined in the section on nursing the soiled patient.

Urine retention
Urinary retention may be due to nerve damage, trauma or obstruction of the lower urinary tract.
Factors to consider:

- Catheterization
- Cystocentesis.

Temperature control
Debilitated patients may not be able to maintain a normal body temperature.

- Recumbent patients are not exercising and therefore do not generate sufficient body heat. Core body temperature and peripheral circulation are reduced, leading to poor perfusion of tissues and cold extremities
- Anorexic patients are at risk due to the lowering of the metabolic rate
- Soiled patients may also be at risk if they are not kept clean, warm and dry
- Post-anaesthetic patients may develop hypothermia, resulting in prolonged recovery.

Prevention
Measures that can be employed to reduce heat loss include:

- Keep the patient out of draughts
- Provide warm and insulative bedding (e.g. synthetic fleece, bubble-wrap, space blankets)
- Keep the kennel area at the correct temperature (e.g. 18–21°C for hospitalized patients)
- Provide a safe heat source (e.g. infra-red heat lamp)
- Physiotherapy – both massage, and passive and active exercise (see section on physiotherapy) can help to maintain body temperature
- Anaesthesia – operation times should be kept to a minimum and supplementary warmth should be provided during and after anaesthesia
- Monitor the patient's body temperature regularly.

Clinical signs of hypothermia
- Abnormally low body temperature
- Pale mucous membranes
- Reduced pulse rate
- Cold extremities
- Depression.

Treatment
Treatment of hypothermia may include the provision of extra warmth and measures to reduce heat loss from the patient (detailed above). The veterinary surgeon may request warmed intravenous fluids.

Musculoskeletal problems

Muscle tone and joint movement are maintained during normal exercise. Due to lack of exercise, recumbent patients lose muscle tone and muscle mass. In addition joint movement may be compromised and limb oedema may occur. The result may be reduced long-term function and mobility. Physiotherapy used from the onset of recumbency enhances the patient's chance of successful rehabilitation.

Prevention and treatment

Physiotherapy techniques used to support recumbent patients include:

- Massage – effleurage, petrissage and friction (see Figure 4.48)
- Passive exercise and active movement (see Figures 4.55 and 4.60–4.63).

Inappetence or inability to eat or drink

Feeding

- Feed a high quality palatable diet, with high digestibility and low bulk
- Ensure that the patient can actually reach the food: offer food by hand if necessary, or try positioning the patient in supported sternal recumbency to allow better access to the feeding bowl
- Appetite stimulation may be tried (see Figure 4.20)
- Enteral tube feeding may be required (see Figure 4.19).

Fluids

- Water should be freely available and offered every 2 h if the patient is unable or unwilling to drink
- Water may be carefully and slowly syringed into the patient's mouth, taking care to avoid aspiration (Figure 4.17)
- Monitor water intake (normal range 40–60 ml/kg/24 h)
- Monitor hydration status – skin tenting, colour and feel of mucous membranes, and capillary refill time (see Chapter 3).

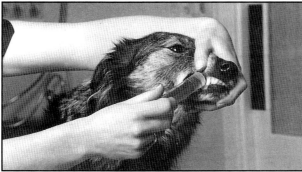

4.17 *Syringe water carefully into the patient's mouth.*

Skin and coat problems

The recumbent patient may be unwilling or unable to groom itself. Matting can occur, and lesions may be undetected. (See also section on grooming the geriatric patient, above.)

Prevention

- Groom regularly
- Look for discharges and bathe eyes, ears, prepuce, or vulva
- Check nail length
- Look for skin lesions or parasites.

Depression

Mental stimulation is vital for the recumbent patient. In a busy surgery it is often difficult to give extra care, but taking time and giving encouragement during nursing procedures can help to prevent depression.

Prevention of depression

- Grooming
- Physiotherapy
- Exercise
- Fresh air
- Varied environment
- Music/radio
- Hand feeding.

The veterinary surgeon may consider sending a depressed patient home to be nursed. It is vital to give the owner an accurate and detailed explanation of nursing care and therapies, with written back-up.

Nursing the soiled patient

The hospitalized patient should be observed regularly and given immediate care when soiling occurs. This will reduce complications and make the animal feel more comfortable.

Patients can be soiled with:

- Food
- Discharges
- Urine
- Faeces
- Vomit
- Blood
- Salivation
- Discharges from the vagina or prepuce
- Wound exudate.

General reduction of soiling

- Provide a large enough kennel so that the animal can move away from the soiled area
- Provide absorbent bedding
- Observe patient regularly
- Remove any soiled bedding immediately
- Clean the soiled kennel appropriately and, when dry, supply fresh bedding
- Sponge down or bathe the patient, dry carefully and return to the clean kennel.

Food and discharges

Any soiling with food should be cleaned and dried immediately. Discharges should be bathed on a regular basis and protective cream applied as required.

Urinary soiling and scalding

Urine soiling may occur during recovery from anaesthesia, with recumbent or incontinent patients, or when patients are given insufficient opportunity to urinate. Repeated soiling can lead to urine scalding.

The general rules above apply, in addition to the following points:

- Opportunity to urinate. Supported towel-walking to the run may be necessary for some patients. Recumbent cats can be assisted to the litter tray at regular intervals with support, and unless contraindicated (e.g. urethral

blockage) gentle steady pressure can be exerted on the bladder to encourage urination
- Record urination on record sheet and note the colour, clarity, odour, straining and frequency
- Catheterization may be indicated
- Look for signs of urine scalding, bathe any affected areas with mild antiseptic solution and dry thoroughly
- Barrier cream can be applied to help to reduce or treat urine scalds.

Faeces

If faecal soiling occurs, adequate and immediate cleansing of the patient are required. Hair may need to be clipped, and barrier cream applied to the perineal region. Monitor hydration status and weight changes. In severe cases intravenous fluids may be prescribed.

The following should be observed and recorded about the faeces when nursing a patient with diarrhoea:

- Content: mucus, blood, endoparasites
- Colour
- Consistency
- Straining.

Vomit

Nursing of the vomiting patient requires good nursing skills in both observation and care of the patient. The following observations should be made:

- Content of vomit (food, bile, blood)
- Frequency of vomiting
- Association with feeding
- Hydration status.

In caring for the vomiting patient:

- General rules for reduction of soiling apply
- The mouth and gums can be bathed with tepid water
- Medication and intravenous fluids may be prescribed by the veterinary surgeon
- When feeding is recommenced it should be introduced slowly, offering small frequent meals of bland food.

Blood, salivation and exudate

General rules of the soiled patient apply, keeping the patient clean, dry and comfortable.

Soiling from exudating wounds can be reduced by using appropriate absorbent dressings with regular dressing changes. Monitor the wound for signs of infection.

Bathing the soiled patient

The first consideration is whether the patient is well enough for a bath. Weak, geriatric or hypothermic patients may be better with a sponge-down to reduce stress and loss of body heat.

Bathing procedures
- Prepare a warm dry kennel for after bathing
- Look for skin lesions, record and report as necessary
- Brush out coat
- Clip any matted hair – with owner or veterinary surgeon's permission
- Select a mild shampoo
- Ensure that the water is at body temperature before the patient is placed in the bath or under the shower hose

- Never leave the patient unattended in the bath
- Rinse out shampoo thoroughly
- Squeeze excess water from the coat
- Dry carefully with towels
- Ensure adequate restraint before using a hairdryer, which should be turned first to low power to ensure toleration by the patient
- Heat lamps may also be used to aid drying
- When the patient is completely dry, barrier cream can be applied to problem areas if required.

 Cats with soiling problems should only be sponged down, as they become very stressed if bathed.

Anorexia and assisted feeding

When an animal that is not eating is admitted to the veterinary practice it may need assisted feeding, ranging from appetite stimulation to parenteral feeding, depending on the clinical condition. It is important to differentiate initially whether the patient is anorexic or dysphagic. Indications for assisted feeding are listed in Figure 4.18, while Figure 4.19 illustrates choice of appropriate feeding procedures. Further details are given in the *Manual of Advanced Veterinary Nursing.*

 Prior to assisted feeding, it is essential that the patient is adequately hydrated and any electrolyte disturbances are corrected.

 With all methods of assisted feeding, it is vital that body weight is monitored carefully.

4.18 **Indications for assisted feeding**

Sign	Cause
Anorexia	Systemic disease
Weakness	Debility
Dysphagia	Oral disease
	Pharyngeal disease
	Oesophageal disease

Anorexia

The anorexic patient has a lack or loss of appetite due to pyrexia, pain, weakness or stress. Animals may refuse to eat because they are hospitalized and in some cases it may be appropriate to send them home for treatment of the disease process. With an anorexic animal, appetite stimulation can be tried initially before progressing to the more complicated techniques.

Dysphagia

The dysphagic animal may have the desire to eat but is physically unable to do so, due to a mechanical or neurological disorder.

 It is inappropriate to use appetite stimulation methods for a dysphagic patient. Enteral feeding should be used until the disorder is repaired or treated.

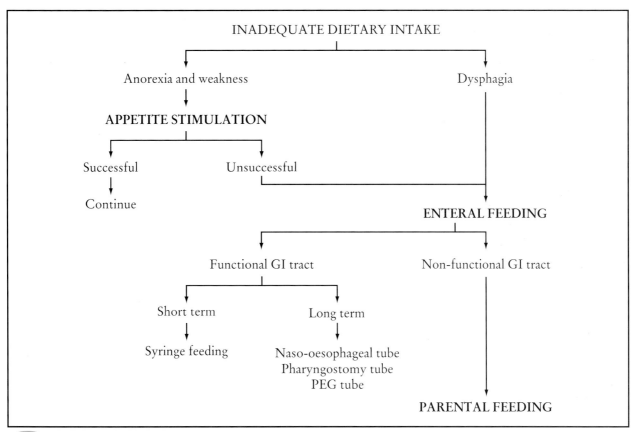

INADEQUATE DIETARY INTAKE

Anorexia and weakness   Dysphagia

APPETITE STIMULATION

Successful   Unsuccessful

Continue

ENTERAL FEEDING

Functional GI tract   Non-functional GI tract

Short term   Long term

Syringe feeding   Naso-oesophageal tube
Pharyngostomy tube
PEG tube

PARENTAL FEEDING

4.19   *Flow chart illustrating appropriate choice of feeding procedures.*

Enteral feeding

This entails using the gastrointestinal tract to provide nutritional support to patients who are unable or unwilling to eat. It is the best choice if the gastrointestinal tract is functioning normally, as it keeps the gut working. If the gut works, use it.

Parenteral feeding

This is administration of the essential nutritional needs of the patient via the intravenous route. Parenteral feeding is used where the gastrointestinal tract is non-functional.

Appetite stimulation

In some cases an inappetent or anorexic patient may be persuaded to eat. Some of the methods listed in Figure 4.20 may be tried.

An animal in pain may be unwilling to eat and *pain relief* may be indicated. Short-term medical appetite stimulants may also be prescribed by the veterinary surgeon.

Syringe feeding (force feeding)

Syringe feeding can be tried with conscious patients who have the ability to swallow normally and a functioning gastrointestinal tract. Syringe feeding can be used on a short-term basis for cooperative patients, to stimulate the appetite and encourage the patient to start eating on its own.

Soft tinned foods can be given into the mouth as a bolus (Figure 4.21), or liquidized food mixed with water (Figure 4.22) can be given carefully with a syringe (Figure 4.23).

For syringe feeding:

- Take care to avoid aspiration
- Never rush the process, as it can increase stress
- Clean the animal after feeding.

4.20 **How to stimulate a patient's appetite**

1. Hand feed, stroke, encourage, reduce stress, spend time with the patient
2. Clear any discharges from nose
3. Dampen oral mucous membranes with water prior to feeding
4. Increase diet palatability, digestibility and biological value
5. Offer favourite foods and a variety of foods
6. Offer strong-smelling foods – particularly for geriatric patients and those with nasal discharge
7. Liquidize food
8. Warm food to body temperature – this increases both aroma and palatability
9. Feed small amounts and often
10. Rub some food round gums, or for cats rub a little food on paws
11. Cats – feed using wide shallow food bowls or plates to avoid interference with whiskers; containers preferably made of plastic as some cats hate stainless steel!

4.21 **How to give a bolus feed to the patient**

1. Place core boluses on the tongue via an adapted 5 or 10 ml syringe (Figure 4.23)
   or
   Food can be placed in the pharyngeal area to stimulate the swallowing reflex
2. Allow the patient to swallow before further feeding.

Medical conditions and medical nursing | **89**

How to give a liquid syringe feed to the patient

1. Liquidize food and mix with water
2. The filled syringe is always directed towards the roof of the patient's mouth and the food introduced slowly. This stimulates the swallowing reflex and reduces the chance of aspiration
3. Place the syringe behind the canine tooth and administer slowly, with the patient's head in a normal/horizontal position

   or
4. Hold the side pocket of the gum open and syringe liquidized food into it, push the gum against the teeth and allow the animal to swallow.

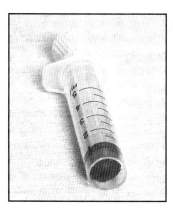

 A syringe for bolus feeding can be made by cutting the end from a syringe and filing the rough edges.

Enteral feeding

When a patient is anorexic or dysphagic and the gastrointestinal tract is functioning normally, the patient's nutritional requirements can be provided by means of a tube passed directly into the caudal oesophagus or stomach.

Three techniques will be described in this section:

- Naso-oesophageal tube feeding
- Pharyngostomy tube feeding
- Percutaneous endoscopically placed gastrostomy (PEG) tubes.

All of these methods are well tolerated by patients. They enable efficient and successful nutritional support of those that are unable or unwilling to eat.

Whichever method is used:

- Blood glucose and urine glucose should be monitored daily
- Hyperglycaemia must be reported immediately.

Feeding requirements

The prepared food must be fine enough to pass through the tube without occluding it. The food must include:

- Water
- Protein of high biological value
- Energy as carbohydrate and fat
- Vitamins and minerals.

Depending on the patient's condition, use veterinary enteral diets, or veterinary diets suitable for the specific debility, liquidized and mixed with water.

Naso-oesophageal tube feeding

A naso-oesophageal tube is introduced via the nose to the nasopharynx and passed carefully down into the caudal oesophagus. While sedation may be required this can be done without a general anaesthetic. The tube is placed and retained in position to allow liquid feed to be administered. The animal can also eat and drink with the tube in place, allowing observation for restored normal feeding behaviour.

Indications and contraindications for naso-oesophageal feeding are listed in Figure 4.24, with the required equipment and feeding method in Figures 4.25–4.27.

4.24 **Indications and contraindications for naso-oesophageal feeding**

Indications

Anorexia
Oral food intake reduced for more than 3 days
Loss of more than 5% of body weight
Where a general anaesthetic is contraindicated
When long-term enteral feeding is required

Contraindications

Non-functional gastrointestinal tract
Oesophageal disease
Persistent vomiting
Unconsciousness

4.25 **Equipment necessary for insertion of a naso-oesophageal tube**

Naso-oesophageal tube – made of polyurethane (PU) or polyvinylchloride (PVC) or silicone. The widest possible tube should be used
3.5–6 FG for cats
5–10 FG for dogs
Sedative if required – under veterinary direction
Local anaesthetic drops/spray
Pen
Water-soluble lubricant
5 ml syringe and 21 g needle
Sterile water
Elastoplast/zinc oxide $^1/_4$ inch tape
Cyanoacrylate glue or suture material
Scissors
Elizabethan collar
20 ml syringe to administer feeding

Complications

Complications resulting from the insertion of a naso-oesophageal tube are:
- Occlusion of the tube
- Regurgitation of the tube (particularly in cats)
- Patient interference
- Ingestion of part of the tube
- Diarrhoea (due to bacterial overgrowth or increased water intake, or feeding too quickly).

Care and maintenance of the tube
- Prior to each feed, flush the tube with 3–5 ml sterile water to ensure that the tube has not been dislodged
- Keep the tube sealed with a cap to prevent entry of air
- Following a feed, flush the tube with 5–10 ml water to prevent occlusion
- Clean the face, eyes and mouth of the patient regularly.

4.26 How to insert a naso-oesophageal tube

1. Apply local anaesthetic drops to one of the external nares (medial aspect) and leave for a few minutes
2. Tubing is pre-measured against the patient to the 9th–10th rib and marked with the pen
3. The patient is restrained in sternal recumbency
4. The patient's head is restrained in a normal position as the tube approaches the pharynx. This helps to prevent tracheal intubation
5. The end of the tube is lubricated and introduced into the anaesthetized naris, directed caudoventrally and medially
6. As soon as the tip reaches the septum (after about 2 cm) the nares are pushed dorsally
7. This opens the ventral meatus of the nasal cavity and ensures passage of the tube into the pharynx
8. The tube is then angled downwards and slightly inwards and advanced slowly into the caudal oesophagus up to the pre-measured line
9. Check that the tube is correctly placed by introducing 3–5 mls sterile water via the tube. If coughing occurs it is probably not in the oesophagus but in the trachea. Pull back tube and reposition. Incorrect placement is more likely if the patient is sedated, due to suppression of the cough reflex. Radiographs of the lateral chest may be indicated to ensure correct placement. If the tube is passed into the stomach there is a risk of reflux oesophagitis and vomiting
10. When the tube is correctly placed apply two elastoplast/zinc oxide butterflies to the external tubing
11. Stick the tapes with superglue to the hair (or suture to the skin) along the bridge of the nose and over the frontal region of the head. With cats the tube/tapes must not interfere with their whiskers as this will reduce their tolerance of the tube
12. Cap the tube
13. Apply properly fitted Elizabethan collar.

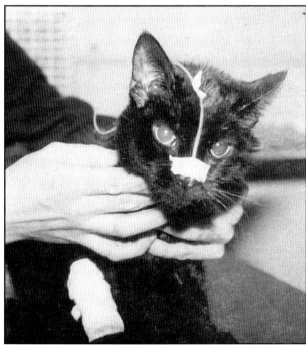

4.27 *Cat with naso-oesophageal tube in place. An Elizabethan collar is subsequently placed to prevent the cat from interfering with the tube.*

Removal of tube

Once the animal has started to eat sufficient amounts of food voluntarily, the tube can be removed. The sutures or glue attachments are released. Keep the tube sealed to prevent aspiration of any contents, with the cap in place or a finger over the end of the tube, and then gently pull it out.

Pharyngostomy tube feeding

A pharyngostomy tube is surgically placed under general anaesthesia through the lateral wall of the pharynx and into the oesophagus. Pharyngostomy tubes have a larger bore than naso-oesophageal tubes, which means that more concentrated food can be passed into the stomach.

Pharyngostomy tubes are less popular in practice, due to the necessity of a general anaesthetic and interference with oropharyngeal function, particularly in cats.

Indications and contraindications for using pharyngostomy tubes are listed in Figure 4.28. The equipment required and technique used for insertion of pharyngostomy tubes are listed in Figures 4.29 and 4.30.

4.28 Indications and contraindications for pharyngostomy tube feeding

Indications
Facial, mandibular or maxillary disease, trauma or surgery
Long-term support required

Contraindications
Pharyngeal trauma
Non-functional gastro-intestinal tract
Persistent vomiting
Unconsciousness

4.29 Preparation and equipment necessary for insertion of a pharyngostomy tube

Pharyngostomy tube
  10–12 FG for cats and small dogs
  5–10 FG for larger dogs
Light general anaesthesia
Aseptic technique
Scalpel handle and blade
Blunt dissecting scissors
Mouth gag
Sutures
Zinc oxide $^{1}/_{4}$ inch tape

4.30 How to insert a pharyngostomy tube

1. General anaesthesia
2. Clip the left side of the neck, caudal to the mandible and aseptically prepare it for surgery
3. Measure the tube and mark it to the 9th–10th rib, so that it will sit in the caudal oesophagus
4. Pass the tube through an incision made in the skin just behind the mandible, through to the oropharynx.
5. With a mouth gag in place, manipulate the tube digitally to redirect it into the oesophagus
6. Sutured it in place through butterfly tapes
7. Cap the tube.

Complications

Complications resulting from the insertion of a pharyngostomy tube are:

- Interference with epiglottal function
- Oedema
- Infection at the site of skin puncture
- Haemorrhage
- Occlusion of the tube
- Aspiration of food
- Patient interference.

Care and maintenance of the tube

- Prior to feeding, flush the tube to check for occlusions
- Keep the incision site and surrounding skin clean and dry
- Keep the tube capped to prevent entry of air
- Following feeding, flush the tube with 5–10 ml water to prevent occlusion.

Removal of tube

- The sutures are released
- Keep the tube sealed to prevent aspiration of any contents, and gently pull it out
- The wound is left to heal by granulation.

Percutaneous endoscopically placed gastrostomy (PEG) tubes

PEG tubes are well tolerated by the patient and have few complications, but specialized equipment is needed. Indications and contraindications are listed in Figure 4.31. Instruments required for placement of a PEG tube following general anaesthesia are shown in Figure 4.32, and the placement method in Figures 4.33 and 4.34.

- Do *not* feed the patient on the day of PEG tube placement
- Check that the tube is in the stomach the next day, *prior* to feeding. this can be done by placing Gastrografin through the tube and taking a radiograph to ensure correct position.

Complications

Complications using PEG tubes are rare but some of the following problems may occur:

- Hyperglycaemia
- Occlusion of the tube
- Infection at the site of skin puncture
- Interference by the patient
- Peritonitis.

4.31 Indications and contraindications for placement of a PEG tube

Indications

The upper gastrointestinal tract must be by-passed
Anorexic patients

Contraindications

Malabsorption in the digestive tract
Non-functional gastrointestinal tract
Persistent vomiting

4.32 Equipment used to insert a PEG tube following general anaesthesia

Mouth gag
Endoscope
Endoscopic forceps/snare
Depezzar mushroom-tipped catheter, 16–24 FG
Dilator (e.g. pipette tip)
Surgical kit
Suture material
14 gauge intravenous (i.v.) catheter
Bandage
Elizabethan collar

4.33 How to insert a PEG tube

1. General anaesthesia
2. Clip and prepare the left costal area for surgery
3. Pass endoscope into the stomach, which is then inflated with air
4. Press tip of the endoscope against the stomach wall so that the light shines through the skin
5. Make stab incision through the skin and pass a 14 G i.v. catheter into the stomach
6. Remove needle and stylet from the catheter
7. Pass suture through the catheter and grasp by the endoscopic forceps
8. One suture end is retained through the i.v. catheter
9. The other end of the suture is then pulled back up the oesophagus and into the mouth by the endoscope
10. Pass suture through dilator
11. Attach depezzar catheter to the suture
12. Push the dilator over the end of the catheter
13. Pull depezzar catheter down the oesophagus and into the stomach with the attached suture, and pull through the stab incision
14. Slightly increase stab incision to allow the tube to be exteriorized
15. Suture depezzar catheter to the skin with a finger trap suture
16. Bandage in place; apply properly fitted *Elizabethan collar*.

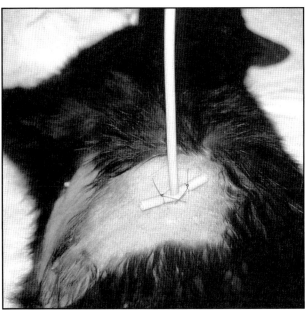

4.34 *A PEG tube in place for enteral feeding of a cat.*

Care and maintenance of the tube
- Prior to feeding, flush the tube to check for occlusions
- Keep the incision and the skin around the catheter clean and dry
- Keep the cap on the catheter to prevent entry of air
- Following a feed, flush the catheter with 5–10 ml water to prevent occlusion.

Removal of the tube
- PEG tubes should be left *in situ* for a minimum of 5–7 days before removal
- Sometimes the tube may be pulled out through the incision intact
- In some cases removal involves a general anaesthetic, cutting off the catheter at skin level, and endoscopy to remove the section left in the stomach
- The wound is left to heal by granulation
- Withhold food for 24 h after removal.

These calculations can also be carried out using figures for Resting Energy Requirements (RER).

Calculation of nutritional requirements for enteral tube feeding
Calculation of the volume of food to be administered over 24 h for naso-oesophageal, pharyngostomy and PEG tube feeding is based on the patient's *calorific requirement* divided by the *calorific content* of the food.

Calorific requirement = basal energy requirement (*BER*) x illness factor (*IF*)

- *BER* is the energy required by an animal in a comfortable stress-free environment without disease
- Patients that weigh less than 2 kg or more than 40 kg must have their *BER* calculated using the following equation:

BER (kcal) = 70 x (body weight in kg)$^{0.75}$

- A simpler *BER* calculation can be used for patients weighing between 2 and 40 kg:

BER (kcal) = [30 x (body weight in kg)] + 70

- *Illness factor* – it is difficult to calculate accurately the energy needs of a patient with a clinical condition. Figure 4.35 gives a general guide to energy requirements
- *Calorific content* of the food is taken as the number of kcal/ml or kcal/g in a selected commercial diet.

Example
For a 20 kg hospitalized Border Collie with neoplasia:

- Body weight (BW) = 20 kg
- *BER* = (30 x BW) + 70 = (30 x 20) + 70 = 670
- *IF* = 1.6
- *Calorific content* of selected food = 1 kcal/ml

The calculation is:

(*BER* x *IF*)/(*calorific content*)
= (670 x 1.6)/1
= 1072 ml food/day required

This patient should be fed as follows.
- Day 1: 357 ml food/24 h, made up to volume 1:3 with water
- Day 2: 715 ml food/24 h, made up to volume 3:1 with water
- Day 3 onward: 1072 ml food/24 h.

Enteral feeding regimes
All daily nutritional requirements over 24 h should be divided into four to six feeds/day. Methods of feeding the patient by enteral means are outlined in Figure 4.36.

When using enteral tubes, food should be introduced gradually and the amounts adjusted initially as follows:

- Day 1: about one-third of the nutritional need, made up to volume with water 1:3
- Day 2: about two-thirds of the nutritional need, made up to volume with water 3:1
- Day 3 onwards: full amount of nutritional need – the total food calculated for a 24 h period
- When commencing bolus enteral feeding a maximum of 20 ml/kg/feed should be given, this can be gradually increased over two to three days
- *Never* exceed the maximum quantities which can be given at a single feed (Figure 4.37).

4.35 Energy requirements for patients with clinical conditions

Clinical condition	BER x illness factor
Hospitalized dog or cat	BER x 1.3
Major trauma/surgery	BER x 1.6
Neoplasia	BER x 1.6
Severe infection	BER x 1.8
Major burns	BER x 2.0

4.36 How to feed a pet by enteral means

1. Use large 20 ml or 50 ml sterile syringes for feeding
2. Warm food to body temperature
3. Position the patient either standing or sitting or in sternal or right lateral recumbency
4. Over the first few days start with frequent small amounts of food. Gradually increase amount and decrease frequency.
5. Feed in boluses slowly over about 15 min to allow for comfort and gastric dilatation and to reduce the chance of vomiting
   or
6. Continuous feeding is thought to be more beneficial (particularly in the acute patient) and this can be done using continuous infusion systems which control the rate of feeding.

4.37 Maximum quantity per bolus feed for anorexic and debilitated patients

Dogs	=	45 ml/kg
Cats, 1–1.4 kg	=	35 ml/kg
Cats, 1.5–4.0 kg	=	30 ml/kg
Cats, 4.1–6.0 kg	=	22 ml/kg

These amounts are half the maximum stomach capacity of the normal dog and cat

Record
For enteral feeding, the following information needs to be recorded:

- The time of the feed, and the volume of food given
- Any regurgitation or vomiting
- Any other observations.

Parenteral feeding

Parenteral feeding (fluid feeding given by the intravenous route, usually into the jugular vein) is a specialized technique.

- It is expensive
- It needs constant monitoring
- Central veins must be used
- Severe metabolic effects can occur.

This subject is dealt with in *BSAVA Manual of Advanced Veterinary Nursing*.

Physiotherapy

Physiotherapy is the use of physical or mechanical agents to treat pain and movement dysfunction as they relate to the muscles, joints and nerves of the body. Pain or dysfunction may be caused by disease, injury or associated inactivity.

Inactivity causes substantial weakness and loss of tissue from all elements of the musculoskeletal system. There is loss of bone, muscle and connective tissue, reduced range of joint movement and a reduction in muscle strength and endurance.

Physiotherapy can be used as a prevention therapy to reduce losses, and as a treatment therapy to promote recovery and build up physical strength and mobility. It must be carried out under the direction of a veterinary surgeon.

- All physiotherapy sessions should be started slowly and built up as the patient improves
- The patient must be in a comfortable position and handled in a quiet and reassuring manner.

Physiotherapy may be carried out at floor or table level. Table level is often most comfortable for the operator but extra restraint of the patient is needed.

Respiratory physiotherapy

Respiratory physiotherapy is particularly useful in the treatment of the recumbent patient and of patients with pulmonary disease. Pulmonary disease or decreased exercise can result in a reduction of lung volume, and reduced ability to clear pulmonary secretions.

The aims of respiratory physiotherapy are:

- To reduce respiratory effort
- To increase the lung volume, therefore increasing oxygen uptake and increasing gaseous exchange
- To increase secretion clearance
- To make the animal more comfortable.

The physiological benefits of respiratory physiotherapy are listed in Figure 4.38.

Respiratory physiotherapy techniques include:

- Positional physiotherapy
- Postural drainage
- Manual techniques.

Patients must be well hydrated before treatment.

4.38 Physiological effects and benefits of respiratory physiotherapy

Physiological effects	Result
Increased lung volume Increased oxygen uptake and gaseous exchange Increased secretion clearance	Increased oxygen supply to the alveoli Reduced pooling of secretions Animal comfort

Positional physiotherapy

The position of the patient can help to increase lung volume, improve ability to clear secretions, and prevent or treat hypostatic pneumonia.

Different positions allow different lung volumes to be attained:

- Standing – maximum expansion of the ribs, diaphragm and lungs
- Sternal recumbency/sitting – reasonable expansion of the lungs
- Lateral recumbency – least expansion of the lungs. If only one lung is affected by disease then the affected lung is positioned uppermost, allowing the lower lung greater expansion. If both lungs are affected then the animal should be repositioned on a regular basis.

The technique of positional therapy is detailed in Figure 4.39.

Treatment sessions

Maintain each position for 10–15 min, three to four times a day.

4.39 How to use positional physiotherapy

1. Encourage the patient to stand at regular intervals
2. Support the patient in sternal recumbency with sandbags, cushions or rolled up towels
3. Maintain each position for between 10 and 15 min, 3–4 times daily.
4. Between treatment sessions turn the laterally recumbent patient on a regular basis, every 2–4 h throughout the day and night.

Postural drainage

Postural drainage uses gravity to assist with secretion clearance. The area of the lungs to be treated is positioned uppermost, and the patient's head should be slightly lower than the body level. Secretions drain into the main bronchial airways and are then coughed up by the patient.

Treatment must be discussed in detail with the veterinary surgeon.

Contraindications

- Recent trauma or surgery to the head, neck, thorax or spine
- Pregnancy
- Obesity
- Breathlessness.

Treatment sessions

Maintain each position for 10–15 min three or four times a day.

Manual techniques

Massage in the form of 'percussions' (coupage) and 'vibrations' can aid clearance of secretions (Figures 4.40–4.44). These should be performed in postural drainage positions.

How to use manual techniques for respiratory physiotherapy

Percussion or coupage (Figures 4.41 and 4.42)	Slow rhythmic clapping with cupped hands and loose wrists on the chest wall, creating an energy wave transmitted to the airways which loosens secretions and allows them to be coughed up
Vibrations (Figures 4.43 and 4.44)	Fine oscillations of the hands on the chest wall directed inwards. These must be performed on *expiration*.
Shaking	Coarse oscillations performed as above.

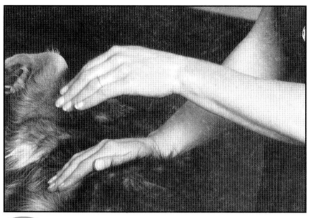

4.41 *Coupage performed on a recumbent patient.*

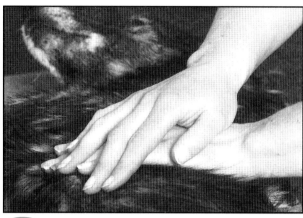

4.43 *Vibrations performed on a recumbent patient.*

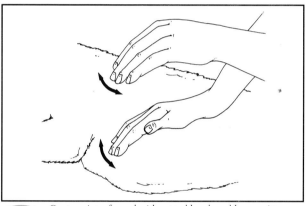

4.42 *Coupage is performed with cupped hands and loose wrists over the chest wall of the debilitated patient.*

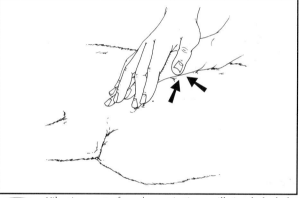

4.44 *Vibrations are performed on expiration, oscillating the heel of the hands.*

> ⚠ Respiration and colour of the mucous membranes must be monitored throughout respiratory physiotherapy.

Following the use of respiratory physiotherapy, a *cough reflex* may be stimulated by tracheal compression, to help to clear loosened secretions.

Contraindications
- Thoracic surgery
- Trauma
- Osteoporosis.

Treatment sessions
5–10 min, four or five times a day.

Orthopaedic and neurological physiotherapy
Orthopaedic and neurological physiotherapy is the treatment of orthopaedic and neurological disease or injury with physical agents such as cold and heat, and with mechanical agents such as massage and exercise. The aim is to increase the blood supply to, and lymphatic drainage from, the affected area and to increase muscle strength and coordination.

The techniques used are:

- Local hypothermia
- Superficial hyperthermia
- Massage
- Passive exercise
- Active exercise
- Hydrotherapy.

Local hypothermia
Local hypothermia is the application of a cold compress to the affected area. It is used in acute phase injury to help to minimize bruising and oedema and to reduce pain in the first 48 h following trauma. Figure 4.45 gives details of the physiological effects of local hypothermia.

Contraindications
- Diabetes mellitus
- Peripheral vascular disease
- Ischaemic injury.

4.45 Physiological effects and benefits of local hypothermia

Physiological effects	Result
Decreased tissue temperature	Analgesia
Vasoconstriction	Reduced oedema
Decreased nerve conduction	Reduced bruising
Relaxation of skeletal muscle	

Treatment sessions
5–20 min every 4–6 h.

Superficial hyperthermia
Superficial hyperthermia is the application of warm compresses to the affected body area. It is used to reduce evident swelling and bruising, and for alleviation of pain, 48–72 h following trauma. The physiological benefits of superficial hyperthermia are listed in Figure 4.46.

Contraindications include bleeding disorders.

4.46 Physiological effects and benefits of superficial hyperthermia

Physiological effects	Result
Increased tissue temperature	Relief of muscle tension
Vasodilation	Analgesia
Increased local circulation	Reduction of oedema
Increased metabolic rate	

Treatment sessions
10–20 min, four to six times a day.

Massage
Massage is used on the limbs to increase arterial, venous and lymphatic flow, facilitating nutrient delivery and waste removal from the tissues (Figure 4.47 gives a list of physiological effects). Massage techniques are described and illustrated in Figures 4.48 to 4.53. Effleurage is used first, to relax the patient, followed by petrissage and friction techniques. When performing massage techniques, the hands should mould to the body contours.

> ⚠ Massage techniques should be used *towards the heart* to encourage venous return.

4.47 Physiological effects and benefits of massage

Physiological effects	Result
Assisted venous return to the heart	Reduced oedema
Increased lymphatic flow	Reduced muscle tension and spasm
Increased muscular motion	Temporary analgesia
Maintained and improved peripheral circulation	Increased muscle tone
Increased tissue perfusion	Increased movement through stretching of adhesions
	Decreased heart rate

4.48 How to use massage techniques

Effleurage (Figures 4.49 and 4.50)	Pass the palms of the hands continuously and rhythmically over the patient's skin with long stroking movements in one direction only. One hand supports the limb and the other massages; alternate the hands with each stroke. Effleurage will stimulate the skin, disperse oedema and promote venous return
Petrissage (Figures 4.51 and 4.52)	Used on muscular areas. Using both hands, lift up the skin and press it down, grasp and squeeze the muscle, roll and release, moving the hands steadily over the area. Petrissage will increase blood supply to the muscles, reduce muscle spasms, and prevent or break down adhesions
Friction (Figure 4.53)	Make a series of small circular movements with the pads of the thumbs, one or more fingers or the heel of the hand, depending on the part of the body under therapy

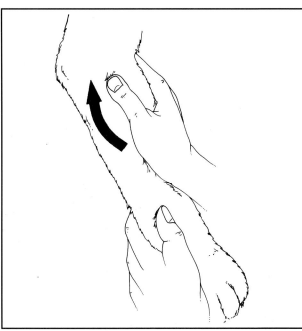

4.49 *Effleurage of the forelimb. One hand supports the limb; the palm of the massaging hand is held flat, with a firm gliding movement pushing up from distal to proximal limb. The massaging hand is lifted off at the axilla and is then placed on the distal limb for support as the second hand starts the next movement.*

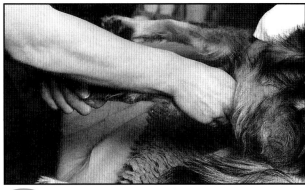

4.50 *Effleurage being given on the hindlimb of a recumbent patient.*

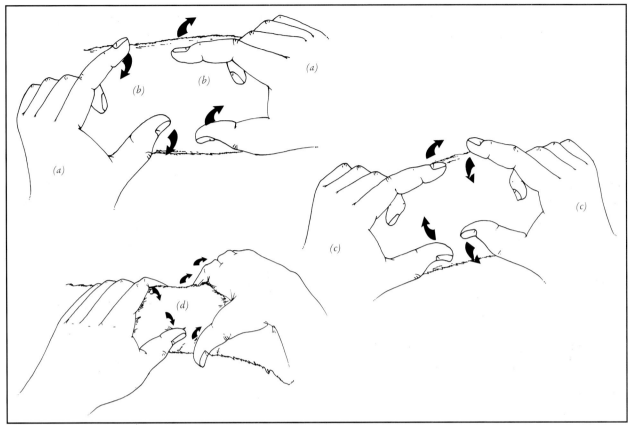

4.51 *Petrissage. With thumbs and index fingers positioned (a), the skin is picked up and pressed down; musculature is grasped, squeezed and rolled, moving each hand in opposite directions (b). The leading digit of each hand rolls down over the muscle, and the trailing digits roll up over the muscle, until the hands are at position (c). Now squeeze and roll back in direction (d) to starting position. The muscle is then released and the process is repeated, moving hands steadily up the limb. Note the muscle is rolled gently and firmly, not twisted.*

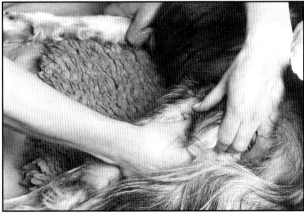

4.52 *Petrissage being given on the hindlimb of a recumbent patient.*

Contraindications

- Infection
- Pyrexia
- Malignancy
- Fracture sites
- Haemoarthrosis
- Acute inflammation.

Treatment sessions
10–20 min, two or three times a day.

Passive exercise/movement
Passive exercise (Figure 4.54) is where there is no active muscle action from the patient. The operator manually moves limbs and individual joints through as full a range as possible.

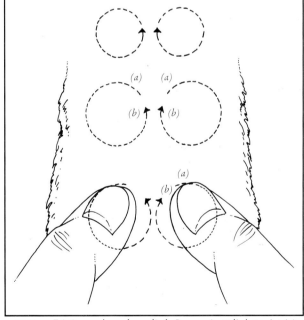

4.53 *Friction used on a lower limb. Pressure is applied at point (a), circular movement is made, and thumbs are removed at point (b); the process is repeated, moving steadily up the limb.*

Passive exercise must be performed with care, as manipulation may initially be painful. The therapy is used for its physiological effects (Figures 4.55–4.58) in recumbent patients, and where movement at a joint has been compromised through injury or treatment – for example, where a limb has been immobilized post fracture, and becomes weak and stiff through lack of use.

4.54 Physiological benefits of passive exercise or movement

Physiological effects	Result
Stretched adhesions Maintained or improved blood and lymphatic flow Stimulated sensory nerves	Maintained or increased range of movement Prevention or improvement of contractures microcirculation to the muscles and joints Improvement of stiffness

4.55 How to use passive exercise on the limbs

The aim is to move each joint individually through its full range

1. The patient should be comfortable, supported in lateral recumbency with the affected limb uppermost. Sandbags can be used to give additional support
2. Use one hand to stabilize the limb above or below the joint during manipulation (Figure 4.56)
3. Use the other hand for manipulation of the joint
4. Manipulate the distal joints of the limb first, i.e. put each toe through its full range of movement (Figure 4.57 and 4.58)
5. Then, working up the limb, put each joint through its full range of movement as far as the hip or shoulder
6. Then move the whole limb passively in a normal ambulatory fashion
7. When the movement at a joint is restricted, gentle overpressure can be used at the end of the range of movement
8. As treatment progresses, range of movement at the restricted joint improves slowly.

In recumbent patients the uppermost limbs are manipulated first. The patient can then be turned and the process repeated on other limbs.

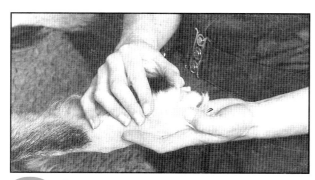

4.56　*Flexion of the distal phalanx.*

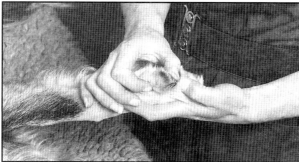

4.57　*Extension of the distal phalanx. Passive exercise is started at the distal limb; each joint of each digit is put through its full range of movement.*

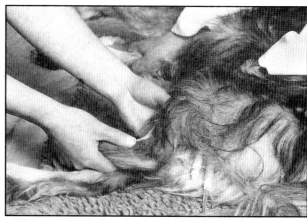

4.58　*Support is given above and below the joint during passive flexion of the hock.*

Effleurage (see Figure 4.49) and petrissage (see Figure 4.51) are used before commencing passive exercise, for their physiological effects and to help to relax the patient.

Contraindications
- Fractures involving the joint
- Congenital joint disease
- Haemoarthrosis (less than 5 days post incident).

Treatment sessions
10–20 min, two or three times daily after massage.

Active movement
Active movement (Figure 4.59) can be divided into three stages in a patient's recovery:

- Active assisted exercise (Figures 4.60 and 4.61) – the patient is weak and unable to stand unaided
- Active exercise (Figure 4.62) – the patient is able to stand on its own but is very weak

4.59 Physiological benefits of active movement

Physiological effects	Result
Increased blood supply and lymphatic drainage Increased muscular tone	Gradual build-up of muscular tone and strength Improved balance and coordination Patient comfort and stimulation

4.60 How to use active assisted exercise

Help the patient to stand

1. Give support with towels slung under the patient's abdomen (Figure 4.61). Two operators may be required for larger dogs, with an additional towel under the chest. Commercial slings are available
2. When progress has been made, start supported walking (e.g. towel walking)
3. The patient is actively working, gaining muscle tone and improving circulation, balance and coordination
4. Each stage may take days to achieve but the patient will eventually be able to stand unsupported and ready to progress to active exercise.

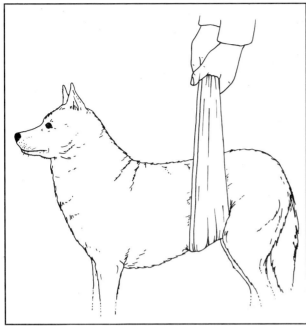

When using active movement, *take things slowly*. Allow the patient to progress with confidence, and observe for signs of distress at all times.

4.61 *Active assisted exercise. A towel can be used to give the patient support.*

4.62 How to use active exercise

1. Commence by standing the patient on its own for a few seconds
2. Progress to encouraging the patient to take a few steps
3. Light support is required initially to make the animal more confident, eventually progressing without support.

4.63 How to use active resisted exercise

The following methods are used progressively as the patient improves.

1. Use manual resistance to movement of the limb
2. Put downward pressure on the pelvis when the patient is standing so it must work to push back up
3. When the animal is walking, put a broom on the floor for it to step over
4. Small weights can be bandaged to the limbs to increase workload further.

- Active resisted exercise (Figure 4.63) – the patient is able to stand and walk alone but is weak. Resistance is applied to movement to increase further the patient's workload and to increase strength, stamina and mobility. Imagination and resourcefulness are needed.

Each stage is started slowly, and must be achieved by the patient before going on to the next stage. The patient builds up strength and coordination (Figure 4.59).

Although enhanced by using these methods, recovery can still be a slow process. Do not rush: allow the patient to regain confidence with its increasing ability.

It should be noted that as 'exercise' therapy is undertaken, the patient will have increased energy requirements and the diet may need to be adjusted accordingly.

Contraindications include recent trauma.

Treatment sessions
From a few seconds, progressing up to 10 min as the patient gains strength.

Hydrotherapy
The patient is exercised in water, which supports the animal while allowing it to move freely without bearing weight. The equipment required and suggested technique are set out in Figures 4.64 and 4.65.

As hydrotherapy treatment progresses and the patient has achieved active exercise in the water, move into resisted exercise: a whirlpool bath is used to offer resistance to movement, thus making the patient work harder.

4.64 Equipment necessary for hydrotherapy

- Sink, tub table or purpose-built pool filled with water – (temperature 37–40°C)
- Waterproof clothing
- Towels
- Hairdryer
- Warm, draught-free kennel

4.65 How to use hydrotherapy

1. Prepare a warm dry kennel for after therapy
2. Gather equipment
3. Check that water temperature is between 37 and 40°C
4. Place the patient in the water, giving initial support
5. Do not leave the patient
6. Remove the patient at the end of the session, or immediately if fatigued
7. Dry the patient thoroughly to reduce the risk of hypothermia before placing in prepared kennel.

Constant monitoring and support must be given while the patient is undergoing hydrotherapy.

Contraindications
- Pulmonary disease
- Epilepsy
- Some skin conditions.

Treatment sessions
Build up sessions slowly, starting with 5 min and (depending on progress) up to a *maximum* of 30 min.

Enemas
An enema is a fluid preparation which is passed through the anus into the rectum and colon to stimulate evacuation of faecal matter, or to introduce fluid preparations for diagnostic or therapeutic purposes. Indications for enemas, enema preparations, equipment necessary and how to give an enema are listed in Figures 4.66–4.69.

Administration equipment
There is a choice of equipment for administration of an enema (Figure 4.68). The most commonly used items in practice are the proprietary micro-enema and the enema pump (Higginson's syringe).

4.66 Indications for enemas

Constipation or impaction due to:
- Nature of faecal matter (e.g. fur balls, bones)
- Obstruction of the faecal passage (e.g. enlarged prostate, rectal neoplasia, anal diverticulum)
- Inability to pass faeces (e.g. recumbency, pelvic nerve damage, gastrointestinal problems – megacolon)

Diagnostic or surgical procedures to:
- Empty colon prior to endoscopy or radiography
- Introduce contrast media for radiographic examination of the colon (e.g. barium enema)
- Empty colon prior to surgery of the pelvis, colon or anal regions

Therapeutic purposes to:
- Administer drugs

4.67 Preparations and suggested quantities for enemas

Preparations used for an enema	Quantities for an enema
Water Soap and water Obstetrical lubricant and water Glycerine and water Olive oil and water Barium sulphate solution	5–10 ml/kg
Liquid paraffin	3 ml/kg
Proprietary brands of micro-enemata, e.g. phosphate enema	Follow manufacturers' instructions

4.68 Equipment used to give an enema

Gloves
Protective clothing
Lubricant
Enema administration equipment or micro-enema
Enema preparation
Litter tray for cats, or outside run for dogs

4.69 How to give an enema

1. Gather all equipment together before starting the procedure
2. Warm enema preparation to body temperature
3. Fill enema administration equipment with enema preparation
4. Lubricate nozzle prior to insertion into the rectum.
5. Ensure adequate restraint. Hindquarters may need to be slightly raised
6. Lift tail
7. Insert tip of nozzle gently
8. Administer enema slowly and gently
9. Stop if there is resistance – never force an enema preparation
10. Allow patient free exercise and observe for evacuation of bowels.

Micro-enema
These come in tubes with long nozzles for direct insertion into the rectum.

Enema pump (Higginson's syringe)
The open-ended tube of the enema pump is inserted into the chosen enema preparation and the bulb squeezed gently to draw the fluid through the pump. This is repeated until the enema preparation starts to come through the rectal insertion nozzle. Once the nozzle is lubricated it is ready for use.

Hose and funnel
The hose is filled with the enema preparation and the funnel is attached to the outer end of the hose. The enema solution is poured in, allowing gravity to fill the rectum.

Hose and 50 ml syringe
The syringe and hose are filled with enema preparation. The hose end is lubricated and inserted into the rectum. The syringe is gently depressed, pushing the enema into the rectum.

Foley catheter
This is used for barium enemas, with attached enema bag. After insertion of the catheter into the rectum the bag is squeezed, forcing the barium into the rectum or suspended above the animal, allowing the barium to flow by gravity. The barium is then allowed to run back into the bag.

Cuffed rectal catheter
This is a device for humans but it can be used to give a barium enema with barium bag attached.

Administering an enema

Enemas should only be given under veterinary direction.

Prior to giving an enema (Figure 4.69), it should be ensured that the procedure will be as stress free and comfortable as possible. Reassurance and encouragement should be given to the patient.

After the procedure:

- Reassure the animal
- Clean and dry the perineal region (oil-based enemas are particularly messy)
- Record the result of the enema on the hospital sheet.

Urinary catheterization

A urinary catheter is a narrow tube inserted via the urethra into the bladder to obtain a sample, maintain drainage or measure urinary output.

Urinary catheterization may be indicated for a number of reasons (Figure 4.70). The equipment required varies depending on the species, size and sex of the patient (Figure 4.71).

Contraindications
- Vaginitis
- Open pyometra
- Complete obstruction of urethra or bladder neck.

Catheters
Types, use, and special features for dogs and cats are listed in Figures 4.72–4.75.

Size of catheter

The catheter must be:

- Sufficient in length to reach the bladder, to ensure good drainage
- Wide enough so that urine will not flow down the outside of the catheter.

The external diameter of a catheter is measured using French Gauge (F, or FG):

1 unit FG = 0.33 mm

For example, a 6 FG catheter has an external diameter of 2 mm.

Storage of catheters and re-use

Catheters should be stored flat in sterile packaging, in a cool dry place. No heavy weights should be placed on top.

Plastic catheters are disposable but some may need to be re-sterilized. Damaged catheters must be disposed of immediately.

4.70 Reasons for urinary catheterization

Diagnostic
Biochemical analysis, when one cannot be obtained by free flow
Bacteriology, where a sterile urine sample is required
Introduction of radiographic contrast media

Surgical
Preoperative bladder drainage
Postoperative bladder drainage to prevent pressure on the bladder wound

Obstruction
Patient comfort – to drain the bladder when there is partial obstruction
To check for urethral patency
Urethral obstruction – hydro-propulsion may be used

Medical
Maintenance of bladder drainage in neurological disorders
Measurement of urinary output
Relief of urinary incontinence, to prevent soiling
Introduction of drugs

4.71 Equipment required for urinary catheterization

General non-sterile
Appropriate restraint, (sedation if required)
Clippers
Antiseptic solution – to clean the vulva or prepuce
Water-based lubricating jelly, or local anaesthetic gel
Kidney dish

General sterile
Gloves
Catheter
Universal container
10 ml or 20 ml syringe
Three-way tap
Positive contrast agent, as required.

If the catheters are to be re-used:

- Check for damage (e.g. kinks)
- Flush forcefully with cold water
- Wash in warm detergent solution
- Rinse
- Dry, pack, label and autoclave (or sterilize using ethylene oxide).

Specula

Specula can be used for catheterization of the bitch, to aid view of the urethral orifice. (Bitches can also be catheterized digitally – see below). Specula that can be used include:

- Auriscope with light source within the auriscope handle
- Catheterization speculum (an adapted auriscope with one edge removed)
- Sim's vaginal speculum
- Human rectal speculum
- Human nasal speculum (two flat blades that separate when the handles are pushed together)
- Home-made speculum from a syringe case.

A light source is useful – use a pen torch if no light source can be attached.

Always clean and sterilize speculums after use. All except the adapted syringe case can be autoclaved.

- Rinse first with cold water, flushing out any debris
- Wash with mild detergent
- Rinse, dry, pack, label and autoclave.

Catheterization technique

General principles for urinary catheterization are listed in Figure 4.76. Sedation under veterinary direction may be required for some patients, particularly cats. Adequate restraint is essential, to minimize contamination and reduce urethral trauma. A good aseptic technique with sterile equipment is essential when catheterizing a patient, to protect staff from zoonosis and the patient from infection.

Catheterization of the bitch

Catheterizing a bitch can be done either by using the *digital method* to locate the urethral orifice (Figure 4.77) or by locating and viewing it with a *speculum* with a light source (Figure 4.78). The digital method can be straightforward in larger bitches, but a vaginal scope may be necessary for those that are too small.

Foley catheter (additional requirements)
Stylet and spigot
Lubricant *must* be water based
Sterile water, syringe and needle (for balloon inflation)
Elizabethan collar
Speculum for bitch catheterization, as required

Jackson cat catheter (additional requirements)
Suture material
Elizabethan collar

Dog and bitch catheters and their use in veterinary practice

Type (Figs 4.73 and 4.74)	Plain plastic (dog)	Foley	Metal (bitch)	Tieman (bitch)
Sizes	6, 8, and 10 FG	8–30 FG	6, 8, 10, and 12 FG	8, 10, and 12 FG
Length	50–70 cm	30–40 cm	20–25 cm	43 cm
Material	Flexible nylon	Soft latex rubber with polystyrene core	Silver-plated brass	Polyvinyl chloride (PVC)
Features	Straight, some rigidity, two lateral eyelet drainage holes	Balloon inflated with sterile water lies behind eyelets at tip of catheter		Curved tip
Luer connector	*Yes*	*No* Spigot adapter required to create luer mount, for attaching syringe or sterile drip administration set. Medical urine collection bags have adapter attached	Some do	*Yes*
Use	*Dog* and *bitch*	*Bitch*	*Bitch*	*Bitch*
Re-use	Disposable	Disposable – the balloon may be weakened after use and catheters must only be used once	Sterilize using an autoclave	Disposable
Advantages	Transparent, ease of use	Indwelling		Transparent
Disadvantages	May be too long for use in bitches	*Very* flexible. Stylet required. Place stylet in eyelet hole at the tip of the catheter and lie it *alongside* the catheter to facilitate placement. Petroleum-based lubricant will damage this catheter	General anaesthesia Urethral trauma	Over-flexible difficult to introduce
Indwelling	*Adaptations for the male dog:* attach zinc oxide butterflies to external catheter for suturing to prepuce	Yes. Held in position by balloon inflated with correct amount of sterile water (written on side arm of catheter). When the catheter is correctly placed the balloon lies at *neck of the bladder* and is then inflated. The water is introduced via a side arm, with one-way valve, which runs up side of the catheter from the balloon to catheter end Resistance to inflation indicates that catheter is not properly placed	*No*	*No*
Notes	If indwelling: flush catheter every 4 h with sterile water to ensure patency	*Deflate* balloon *before* removing catheter *Flush* catheter every 4 h with sterile water to ensure patency. Urine will not flow down the catheter until *stylet is removed* after placement	Rarely used	

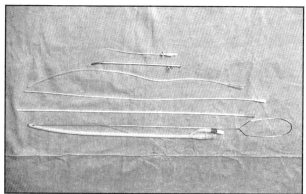

4.73 *Types of urinary catheter. From top to bottom: Jackson cat catheter; metal bitch catheter; Tieman bitch catheter; Portex dog catheter 6FG; Portex dog catheter 8FG; Foley catheter with stylet in place.*

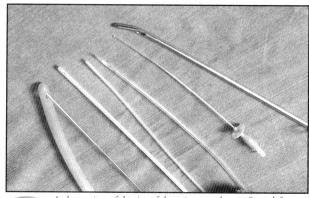

4.74 *A closer view of the tips of the urinary catheters. From left to right: Foley catheter with stylet in place; two plain plastic dog catheters; Tieman bitch catheter (with curved tip); Jackson cat catheter; metal bitch catheter.*

4.75 Cat catheters and their use in veterinary practice

Type	Plain plastic	Jackson (cat) (Figures 4.73 and 4.74)
Sizes	3 FG and 4 FG	3 FG and 4 FG
Length	30 cm	11 cm
Material	Flexible nylon	Flexible nylon
Features	Straight, some rigidity, two lateral eyelet drainage holes	Metal stylet in the lumen of the catheter to aid placement. It is removed once the catheter is correctly placed
Luer connector	*Yes*	*Yes*
Use	*Tom* and *queen*	*Tom* and *queen*
Indwelling	*No*	*Yes in tom cats*. A circular nylon flange at the proximal end enables the catheter to be sutured to the prepuce
Advantages	Transparent, ease of use	Indwelling
Disadvantages	More flexible	
Re-use	Disposable	Disposable

4.76 General principles for urinary catheterization

- Gather all equipment together before starting the procedure
- Clip hair and clean skin around vagina or prepuce with antiseptic solution
- Before removing catheter from packaging, measure against the patient the length needed to reach the bladder
- Wash/scrub hands and put on gloves
- Assistant opens outer packaging of catheter
- Operator removes catheter in inner sterile packaging
- Operator must snip the end off the inner packaging and push the tip of the sterile catheter out
- Assistant lubricates the end
- Operator pushes back the inner packaging as the catheter is advanced into the urethra, maintaining sterility
- *Never force a catheter:* if there is any resistance, *stop*
- When urine starts to flow down the catheter, stop
- Depending on the reason for catheterization, attach either syringe or three-way tap, suture in place, inflate balloon, or collect urine sample.

4.77 How to catheterize a bitch, using the digital method (described for a right-handed person)

1. General principles as in Figure 4.76
2. Position patient either standing or in lateral recumbency, with the tail held securely deflected
3. Scrub hands and put on sterile gloves
4. Lubricate the gloved left index finger and insert between the lips of the vulva into the vestibule in a dorsal then cranial direction
5. Locate the urethral orifice as a raised pimple on the ventral floor
6. Move finger just cranial to the urethral orifice
7. Use right hand to guide the catheter under the left finger along its length and into the urethral orifice
8. Advance catheter into the bladder.

4.78 How to catheterize a bitch using a speculum

Standing position	Dorsal recumbency
- General principles as in Figure 4.76 - Position patient, the tail securely deflected - Lubricate *speculum*	
	- Draw the *hindlimbs* in a *cranial direction*
- Insert speculum in a dorsal and then cranial direction	
- Visualize the *urethral orifice* on the ventral floor of vestibule	
- *Advance catheter* through speculum into urethral orifice and then into bladder	- *Advance catheter through speculum into urethral orifice*
	- Draw *hindlimbs caudally*
	- Advance catheter into the bladder

Whatever method is used, care should be taken to reduce trauma by lubricating equipment and handling the patient gently.

Catheterization of the male dog and the cat
Catheterization of the male dog is described in Figure 4.79 and of the cat in Figure 4.80.

4.79 How to catheterize a male dog

1. General principles as in Figure 4.76
2. Restrain patient in lateral recumbency or standing
3. Extrude penis by retracting the prepuce
4. Prepare catheter
5. Insert catheter gently but firmly into extruded penis
6. Advance into the bladder – stop if there is any resistance.

Resistance may be found at any of the common sites of urethral obstruction: neck of bladder, prostate, ischial arch, and caudal to os penis

4.80 How to catheterize a cat

Queen	Tom cat
• General anaesthesia or heavy sedation • Position in lateral recumbency • Lubricate catheter • Pass blind along vaginal floor and guide ventrally into urethral orifice • Advance catheter into bladder	• General anaesthesia or heavy sedation • Position in right lateral recumbency, tail deflected • Extrude penis by applying gentle finger pressure on either side of prepuce • Advance catheter tip with slight rotation, along urethra, parallel to vertebral column • Advance catheter into bladder • Suture in position if appropriate

Complications

Complications that may occur following urinary catheterization include:

• Infection
• Cystitis
• Bladder/urethral trauma.

If blood is seen at catheterization, when multiple catheterization is used, or when an indwelling catheter is placed, *prophylactic antibiotics* may be prescribed by the veterinary surgeon.

After catheterization, observe urine for colour, odour, clarity and haematuria, and any straining or frequent urination with little urine produced. Record and report to the veterinary surgeon.

Measuring urine output

Urine output can be monitored by placement of an indwelling catheter and collecting and measuring urine produced by the patient.

• A urine collection bag (Figure 4.81 and Chapter 3) can be attached to the catheter
• The catheter can be sealed with a bung and the bladder emptied at regular intervals.

The urine collected is measured and recorded:

• Normal urine output is calculated at 1–2 ml/kg/h
• A urine output of less than 1 ml/kg/h should be reported immediately to the veterinary surgeon

4.81 Urine collection bags

Urine collection bags	Catheter attachment
Medical urine collection bag (intended for human use)	Foley catheter – these collection bags have an incorporated spigot, which fits directly into the Foley catheter
Sterile administration set and empty drip bag	Can be attached to any catheter with a luer connector (Figures 4.73 and 4.74). A Foley catheter must have a spigot adapter (either plastic or metal) for connection

• A collection bag should be of adequate size for the potential urine output of the patient, and the contents of the bag should be measured and emptied at regular intervals
• Patients who have sealed indwelling catheters must have the bladder emptied at regular intervals
• Record details of urine collected and time of emptying bag/bladder
• Indwelling catheters can remain *in situ* for up to 10 days unless problems arise.

Further reading

Chandler EA, Gaskell CJ and Gaskell RM (eds) (1994) *Feline Medicine and Therapeutics*, 2nd edn. Blackwell Scientific Publications, Oxford

Cox C (1997) Naso-oesophageal tube feeding in dogs and cats: practice tip. *In Practice* **19**(1), 30–32

Gorman N (ed.) (1998) *Canine Medicine and Therapeutics*, 4th edn. Blackwell Science, Oxford

Hill RC (1994) Critical care nutrition. In: Wills JM and Simpson KW (eds) *The Waltham Book of Clinical Nutrition of the Dog and Cat*, pp. 39–61. Elsevier Science, Oxford

Lane DR and Cooper B (eds) (1999) *Veterinary Nursing, 2nd edn.* Butterworth-Heinemann, Oxford

Lewis LD, Morris ML Jr and Hand MS (1989) *Small Animal Clinical Nutrition III*. Mark Morris Associates

Simpson KW and Elwood CM (1994) Techniques for enteral nutritional support. In: Wills JM and Simpson KW (eds) *The Waltham Book of Clinical Nutrition of the Dog and Cat*, pp. 63-74. Elsevier Science, Oxford

Simpson JW, Anderson RS and Markwell PJ (1993) *Clinical Nutrition of the Dog and Cat*. Blackwell Science, Oxford

Tennant B (1993) Tube feeding in small animal medicine: exam help. *Veterinary Practice Nurse* **5**(1), 13–17

BSAVA Manuals covering relevant systems and disease in small animals, including:
Canine and Feline Nephrology and Urology
Companion Animal Nutrition and Feeding
Small Animal Endocrinology
Small Animal Neurology, 2nd edition
Small Animal Oncology
Small Animal Diagnostic Imaging
Canine and Feline Gastroenterology
Canine and Feline Cardiorespiratory Medicine and Surgery

5 Laboratory tests

Clare M. Knottenbelt and Wendy Busby

This chapter is designed to give information on:

- Health and safety in the practice laboratory
- Maintenance and use of a microscope
- Collection, preparation and preservation of samples
- Blood sampling techniques
- Techniques for the laboratory tests commonly performed in veterinary practice
- Identification of white blood cells, urine crystals and common external parasites

Introduction

Laboratory tests are usually performed as part of an investigation of a clinical problem or as a routine health screen. Many laboratory tests can be performed 'in house' with relatively simple equipment, whilst others need to be sent to external laboratories for analysis. This chapter will describe how to perform the common in-house tests and procedures for external submission.

Health and safety

Before using the laboratory all staff should be advised of potential hazards and should understand how to use the laboratory equipment. The following basic laboratory rules should be adhered to.

- Establish fire prevention and fire drill routines
- Provide a first aid kit and train a staff member to act as a first aider
- Always wear adequate protective clothing, including a white coat
- Wash hands frequently and before leaving the laboratory
- Do not eat or drink in the laboratory and do not mouth-pipette
- Label all hazardous materials, clean up spillage immediately, dispose of waste correctly and keep the laboratory tidy.

Waste disposal

- Spillages should always be cleaned immediately
- The laboratory should be kept tidy

- Clinical waste should be disposed of appropriately
- Glassware should be soaked in suitable disinfectants before disposal
- Sharp objects, including disposable plastic instruments, should be placed in a sharps bin
- Samples and culture plates should be autoclaved and placed in yellow clinical waste bags.

Waste in clinical waste bags, glass bins and sharps bins is sent away to be incinerated at the appropriate temperature (see *BSAVA Manual of Veterinary Care*, Chapter 5).

Collection and submission of samples

Veterinary investigations frequently involve the collection and preservation of various samples. Veterinary nurses may conduct or assist in sampling techniques, and should ensure that samples are collected and preserved in a reliable and safe manner.

When collecting samples from any patient the following points should be remembered.

- Health and safety rules must be adhered to, ensuring cleanliness and personal hygiene for protection of both the patient and the handler
- Sterile equipment, including needles, catheters and containers, should be used
- All equipment should be gathered before starting the procedure
- The patient should be adequately restrained
- Samples should be labelled immediately after collection, stating the owner's name, animal identification, date, and nature of sample

- Whenever possible, fresh samples should be examined
- Samples should be stored correctly if they cannot be examined immediately
- A laboratory submission form should be completed for each case with details of the patient, type of sample, a full clinical history and details of tests required
- Regular quality control tests should be carried out on in-house laboratory equipment and the results should be recorded
- Samples for an outside laboratory must include a laboratory analysis form and be prepared, packaged and posted correctly.

Preservation

The preferred method of sample preservation should always be confirmed with the external laboratory prior to sample collection. The methods of preservation that are commonly used are outlined in Figure 5.1.

Anticoagulants

Figure 5.2 lists the anticoagulants required for various blood tests. A range of anticoagulant tubes is available and each tube is manufactured with the appropriate amount of anticoagulant for a given amount of blood. Tubes should therefore be filled to the level indicated by a line or arrow on the side of the tube.

- Overfilling can result in clot formation
- Underfilling may affect some blood parameters.

Once filled, the tube should be gently rolled to ensure that blood is thoroughly mixed with the anticoagulant. Shaking the tube may result in *haemolysis* (rupture of red cell membranes).

Serum or plasma separation

Separation prevents contamination by red cell contents due to haemolysis. Exposure to heat, cold or violent shaking enhances haemolysis. If a sample is to be posted to a laboratory, separation of serum or plasma is recommended (Figure 5.3).

Smears

Preparation of a good quality smear is often difficult and requires practice. The smear should be dried rapidly, or fixed by immersion in absolute methanol for 5 minutes, to prevent changes in cell morphology. Once dried or fixed the smear can be stored for 2 weeks or indefinitely, respectively. Slides should be transported in slide holders to prevent breakage.

5.1 Preservation of common samples

Sample	Type of analysis	Preservation required
Blood	Whole blood or plasma Serum Blood smear	Anticoagulant (Figure 5.2) essential None, separate once clot has formed (Figure 5.3) Air-dried smear essential
Urine	Urinalysis Sediment analysis Culture Reagent strip test	Thymol, toluene or HCl unless examined within 30 min Formalin or thymol Boric acid No preservation – perform as soon as possible and read
Faeces	Routine faecal analysis Culture	Refrigerate if cannot be performed immediately Refrigerate if cannot be performed immediately
Body tissue	Histopathology Fine needle aspirate	10% formalin essential Air-dried smear essential

5.2 A guide to anticoagulants in Vacutainer™ and universal blood sample tubes

Anticoagulant	Universal lid	Vacutainer™ colours	Sample
EDTA (ethylene diamine tetra-acetic acid) which combines with calcium to prevent clotting and causes least distortion of cells	Pink/red	Lavender	Whole blood for haematology
Lithium heparin	Orange	Green or green/orange	Plasma for clinical chemistry and electrolytes
Fluoride oxalate/fluoride (inhibits glucose-using enzymes)	Yellow	Grey	Whole blood for blood glucose
Sodium/potassium citrate	Lilac		Whole blood for clotting and coagulation tests
No anticoagulant	White/clear	Red	Serum for clinical chemistry and bile acids, serum enzymes
Serum gel	Brown		As above

Colour codes should always be checked as some manufacturers may differ. Vacutainers™ were originally designed for human and large animal use with the blood taken directly from the patient into the container. In small animals this process increases haemolysis and the excessive vacuum may collapse the vein against the needle. Vacutainers™ are therefore not recommended for use in this manner in small animal sampling.

5.3 Preparation of plasma and serum samples

1. Collect at least 2 ml of whole blood and place in heparin tube (for plasma) or plain tube of correct size (containing no anticoagulant) (for serum)
2. Serum samples should be left for at least 1 hour at room temperature to ensure clot formation and separation (15 minutes is usually adequate). Plasma samples can be centrifuged immediately
3. Carefully detach clot from the side of the tube with a swab stick

> Clot disruption, sample warming or violent shaking will increase the risk of haemolysis

4. Centrifuge at 3000 rpm for 5 minutes
5. Remove the supernatant (serum or plasma) and place into a tube containing no anticoagulant
6. If the sample is to be frozen, ensure that there is sufficient space in the tube for expansion during freezing.

Slide storage
Unfixed slides of blood smears that cannot be examined immediately should be stored to prevent desiccation. This can be done by sealing the sample in a plastic bag or by using a Petri dish (Figure 5.4).

5.4 Storing slides using a Petri dish

Equipment: Petri dish, tissues, sterile water, matchsticks, sealing tape

1. Remove lid of Petri dish and place upside down on a bench
2. Place tissue/blotting paper in lid of Petri dish
3. Dampen with sterile water
4. Place two sticks or matchsticks on top of tissue
5. Place slide on sticks, cover with base, seal with tape
6. Label clearly, store in cool and dark place.

Refrigeration
Storage at 4°C preserves whole blood and fresh tissue samples in the short term and is preferable to storage at room temperature. Storage for longer than 24–48 hours should be avoided whenever possible.

Freezing
Freezing preserves serum and plasma samples indefinitely. Freezing is the method of preservation for some histological examinations and for some non-routine blood tests, such as measurement of ACTH levels. Checks should be made with the laboratory before freezing a sample. Storage at –10°C will preserve samples for up to 1 week but lower temperatures (–15°C to –20°C) will preserve samples indefinitely. Frozen samples should be thawed slowly at room temperature.

Formol saline and formalin
These chemicals preserve cell structure after collection and are therefore used for tissue samples for histopathology. Skin contamination and inhalation must be avoided when handling these chemicals.

Transport media
Specific transport media are required to preserve certain virology and bacteriology samples. The correct transport medium must be used and so the external laboratory's requirements should always be checked beforehand.

Sediment preparation
Sediment is a concentrated sample of the solid components within a liquid sample (Figure 5.5) – for example, cells or crystals in a urine sample. Smears of the suspension can be examined microscopically. If cytological examination is required, air-dried smears are stained; for urine, a wet preparation is examined microscopically.

5.5 Preparation of a sediment

1. Place fluid in a test tube and centrifuge at 3000 rpm for 10 minutes
2. Remove supernatant (fluid lying above the sediment) with a pipette
3. Resuspend sediment in the small amount of supernatant that remains by gently tapping the base of the test tube.

Labelling of samples
Each sample should be labelled with the owner's name, the animal's name or reference number, the type of sample collected and the date of collection (for example: 'Bobby Smith – Urine 24/8/98').

Paperwork
An appropriate submission form should accompany every sample submitted to an external laboratory. If a submission form is not available, similar information should be provided in an accompanying letter (Figure 5.6). This information ensures that the laboratory performs the appropriate test and is able to interpret the results. Forms should be placed in a plastic envelope to prevent contamination if the sample breaks in transit.

5.6 Information required by external laboratories

- Name and address of submitting veterinary surgeon
- Owner's name
- Animal's name or reference number
- Species, breed, age and sex (M, MN, F, FN)
- Date of sampling and time of collection
- Clinical history, including presenting signs and current treatments
- Types of samples collected, including type of preservatives used
- Site(s) of sample collection
- Test or examination required.

Postage and packaging
Samples that are not preserved, packed or posted appropriately may be damaged in transit. Damaged samples can produce inaccurate results and it is therefore extremely important to ensure that samples arrive in the best possible condition.

- The information supplied by the laboratory should be checked to ensure that the correct types of samples are being sent

- Samples should not be posted on a Friday, as they will sit in a warm post box all weekend.

The following are Royal Mail rules for postage of pathological samples and must be adhered to:

- The sender must ensure that the sample will not expose anyone to danger (COSHH, 1988)
- A maximum sample of 50 ml is allowed by post, unless by specific arrangement with the Royal Mail
- Sample must be labelled correctly with time, date, owner, animal identification and nature of the sample (e.g. 'Heparinized plasma')
- The *primary container* must be:
  - Leak-proof
  - Wrapped in enough absorbent material to absorb the complete sample if leakage or breakage occurs
- The wrapped sample is placed in a leak-proof plastic bag and then in a rigid *secondary container* (e.g. polypropylene clip-down container or cylindrical metal container)
- A correctly completed laboratory form should be sealed in a plastic bag for extra protection and placed with sample
- The whole package should then be placed in a *tertiary container* (strong cardboard or grooved polystyrene box), approved by the Royal Mail, and sealed securely. External laboratories usually provide these containers
- Outer packaging must be labelled conspicuously:
  - FRAGILE WITH CARE
  - PATHOLOGICAL SPECIMEN
  - ADDRESS OF LABORATORY
  - ADDRESS OF SENDER
- The package should be sent by first-class letter post (*not* parcel post).

 If the Royal Mail's conditions are not complied with, the sender is liable to prosecution.

Laboratory equipment

Using a microscope

Figure 5.7 describes the setting up and use of a microscope; Figure 5.8 shows how to read the Vernier scale.

Care of laboratory equipment

- The wiring (including the plug and fuse) of all electrical machinery should be checked regularly
- Servicing, cleaning and lubrication should be performed following the manufacturer's guidelines. Recording details of usage and servicing will ensure that all equipment is safe and reliable
- Microscopes should receive special attention (Figure 5.9)
- Microhaematocrit centrifuges should be cleaned regularly, because when capillary tubes break they contaminate the rubber cushion with blood and glass
- Cleaning and disinfection procedures must be established for incubators to ensure that bacterial contamination does not occur
- Quality control procedures should be performed on a regular basis to ensure that results continue to be accurate.

5.7 Using a microscope

1. Place the lowest power objective into position and turn the light intensity switch (rheostat) to a low setting before switching on the light
2. Place the slide or counting chamber into the mechanical stage and adjust the position so that the lens lies over the area to be examined
3. Adjust the distance between the two eyepieces so that a single image can be seen. Increase the light intensity as necessary
4. Use the coarse and fine focus to bring the object into focus
5. Adjust the condenser and diaphragm to ensure optimal illumination
6. Examine the whole slide by moving the knobs on the mechanical stage
7. Once an area of interest has been identified, rotate the objective lenses to the next power and adjust the fine focus. It may be necessary to adjust the condenser, diaphragm and light intensity
8. Oil immersion provides maximum magnification. If this is required:
   - Focus the object on a lower power then rotate the objective lens out of position
   - Place a drop of immersion oil over the area of interest and rotate the oil immersion lens into position

Always ensure that the lens is lying within the oil, otherwise the image will be distorted. Avoid contaminating the dry lenses with oil

9. Areas of interest can be recorded using the two Vernier scales (Figure 5.8) at any magnification.

5.8 Reading the Vernier scale

Each scale consists of a main scale divided into millimetres and a smaller Vernier plate with 10 divisions.

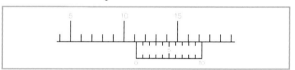

1. First read opposite zero on the Vernier scale the lower number from the upper scale (in this diagram 11)
2. Then read on the bottom scale where lines from top and bottom are directly in line (in this diagram 3)
3. Therefore the reading is 11.3
4. Repeat the reading for the scale at right angles
5. The readings are reported in the same way as grid references on a map (usually horizontal then vertical reading)
6. Always place the slide with the label to the right so that points can be relocated.

5.9 Maintenance and care of a microscope

- Identify a position in the laboratory appropriate for the microscope, i.e. away from direct sunlight, sinks and vibrating machinery
- Avoid moving the microscope from the chosen site if possible
- Keep the microscope covered when not in use
- Turn the light intensity switch (rheostat) down to minimum if the light is left on for a prolonged period and before switching it off
- Clean the lenses with lens paper after using oil immersion
- Lower the stage and turn the lowest power objective into position after use.

Technique	Reasons
Gather and correctly prepare equipment	To avoid unnecessary delay
Appropriate restraint	Safety and good access to vein
Clip skin over vein and apply 70% alcohol (surgical spirit)	To prevent introduction of infection and improve visualization of the vein
Raise vein by occluding the movement of blood towards the heart	To allow the vein to fill up and swell to make sampling easier
Sample from the part of the vein exposed furthest from heart	Minimizes damage to the vein, making it suitable for later use if required
As blood starts to come back, apply gentle pressure on plunger	Too much pressure allows the blood to flow too fast and cells may haemolyse or the vein may collapse against the bevel of the needle
Once the sample is obtained, the vein is released and pressure put on the insertion site for at least 15 seconds	To reduce haemorrhage or haematoma
Remove the needle from the syringe and the tops from the required blood tubes and decant the blood gently	Pushing blood back through the needle and overzealous evacuation of the syringe cause haemolysis
Fill serum samples last	Serum is obtained from a clotted sample
Fill anticoagulant tubes accurately and replace cap firmly	Overfilling may induce clotting. Underfilling may give unreliable results, or alter cell size and morphology
Gently mix/roll	Overenthusiastic mixing causes haemolysis
Label containers immediately	So that they do not get mixed up
Dispose of all pathological and hazardous waste appropriately	In accordance with Health and Safety regulations
Complete laboratory forms as necessary	To ensure accurate communication

Blood samples

Blood samples for biochemical or haematological analysis are often required for diagnostic or monitoring purposes.

Sampling, storage and postage procedures must be appropriate otherwise inaccurate and unreliable results may be obtained. Some general rules for blood sampling are outlined in Figure 5.10.

Equipment
Equipment required for blood sampling (Figure 5.11) includes:

- Sterile needle and syringe
- Cotton wool/swab
- Surgical spirit
- Curved blunt-ended scissors or clippers
- Sample tube(s).

Choice and preparation of needle and syringe
Use as large a needle as practical (Figure 5.12) as this allows more efficient evacuation of blood and reduces haemolysis of the sample. The syringe size is determined by the amount of

5.11 Blood sampling equipment

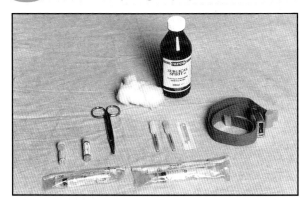

Blood sample tubes, scissors, cotton wool, surgical spirit, sterile needles, tourniquet (optional) and syringes.

5.12 Needle sizes for blood sampling

Species	Needle size
Cat	21 G x $^5/_8$ in
Dog	20 G or 21 G x $^5/_8$ in or 1 in

blood required for analysis. The needle and syringe should be both sterile and dry: dirty equipment will cause contamination of the sample; wet equipment will cause haemolysis.

- The syringe and needle must be put together aseptically
- The bevel of the needle should be turned uppermost, in line with the graduations on the syringe, so that it is possible to see the amount of blood obtained
- The seal on the syringe should be broken before taking the sample so that it is easier to draw the blood once in the vein
- The syringe and needle (with needle guard in place) are now prepared and are placed with the other blood sampling equipment.

Choice of vein
The jugular is the best vein for obtaining a blood sample from dogs and cats. The cephalic vein and the lateral saphenous vein (which runs across the lateral aspect of the hock) can also be used. In general, collection from a larger vein results in a better quality sample (Figure 5.13). Collection from the cephalic vein is suitable for collecting small samples from large patients.

Techniques
Techniques for collecting blood samples from the jugular vein and from the cephalic vein are given in Figures 5.14–5.17.

Restraint
To ensure adequate restraint of the animal, a handler should be present. Good restraint is essential to:

- Gain best exposure of the vein
- Prevent or reduce patient movement during sampling
- Ensure minimal trauma to the patient.

5.13 Choice of vein for obtaining a blood sample

Jugular vein

One of a pair of large veins which return blood from the head and neck region to the heart; they run down either side of the neck from approximately the point of the mandible to the point of the shoulder, with strong venous return

A larger needle can be used when sampling from the jugular vein than from the cephalic vein; this reduces haemolysis and the risk of clotting

A large volume of blood can be obtained relatively quickly

Quick and efficient method causing very little stress to the patient

Enables the cephalic to be left free for anaesthesia or fluid therapy

Useful in animals with shock

Cephalic vein

Runs down the cranial aspect of each forelimb and is accessible distal to the elbow

Familiar vein for venepuncture

Suitable for small samples from large dogs

5.14 Collecting blood samples from the jugular vein

1. The handler stands on the left of the patient
2. The patient is restrained sitting at the front of the table to allow good access to the vein (particularly important in smaller patients)
3. The handler's right arm is passed over the patient's back and round the front of the patient to encircle and control the forelimbs
4. The left arm is used to control and support the head
5. The area over the vein is clipped and swabbed
6. The vein is raised with the thumb, holding excess skin taught with the fingers of the same hand (Figure 5.15)
7. The sample is obtained using a sterile needle and syringe
8. Occlusion on the vein is released before the needle is removed from the vein
9. Thumb pressure is exerted immediately over the needle insertion site.

Cats and small dogs can be sampled in dorsal recumbency on the handler's knee.

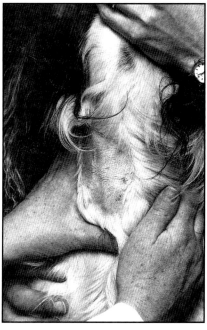

5.15

Technique of raising the vein for a jugular sample.

5.16 Collecting blood samples from the cephalic vein

1. The handler stands on the left of the sitting or sternal–recumbent patient
2. The left hand is passed under the patient's neck and holds the head turned slightly away from the sampler against the handler's shoulder
3. The right arm is passed over the patient's body, the right hand cups the elbow and extends the patient's right forelimb. The handler's upper arm and body are used to support the patient
4. The area over the vein is clipped and swabbed
5. The handler's right thumb is then placed across the right forelimb just below the elbow and gentle pressure is applied to raise the vein (Figure 5.17)
6. The sampler places a thumb alongside the vein to stabilize it and stop the vein moving away on needle entry
7. The needle is inserted to pick up vein and the sample is obtained
8. Occlusion on the vein is released before the needle is removed from the vein
9. Thumb pressure is exerted immediately over the needle insertion site.

This technique is only suitable for collecting small volumes of blood from large patients.

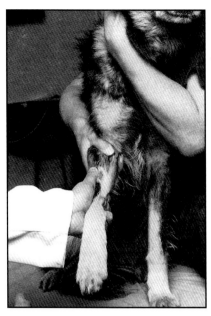

5.17

Technique of restraint for cephalic blood sampling.

Sample preparation

Once the sample has been collected it may need to be processed further before analysis can take place. If it cannot be examined immediately it will need to be stored. The type of sample collected depends on the type of analysis required.

Whole blood samples

Whole blood is used for haematological analysis (red blood cells, white blood cells, platelets). Whole blood must be collected into a specific anticoagulant before analysis. It should not be frozen, but can be stored in a refrigerator at 4°C for up to 48 hours. Previously chilled samples must be returned to room temperature before analysis.

Plasma samples

Plasma is produced by removing the cellular components from whole blood in anticoagulant. Blood is placed into heparin anticoagulant and the heparinized plasma is separated from the red cells (see Figure 5.3). The sample should be labelled with the usual details and the words 'heparinized plasma'.

Serum samples

Serum is produced by allowing blood to clot and removing the cellular components. Blood is placed in a plain tube (with no anticoagulant) and left to clot at room temperature, out of the sun. Once the clot has retracted (approximately 1–2 hours) the serum can be separated from the clot (see Figure 5.3). The sample should be labelled with the usual details and the word 'serum'.

Storage of plasma and serum

Serum and plasma can be stored in the refrigerator at 4°C for up to a maximum of 48 hours or frozen for longer periods. Different analytes are stable in samples for variable periods. Always check with the laboratory to determine how long a sample can be stored. Samples that have been frozen or chilled should be returned slowly to room temperature before examination.

Problems with blood samples

The following factors affect blood sample analysis and may cause erroneous results.

Icteric samples

The sample is yellow, due to large amounts of bilirubin in the blood. This is unavoidable in certain clinical situations, such as liver disease, but nevertheless will affect results of other parameters.

Lipaemic samples

The sample is cloudy, due to large amounts of lipid in the blood. Collect a fasting sample (at least 12 hours). Sample may clear on standing.

Haemolysed samples

The serum is pink or red, due to damage to red cell membranes and release of haemoglobin. To reduce haemolysis:

- Use dry sterile equipment
- Take a jugular sample with a large needle
- Reduce the vacuum on the syringe
- Remove the needle before decanting the blood
- Do not crush the last cells in the syringe
- Mix sample tube carefully
- Separate serum or plasma before posting.

Haemolysis will affect haematological and biochemical results.

Haematology

Important terms are given in Figure 5.18.

5.18 Measurement of red cell parameters in a practice laboratory

Red cell parameter	Definition	Unit	Method of measurement
Packed cell volume (PCV)	Proportion of blood volume which comprises red cells	% or l/l	Microhaematocrit centrifuge Automated haematology analyser
Red blood cell count (RBC)	Number of red cells per litre of blood	$\times 10^{12}$/l	Haemocytometer Automated analyser
Haemoglobin (Hb)	Weight of haemoglobin per decilitre of blood	g/dl	Automated analyser
Mean cell volume (MCV)	Average volume of a single red cell	fl	$MCV = \dfrac{PCV\ (\%) \times 10}{RBC}$
Mean cell haemoglobin concentration (MCHC)	Percentage of haemoglobin in 100 ml of red cells	%	$MCHC = \dfrac{Hb\ (g/dl) \times 100}{PCV\ (\%)}$

5.19 Measurement of PCV using a microhaematocrit centrifuge

1. Invert blood tube to ensure that contents are thoroughly mixed
2. Three-quarters fill two capillary tubes by holding both the blood tube and the capillary tubes at an angle to enhance flow
3. Place a finger on the end of the capillary tube to prevent blood flowing out. Plug the opposite end of the tube with soft clay
4. Place both capillary tubes on opposite sides of the centrifuge, with the plug against the rubber rim of the centrifuge. Note the numerical position of each patient's samples
5. Replace the metal cover and lock the centrifuge lid. Centrifuge at 10 000 rpm for 5 minutes and allow machine to come to a halt
6. Remove capillary tubes and measure PCV manually or using a microhaematocrit reader. The sample will be divided into three layers: red cells, white blood cell layer (buffy coat) and plasma
7. The PCV is calculated, in litres per litre (l/l), by measuring the length of the red cell layer and dividing it by the total length of all three layers. This figure is then multiplied by 100 to give PCV as a percentage
8. Note the size of the buffy coat and the colour of the plasma (red = haemolysis, yellow = jaundice).

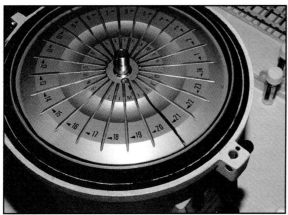

Microhaematocrit centrifuge. Tubes are placed on opposite sides of the centrifuge to ensure that the drum is balanced during spinning.

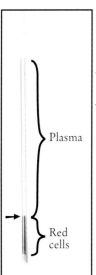

Appearance of a capillary tube after centrifugation. The buffy coat is marked with an arrow. Note the size of the red cell layer and the colour of the plasma layer. This sample was collected from a dog with severe anaemia and jaundice. The PCV can be calculated by measuring the length of the red cell layer and dividing it by the length of all three layers. This figure is then multiplied by 100 to give PCV as a percentage.

Plasma

Red cells

Packed cell volume (PCV)

The PCV is the percentage of whole blood volume that is taken up by the red cells. The PCV will fall in patients with anaemia and may be elevated if the patient is dehydrated or has abnormally high red cell production.

The PCV is measured by centrifuging a capillary tube of whole blood using a microhaematocrit centrifuge and then calculating what percentage of the blood volume is red cells. PCVs are usually measured using blood collected into EDTA anticoagulant, but heparinized capillary tubes are available to allow blood to be collected directly into the capillary tube from a small nick made in the patient's skin. Figure 5.19 describes the method of determining PCV.

Blood smears

Smears should be performed as soon as possible after blood collection. Preparation of a blood smear and common faults are described in Figures 5.20–5.22.

Examination of a stained blood smear provides information about red and white cell morphology (structure), differential white cell counts and platelet counts and may identify blood parasites such as *Haemobartonella felis* (the organism responsible for feline infectious anaemia).

Blood smears are commonly stained with Leishman's (Figure 5.23) or Diff-Quik™ (Figure 5.24). The use of different stains such as Giemsa (Figure 5.23) may identify particular types of cells, such as reticulocytes (immature red cells), or parasites, such as *H. felis*. Once stained, the slide is examined microscopically under both low power and oil immersion (Figures 5.25 and 5.26). Figure 5.27 explains how to preserve a blood smear permanently.

5.20 Preparation of a blood smear

Equipment required: two clean glass slides (A = smear slide, B = spreader slide; see Figure 5.21), one capillary tube, blood sample in anticoagulant (usually EDTA)

1. Invert the blood tube to ensure that the contents are thoroughly mixed
2. Using a capillary tube, place a single small drop of blood at one end of glass slide A
3. Holding glass slide A firmly on the work surface, place one end of slide B on the opposite end of slide A at an angle of 30–45 degrees
4. Draw slide B back to the drop of blood and allow blood to spread out
5. Push slide B away from blood drop in a single rapid motion
6. Rapidly air-dry slide A
7. Check the quality of the smear. If it is adequate, store or stain immediately.

How to recognize a good blood smear

1. Does it air-dry rapidly? Thick smears will take longer to dry.
2. Does it have a feathered (irregular) edge in the shape of a semi-circle? Both these factors indicate that the blood has been spread out sufficiently to produce a monolayer (i.e. one cell thick), which makes examination of cell structure easier.

Good smears are a result of lots of practice. Always prepare a number of smears and only submit the best.

5.21 Preparation of a blood smear

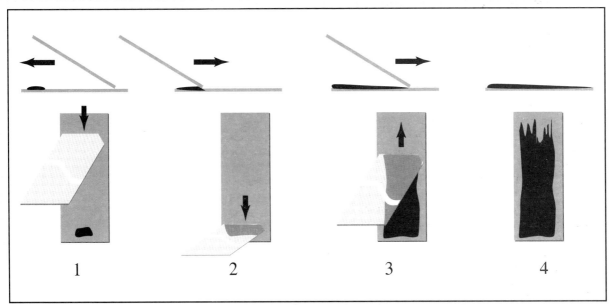

Draw back and push away method for blood smears.

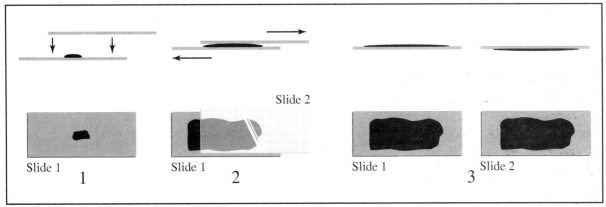

Pull-apart method for blood smears.

5.22 Common faults in blood smears and how to avoid them

Fault	Remedy
Too thick	Use a smaller drop of blood
Too thin	Use a larger drop of blood and/or use a faster spreading motion
Alternating thick and thin bands	Ensure that spreading motion is smooth, and avoid hesitation
Streaks along the length of the smear	Ensure that the edge of the spreader is not irregular or coated with dried blood and that there is no dust on the slide or in the blood
'Holes' in the smear	Ensure that the slide is free of grease
Narrow thick smear	Ensure that the blood is allowed to spread right across the spreader slide before making the smear

5.23 Common stains for blood smears

Leishman's stain

1. Place the air-dried slide on a slide rack and cover with Leishman's stain. Leave for 1–2 minutes to fix
2. Pour on distilled water (using twice the volume of the stain present on the slide) and gently rock the slide to mix the water with the stain
3. Leave for 15 minutes before washing and flooding the slide with distilled water
4. Leave the distilled water on the slide for 1 minute (the smear should start to appear pink)
5. Pour off the water and allow to dry in an upright position.

Giemsa stain

1. Dip the air-dried slide in methanol for a few seconds to fix the cells
2. Flood the slide with Giemsa and leave for 30 minutes
3. Wash the slide in distilled water and allow to dry in an upright position.

5.24 Diff-Quik™ stain

1. Dip the air-dried slide into the fixative solution (fast green in methanol) five times
2. Dip the slide five times into stain solution one (eosin) and then stain solution two (thiazine dye)
3. Rinse the slide with distilled water and leave to dry
4. When performing a platelet count, it may be necessary to dip the slide seven times in the second stain solution to achieve adequate staining.

5.25 Examination of a blood smear

1. Examine the smear under low power:
   - Assess the quality of the smear and find an area where the red cells rarely touch each other (monolayer)
   - Get a general impression of the numbers of white cells present
   - Check for clumping of white cells and platelets at the feather edge
2. Place a drop of immersion oil on the smear
3. Examine the smear under oil immersion:
   - Count the numbers of neutrophils, lymphocytes, eosinophils, basophils and monocytes in 200 white cells. The percentage of each cell type is calculated by dividing the number counted by 2. (For differential white cell count, see *BSAVA Manual of Advanced Veterinary Nursing*, Chapter 6)
   - Assess red cell morphology (strength of colour, size and shape of cells, size and shape of central pallor)
   - Perform platelet count (count number of platelets in 10 microscopic fields and multiply by 1.5 – see *BSAVA Manual of Advanced Veterinary Nursing*, Chapter 6).

5.26 The battlement technique for differential blood films

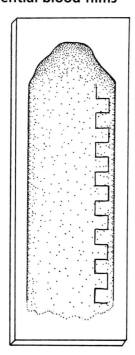

5.27 Permanent preservation of a blood smear

- Place DPX glue on the tail section of the smear and place a coverslip on top
- Or use acrylic spray to preserve the whole smear.

Note: If glue is used to hold the coverslip, then the glue must be allowed to dry before the slide is examined.

White blood cells

White blood cell counts can be performed in the laboratory using dilution in a 'Unopette™' to destroy the red cells (Figure 5.28). A haemocytometer is used to count the white cells (Figure 5.29). The percentages of the different types of white cells and other nucleated cells (such as normoblasts) are established by counting the numbers of each cell type in 200 nucleated cells found on a blood smear stained with Leishman's.

Differential counts can be calculated using the following equation for a neutrophil count:

Number of neutrophils counted/200 x total white blood cell count

Figure 5.30 demonstrates the appearance of various white cells found in routine blood smears. White cell morphology or appearance varies between species and with the type of stain used (Figure 5.31).

5.28 White blood cell count using a Unopette™

Equipment required: Unopette™ disposable pipette (correct size for WBC), Unopette™ reservoir of diluent, haemocytometer, blood sample in anticoagulant (EDTA)

Note: The diluting fluid for a WBC is 2 ml acetic acid mixed with 1 ml of 1% gentian violet and 97 ml of saline (this fluid results in destruction of the red blood cells).

1. Draw up 25 μl blood (i.e. fill the WBC Unopette™ pipette), holding the pipette at an angle of 45 degrees

2. Place the pipette in the Unopette™ reservoir of diluent (produces a dilution of 1 in 20)

3. Invert the reservoir to rinse the pipette and thoroughly mix the contents. Leave for at least 10 minutes to ensure that all the red cells are haemolysed

4. Reverse the pipette and discard the first few drops

5. Fill the haemocytometer. Using low power (x 10), count all white cells seen in squares W, X, Y and Z on the haemocytometer (Figure 5.29). Ignore any white cells touching the bottom and right-hand sides of the square but include those touching the top and left-hand sides

6. Multiply the total count for all four squares by 50 to get the number of white cells per mm³ (equivalent to the number x 10⁹ /l).

5.29 Haemocytometer grid

To perform a white cell count, the numbers of white cells in the squares marked W, X, Y and Z are totalled and multiplied by 50. When a red cell count is being performed the squares marked A, B, C, D and E are totalled and divided by 100. (When performing a red cell count, dilute blood to 1 in 200 with 3% sodium citrate and 40% formol saline.)

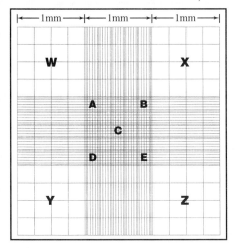

5.30 Appearance of the common white blood cells following staining with Leishman's

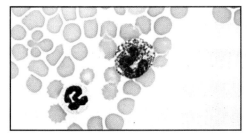

Canine eosinophil and neutrophil stained with Leishman's stain. Note the granular appearance in the cytoplasm of the eosinophil. Both cells have a segmented nucleus.

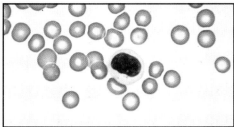

Canine lymphocyte stained with Leishman's stain. Note the large rounded nucleus with little cytoplasm.

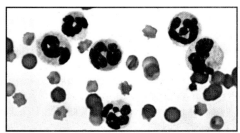

Feline neutrophils stained with Leishman's stain. Note the segmented nuclei. Some of these neutrophils are giant neutrophils, which are produced in association with severe inflammation.

5.31 Blood smear (from a cat) stained with Diff-Quik™

Note the appearance of the neutrophils and platelets of the cat. Platelets can sometimes be hard to see on smears stained with Diff-Quik™. If this is a problem dip the slide into the final stain (purple) seven times instead of five, as this increases platelet staining.

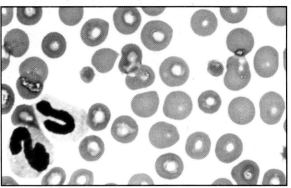

Biochemistry

Biochemical analysis is usually performed on serum or heparinized plasma, which has been separated. Since stress or recent feeding can significantly affect the results of biochemical tests, samples should be collected after a 12-hour fast and patient handling should attempt to minimize stress. The presence of lipaemia and haemolysis results in a number of parameters being falsely elevated or decreased. Wherever possible, serum or plasma for biochemical analysis should be separated and examined to ensure that lipaemia and haemolysis are not present. Cats are particularly prone to stress associated with blood collection, resulting in high blood glucose and an increase in white blood cells (neutrophils and lymphocytes).

Urine

Urine collection is a commonly used diagnostic tool in veterinary practice. Veterinary nurses need to be able to:

*   Advise an owner on how to obtain a free flow sample
*   Assist the veterinary surgeon with catheterization and cystocentesis.

Collection of urine samples

Free-flow samples
This technique is useful for many parameters, but it is unsuitable when a sample is required for bacteriology. As the initial flow is likely to contain surface bacteria, preputial, prostate or vaginal fluids, a mid-stream sample gives the best representation of bladder contents and reduces contamination.

Equipment

*   Gloves
*   For dogs – a clean shallow dish (kidney dish) or commercial urine-collecting receptacle
*   For cats – a litter tray, either empty or with 'washable litter' (pre-washed and disinfected fish-tank pebbles or commercial pebbles)
*   Sterile universal container.

Ensure that containers and litter trays used for urine sample collection have been thoroughly rinsed and have not been cleaned with bleach, as this will alter the pH.

Technique

- For dogs: keep the dog on a lead and attempt to catch a mid-stream sample of urine in the dish
- For cats: from the litter tray, decant the urine into a universal container and test it as soon as possible.

If a urine sample cannot be obtained in this manner, gently squeezing the bladder (manual expression) may encourage patients to urinate:

- Palpate the caudal abdomen to locate and determine the size of the bladder
- Apply gentle constant pressure (this may be required for a few minutes before the patient will urinate)
- Collect the urine.

Patients must have at least 10–15 ml of urine in the bladder if this technique is to be successful.

 Always check with a veterinary surgeon before using this method, as it is contraindicated in cases of urinary obstruction or local trauma.

Catheterization

A urinary catheter is passed up the urethra and into the bladder to obtain a urine sample. Catheterization minimizes contamination from the external genitalia and urethra and is therefore preferred over free-flow samples if bacteriological examination is required. This method can also be used when there are small amounts of urine within the bladder or when complete emptying of the bladder is required.

 Catheterization is contraindicated if vaginitis or open pyometra are evident, as infection may be introduced into the bladder.

Equipment

- Gloves
- Sterile catheter
- Cotton wool and antiseptic
- Kidney dish
- Speculum (bitches – optional)
- Sterile urine sample bottle.

Technique

- Once the patient has been catheterized, direct the initial flow of urine into a kidney dish
- Take a mid-stream sample directly into a sterile universal
- Label the sample appropriately.

Cystocentesis

Cystocentesis is the removal of urine directly from the bladder, using a needle, and is performed by a veterinary surgeon.

Cystocentesis prevents the sample becoming contaminated by the urethra or genitalia and is therefore used to obtain a sample for bacteriology. It can also be used to drain the bladder in an obstructive emergency.

Equipment

- Gloves
- Clippers
- Sterile syringe
- Three-way tap
- Sterile needle, usually 23 g/25 g x 1–1$\frac{1}{2}$ inch, depending on size and obesity of the patient
- Sterile urine sample containers.

Patient preparation

- For cats:
  - Position and restrain the animal, usually in lateral recumbency or standing
  - Clipping is not routinely performed for this procedure in cats
- For dogs:
  - Position and restrain the animal, usually in dorsal recumbency
  - Clip an area 50–75 mm square around the midline of the caudal abdomen
  - Prepare skin aseptically.

Technique

The veterinary nurse's role is to assist prior to and following the actual procedure.

- The bladder is palpated, and held steady through the abdominal wall
  - In cats, the bladder is stabilized and the needle is inserted into the body of the bladder
  - In dogs, the needle is inserted to one side of the midline and slightly caudally into the bladder
- The plunger is withdrawn to obtain a sample
- The needle is removed from the skin, and pressure is applied at the site of penetration to prevent leakage of urine
- The contents of the syringe are evacuated into sterile universal containers and labelled immediately.

 Bladder palpation should be avoided after cystocentesis.

Preservation and storage

Urine samples should be examined immediately, or within 30 minutes of collection. Storage of urine results in increased pH and bacterial number and the spontaneous formation of crystals. Bacteria in the urine utilize any glucose present and may therefore mask glucosuria.

Crystals multiply and cells lyse in samples stored in a refrigerator (4°C). Samples can be preserved with the use of certain chemicals (Figure 5.32).

Urine examination

A number of tests are routinely performed on urine. The method of each test is shown in Figure 5.33.

A refractometer should be used to measure urine specific gravity. Dipstick estimations of specific gravity give a guide but are inaccurate (Figure 5.33).

Microscopic examination should be performed on a freshly prepared sediment, as described Figure 5.33. The common microscopic findings and their clinical significance are described in Figures 5.34 and 5.35.

5.32 Preservatives that can be used in urine samples (urine samples should preferably be examined fresh)

Urine preservatives	Comments	Type of analysis
Thymol	Will preserve urine for 24 hours	Biochemistry (except glucose) and sediment – but kills bacteria
Toluene or HCl	A thin layer over the surface – TOXIC	Biochemistry
Boric acid	Provided in commercial sample bottles 200 mg to 10 ml of urine	Bacteriology
Formalin	1–2 ml formalin to 15 ml urine – TOXIC	Sediment (kills bacteria and alters protein results)

5.33 Summary of the tests used in routine urinalysis

Examination	Method
Visual inspection	Assess colour and turbidity (cloudiness)
Specific gravity (SG)	To calibrate refractometer place water beneath plastic cover of refractometer Adjust until SG = 1.000 and then dry refractometer Place urine under plastic cover of refractometer Read SG (the point where blue area turns to white) Rinse and dry refractometer Note: Dipstick assessment of SG is inaccurate
Dipstick analysis (pH, glucose, ketones, protein, bilirubin)	Invert urine sample to ensure thorough mixing Cover all squares on dipstick with urine and note time Read dipstick results at times indicated on barrel Note: Dipstick SG is inaccurate and dipsticks will not detect all types of ketones
Microscopic examination of sediment	Examine as soon as possible after collection Centrifuge 10 ml at 2000 rpm for 5 minutes Remove supernatant and resuspend sediment by tapping tube Wet preparation: Place a drop of suspension on a slide and stain with new methylene blue if necessary Place a cover slip over the urine Dry preparation: Make a smear using a drop of resuspended sediment Rapidly air-dry and stain with Leishman's stain

5.34 The appearance of common findings on microscopic examination of urine sediment and their clinical significance

Abnormalities	Appearance	Significance
Cells		
Pyuria	Large numbers of WBCs usually neutrophils	Suggests urinary tract inflammation. Look for bacteria
Haematuria	Large numbers of RBCs. May be crenated or lysed, depending on urine concentration	Bleeding into the urogenital tract
Epithelial cells	Flat irregular squamous cells with a small nucleus	Normal cells shed from the urethra, vagina or vulva
Transitional cells	Round small epithelial cells	May suggest urinary tract infection or neoplasia if found in large clumps
Casts	'Worm-like' structures	
Hyaline	Colourless, cylindrical	Mild tubular inflammation, pyrexia Least significant type of cast
Cellular	Contain RBCs, WBCs, epithelial cells or a mixture	Renal tubular disease
Granular	Contain remnants of epithelial cells and WBCs resulting in a granular appearance	Significant inflammation
Waxy	Opaque and wider than hyaline casts	Various renal diseases
Crystalluria (See Figure 5.35)		
Struvite (triple phosphate)	Colourless 'coffin-lid' Found in alkaline urine	Common in normal cats and dogs Associated with infection or calculi in some cases
Calcium oxalate	Colourless 'envelopes' or small stars Found in acid urine	May be normal Associated with calculi or ethylene glycol toxicity
Calcium carbonate	Yellow/colourless spherules or dumb-bells	Rare in dogs and cats Common in herbivores
Ammonium urate	Yellow-brown 'thorn apples'	Normal in Dalmatians Associated with calculi and liver failure
Uric acid	Prisms or rosettes	Common in Dalmatians, may be normal in other pets Associated with calculi

Microscopic examples of some of the common urinary crystals

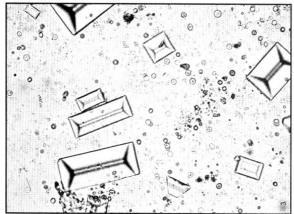

Struvite (triple phosphate) crystals.

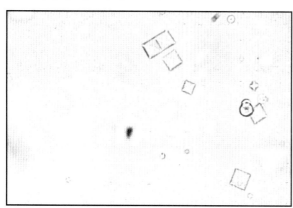

Calcium oxalate crystals.

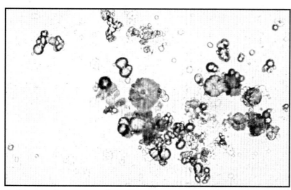

Calcium carbonate crystals.

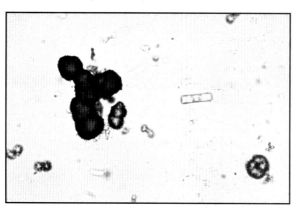

Ammonium biurate crystals.

Faeces

Faecal samples may be required to aid diagnosis in gastrointestinal disease and it is important that samples are collected and examined fresh to obtain accurate results.

Faeces are routinely examined for undigested food material and endoparasites. Faecal culture is performed to identify selected faecal pathogens such as *Salmonella* and *Campylobacter* species.

Collection

The sample can be obtained per rectum or, more commonly, freshly passed faeces are collected (Figure 5.36).

5.36 **Collection and storage of freshly passed faeces**

1. By the owner at home:
   - Provide the owner with a sterile faecal pot (commercially available complete with spatula)
   - The container should be filled as full as possible – this reduces desiccation of faeces or parasites, and reduces bacterial growth
   - The owner should bring the sample to the surgery immediately, or refrigerate and bring in as soon as possible
   - Request that the equipment be returned for disposal as clinical waste if infectious disease is suspected
2. By the nurse in hospital:
   - Collect a *fresh* sample; fill container full and label
   - Collect a sample per rectum.

Equipment

- Sterile faecal pot (commercially available complete with spatula)
- Gloves
- Spatula
- For cats: litter tray, either empty or with washable (non-absorbent) litter
- Lubricant.

Collection of samples per rectum

Per rectum collection of faecal samples ensures that fresh uncontaminated faeces are obtained for immediate examination but the procedure is uncomfortable for the patient. Adequate restraint will be required.

- Clean and lubricate the perineal area (to prevent introduction of skin cells/bacteria)
- Wearing a sterile glove, lubricate a gloved finger and advance it gently into the rectum – do not use force
- Obtain the sample
- Fill and label the container.

Storage

If faeces cannot be examined immediately, they should be stored in an airtight container or in the refrigerator. Faecal swabs for bacteriology can be stored in the refrigerator prior to despatch to an external laboratory. Faecal material is preferred to a swab.

Examination

Figure 5.37 describes the method of in-house tests performed on faeces. Figure 5.38 gives a guide to the identification of common intestinal parasites of cats and dogs in faecal samples.

5.37 Common faecal examinations

Preparation of a faecal smear

1. Place a few drops of water or saline on a clean microscope slide
2. Mix a small quantity of faeces into the fluid, using a spatula
3. Add a drop of iodine. Starch granules will stain dark blue or black
   - This will stain undigested muscle fibres, whose striations and nuclei can be clearly seen
   - Note that muscle from tinned food will appear as if digested
4. Add a drop of Sudan III. This will stain fat globules orange-red
5. On a separate faecal smear, add a drop of eosin to detect muscle fibre
6. Use a cover slip to cover the preparation
7. View under x 40 objective
8. The presence of undigested food particles in the faeces is suggestive of digestive enzyme deficiency, e.g. pancreatic insufficiency.

Detection of parasitic ova

To identify ova, carry out a faecal flotation in a saturated solution of salt, glucose, zinc sulphate or sodium nitrate.

1. Thoroughly mix 3 g of faeces with 42 ml water. If necessary, pass the solution through a strainer. Pour the filtrate into a 15 ml test tube
2. Leave the solution to settle for 15 minutes, or centrifuge at 1500 rpm for 3 minutes
3. Discard the supernatant and fill the test tube with saturated solution
   - Roundworm eggs will float to the surface of the solution
   - Coccidian oocysts float more slowly and it is necessary to wait for 10 minutes for them to come to the surface
   - Using a flat bottomed glass rod, touch the surface of the solution and transfer to a glass slide
   - Add a cover slip to the slide
   - Examine under low or high power objective

Note: Tapeworm segments do not float and the faeces should be examined microscopically for gravid segments.

5.38 Identification of the common intestinal parasites of cats and dogs

Roundworms

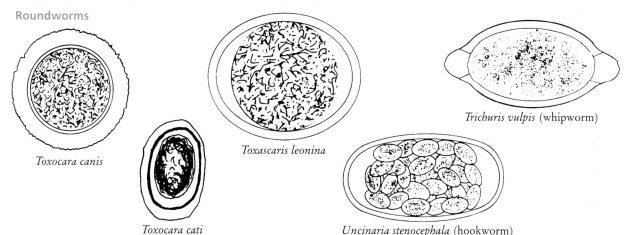

Trichuris vulpis (whipworm)

Toxocara canis

Toxascaris leonina

Toxocara cati

Uncinaria stenocephala (hookworm)

Tapeworms

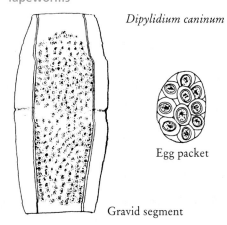

Dipylidium caninum

Egg packet

Gravid segment

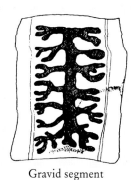

Taenia spp.

Egg

Gravid segment

Body fluids

Body fluids are often needed for diagnostic purposes and the veterinary nurse's role is to help to prepare the patient and assist the veterinary surgeon. Samples may be submitted for cytology (EDTA), protein analysis (heparin or plain) or bacteriology (sterile plain tubes). To avoid introducing infection, the collection of all body fluids must be performed aseptically and gloves should be worn for all techniques.

Abdominal/peritoneal paracentesis

Equipment

- Sterile 19–20 G needle x 1–2 inch
- Sterile 10–20 ml syringe
- Three-way tap
- Sample tubes
- Kidney dish to drain fluid for therapeutic reasons
- Clippers.

Patient preparation

- Clip the ventral abdomen from the umbilicus caudally about 75 mm and about 50 mm either side of the midline
- Scrub, using aseptic surgical technique
- Position the patient in dorsal or lateral recumbency, or standing
- To gain a sample, the needle is inserted to one side of the midline slightly behind the umbilicus.

Thoracentesis

Equipment

- Sterile 18 G x $^3/_4$–1 inch needle (or over-the-needle catheter)
- Sterile syringe and three-way tap
- Tube to feed from drainage luer of three-way tap into a bowl of sterile saline (recommended, to reduce chance of air entering the chest)
- Clippers
- Scalpel blade and suture (for over-the-needle catheter only)
- Kidney dish for removal of fluid for therapeutic reasons
- Sample tubes.

Patient preparation

Local anaesthetic/sedation is sometimes required.

- Position the patient in lateral or ventral recumbency or standing
- Clip the costal area on the right side two-thirds of the way down the chest for fluid, over the sixth to eighth ribs
- Local anaesthetic is injected subcutaneously and into the intercostal space
- Scrub, using aseptic surgical technique
- The site for thoracentesis is the seventh intercostal space (entering the skin over the eighth intercostal space).

Cerebrospinal fluid (CSF)

Cerebrospinal fluid samples are sometimes taken to aid diagnosis of neurological problems.

The area most commonly sampled is between the occipital crest and the first cervical vertebra, and less commonly between the sixth and seventh lumbar space (dog) and lumbosacral space (cat).

Equipment

- Hypodermic or spinal needle, 22 G x 1–3 inch, depending on patient size
- Clippers
- Sample tubes (EDTA and plain).

 This technique is contraindicated in cases of head trauma and increased intracranial pressure.

Patient preparation
General anaesthetic is required.

- Position the patient in lateral recumbency
- Clip from the occipital protuberance of the skull to behind the lateral wings of C1
- Prepare the site aseptically
- The neck should be flexed without twisting.
- Author to add sentence

Arthrocentesis
This technique is used to collect joint fluid, which is normally clear or slightly yellow in colour.

Equipment

- Sterile needle 21–23 G x 1 inch
- 2 ml syringe
- Clippers
- Sample tubes and clean slides.

Patient preparation
General anaesthetic is required.

- Position the patient in lateral recumbency with the joint in flexion
- Clip adequately around the joint
- Prepare the clipped area aseptically.

Sample submission

- Decant the sample from the syringe into selected sample tubes
- Label appropriately, including the source of the sample
- For in-house cytology analysis, smear the sample on to a slide, air-dry and stain with Leishman's or Diff-Quik™
- For an external laboratory, centrifuge the sample, pipette off the supernatant and decant the deposit (concentrated cells and bacteria) into a suitable tube and prepare for dispatch.

Skin sampling

Skin sampling is used both for definitive diagnosis and for assessment of treatment protocols in dermatoses. Dermatological diagnosis is frequently achieved by performing a number of diagnostic tests to eliminate various causes. The common dermatological tests and diagnoses are described in Figures 5.39–5.47.

Since some external parasites and fungal infections are zoonotic (i.e. can be transmitted from animals to humans), knowledge of the life cycle, host specificity and zoonotic risk (Figure 5.48) allows appropriate advice to be given to persons likely to come into contact with the affected animal.

Common skin sampling procedures

Test	Indications	Equipment	Technique
Hand-held lens examination	Fleas, flea dirt, lice, and *Cheyletiella*	Low-power hand-held magnifying lens	Examine skin and hair with lens
Coat brushing	Fleas, lice, *Cheyletiella*, dermatophytes (ringworm)	Fine toothed comb Paper for collection of material Microscope slides Liquid paraffin Pipette Cover slips Microscope	Stand the patient over paper Groom animal's coat with comb Examine debris with hand-held magnifying lens Place some debris on a slide with a drop of liquid paraffin and apply a cover slip Examine under low-power microscope Use damp cotton wool to examine suspected flea dirt (turns reddish brown at edge of dirt) Samples for an outside laboratory should go into paper packs
Mackenzie brush	Dermatophytes or spores of dermatophytes	Mackenzie brush Growth medium	Sterile toothbrush is brushed through coat to collect hairs Press toothbrush on to dermatophyte test medium or Sabouraud's medium for culture
Skin scraping	For detection of all mites, particularly those living deep in the skin	Scissors or clippers liquid paraffin or10% potassium hydroxide (KOH) (Figure 5.40) Pipette Scalpel blade (size 10 or 15) Microscope slides, cover slips, microscope	See Figure 5.41
Wood's lamp	Some strains of *Microsporum canis* fluoresce when exposed to ultraviolet light	Wood's lamp (ideally double tube) Gloves Protective clothing Dark room	Allow lamp to warm up (5–10 minutes) In a dark room, expose hairs for 3–5 minutes (some are slow to respond) 50% of *Microsporum canis* will fluoresce apple green in colour If positive, perform hair plucking and culture on dermatophyte test medium, Sabouraud's medium, or send to outside laboratory **Note:** Some bacteria, skin debris or certain drugs may fluoresce and give false positive results
Hair plucking	Samples for fungal culture or trichograms, dermatophytes (ringworm) or occasionally *Demodex* mites	Broad-rimmed epilation forceps Slides Liquid paraffin Gloves	Look for hairs immersed in scale and crust Pluck single, entire hairs from the edges of lesions, using epilation. **For in-house examination:** Place hair on slide Add liquid paraffin or stain (lactophenol cotton blue or Quink black/blue ink) Examine under microscope Affected material including hair shaft will stain blue **For an outside laboratory:** Place hair sample in clearly labelled, paper envelope
Sticky tape preparation	Lice and *Cheyletiella*	Scissors or clippers Clear sticky tape (19 mm wide) Liquid paraffin Microscope slides Microscope	See Figure 5.43
	Malassezia and bacteria	As above plus Scotch™ tape 19 mm – other tapes unsuitable for staining Diff-Quik™ or Rapi-Diff™ stains Tissues Microscope Immersion oil	See Figure 5.43
Impression smears	Cytological assessment or *Demodex*	Microscope slide Microscope	Slide is pressed directly against lesion and smeared Air-dry slide Stain for cytology Examine under microscope
Fine needle aspirate	*Demodex*, bacteria, cytology	Sterile 5 ml syringe Sterile 21 G needle Microscope slides Cover slip Microscope	Aspirate pustule or nodule contents using a sterile syringe and needle Express contents on to slide Smear or place cover slip on top Examine under microscope
Skin biopsies	Histopathology, dermatophytes, *Malassezia*, bacteria, and occasionally mites	Biopsy punch or scalpel blade and handle Sterile swabs 10% formalin in wide-mouthed container Shiny card Sterile needle Suture material and instruments	See Figure 5.42

5.40 Comparison of liquid paraffin and 10% KOH for use in skin scrapes

Liquid paraffin	10% KOH
Non-caustic, quick and easy	Caustic to skin (both animal and human)
Live mites can be seen, particularly important when re-scraping demodectic mange cases during treatment	Kills mites
	Useful to clear/decolorize skin and hair debris
Preserves mites for several days	Clears sample at room temperature in 30 minutes or faster if warmed for a few seconds with a bunsen burner
Will not clear debris, and difficult to clear using KOH subsequently	Mites desiccate quickly using this medium

Note: Choose one type of medium and stick with it.

5.41 Preparation and examination of a skin scraping

1. Sedate under veterinary direction if required (e.g. for scrapes from face, feet or painful lesions)
2. Select areas of affected skin (erythema, papules, scaling, alopecia)
3. Clip hair carefully with scissors or clippers, taking care not to touch the skin surface
4. Pipette a drop of liquid paraffin on to the skin or scalpel blade
5. Gently pinch up skin at the selected site to help to extrude mites/bacteria
6. Hold the skin flat and taut and scrape with the scalpel blade at an angle of 90 degrees to the skin until capillary ooze is seen. Always scrape several sites
7. Transfer scraping on to microscope slide(s). If the material on the slide is too thick it will be difficult to see anything – divide material between slides
8. Add a small amount of liquid paraffin and apply cover slip

   OR

   Using a Pasteur pipette transfer a few drops of 10% KOH on to the slide and mix with the skin scraping. Leave for 30 minutes or heat gently over a Bunsen burner. Apply a cover slip

   > KOH is caustic. Remember to wear gloves.

9. Clean scrape sites with dilute antiseptic
10. Examine slide(s) first under low power (x 4) magnification to increase scanning speed. Use with condenser low, and light beam diaphragm half-closed to closed to optimize contrast
11. Increase magnification to x 10 and systematically examine slide.

Note: Some types of mite are found in small numbers in normal animals. Some mites require collection by deep skin scrapes, whilst others can be detected on superficial skin scrapes. The appearance of the common mites is described in Figure 5.46 and illustrated in Figure 5.47.

5.42 Performing a skin biopsy

1. Clip hair carefully, avoiding the skin surface. Do not scrub
2. Collect a sample using a biopsy punch or an elliptical incision
3. Blot off excess fluid with a sterile swab (so that it does not slip off the card)
4. Using a sterile needle, place the dermal layer in contact with a piece of card, to prevent curling
5. Place in 10% formalin immediately – cells deteriorate very quickly if left exposed to air
6. Close skin with a single suture.

5.43 Sticky tape preparation

For lice and *Cheyletiella*

- Select areas of dry scaly skin and scurfy hair
- Clip the hair carefully, avoiding the skin surface
- Apply the sticky surface of the adhesive tape to the skin and base of hairs
- Add a small drop of liquid paraffin to a microscope slide
- Place the tape (sticky side down) on to the microscope slide
- Examine immediately, using low power objective

For *Malassezia* and bacteria

- Select areas of greasy erythematous skin (axillae, inguinal and interdigital regions)
- Clip hair carefully
- Apply the sticky surface several times to the skin
- Stain the sticky tape with Diff-Quik™ (Figure 5.24)
- Attach the tape (sticky side down) to a microscope slide
- Cover with tissues and exert gentle pressure to remove excess fluid
- Examine immediately, using x 40 or x 100 under oil immersion.

Skin swabs

A swab is a small piece of absorbent cotton wool wrapped firmly around the end of a long stick. The swab is sterilized and sealed in a plastic outer tube with a non-absorbent cotton wool plug at the bottom. Transport media (provided by the external laboratories) such as activated charcoal can be used to reduce bacterial growth.

Swabs are used to detect the presence of bacteria, *Malassezia* or *Demodex* species in skin lesions. Figure 5.44 describes collection of a skin swab.

5.44 Collection of skin swabs

Equipment required: Sterile 22–27 G needle (for pustules), sterile bacteriological swab, slides (for in-house examination)

1. Select lesions or areas which may be suspected of bacterial infection (e.g. pustules)
2. Select correct type of swab with transport medium if submitting for bacteriology
3. Rupture the pustule first with a sterile needle
4. Break the seal and remove the swab without touching the edges, handling the lid only
5. Rub the tip over or into the affected area
6. Replace in the tube immediately and label
7. Make a smear sample for examination or package and dispatch to outside laboratory.

5.45 Diagnosis and significance of mites of the dog and cat

Mite	Host	Diagnostic test	Significance
Demodex canis	Dog	Found deep within the follicles so the skin should be squeezed before performing a deep skin scraping	Small numbers found in normal dogs. Many mites and immature forms confirms infection
Demodex cati	Cat	Found deep within the follicles so the skin should be squeezed before performing a deep skin scraping	Rare
Sarcoptes scabiei	Dog	Lives in epidermal burrows, therefore multiple deep scrapings required. Take multiple skin scrapings from the elbow, ear or sites with papules	Presence of even one mite is diagnostic
Notoedres cati	Cat	Single skin scrape of eyes, ear or face	Rare
Cheyletiella	Cat Dog	Can be seen as 'walking dandruff' with the naked eye Superficial skin scrapes or sticky tape preparations or coat brushings useful	Common cause of pruritus and skin scaling
Otodectes	Cat Dog	Mites visible with the naked eye. Superficial scrapings, smears of ear wax or sticky tape preparations helpful	Common cause of ear problems, but can also cause a generalized problem

5.46 The microscopic appearance, distribution and clinical signs of the common external parasites

Parasite	Parasite appearance	Clinical signs	Usual distribution
Ctenocephalides (flea)	Eggs: small brown laterally compressed Flea dirt: brown granules turn red when wet	Pruritus Acute: wheals and erythema Chronic: seborrhoea, lichenification, alopecia	Dogs: dorsum (especially lumbosacral area) and ventrum Cats: Miliary (generalized) dermatitis or focal eosinophilic granuloma (pink plaque)
Dipteron (fly)	Larvae: many forms	Mild: local wheal Severe: 'fly-strike'	Perimeum, genitalia, wounds etc.
Lignognathus (louse)	Eggs: small, white and attached to hair ('nits') Adults: sucking lice with typical fixed piercing mouth-parts	Mild: carrier showing no sign Severe: papules, crusts, seborrhoea sicca	Under matted hair and around body orifices
Trichodectes (louse)	Adults: biting lice with broad head Chewing mouth-parts on ventral aspect	Mild: carrier showing no sign Severe: papules, crusts, seborrhoea sicca	Under matted hair and around body orifices
Cheyletiella (mite)	Eggs: loosely attached to hair Adults: large white 'walking dandruff'	Mild: carrier showing no sign Severe: mild, non-suppurative dermatitis and scurf	Diffuse although usually more dorsal
Ixodes (tick)	Adults: flattened, ovoid, yellow-white to red-brown.	Carrier showing no sign or mild local irritation (especially if incompletely removed)	Ears, face and ventral body
Sarcoptes scabiei (canine scabies)	Adults: round-bodied mite	INTENSE PRURITUS. Alopecia, scales and crusts	Ventrum, ears and elbows
Otodectes (ear mite)	Adults: white dots visible with the naked eye	Ears: otitis externa Generalized: may mimic flea allergic dermatitis	Ears, occasionally generalized
Notoedres cati (feline scabies)	Resembles *Sarcoptes*	PRURITUS Lichenification, crusting, alopecia	Head, ears and neck, occasionally generalized
Demodex (mite)	Adults: small cigar-shaped mites Four stages of life cycle may be present	Mild erythema, alopecia. May be pruritic if secondary pyoderma present	Localized (especially face and forelimbs) or generalized

5.47 Appearance of the common mites of the dog and cat

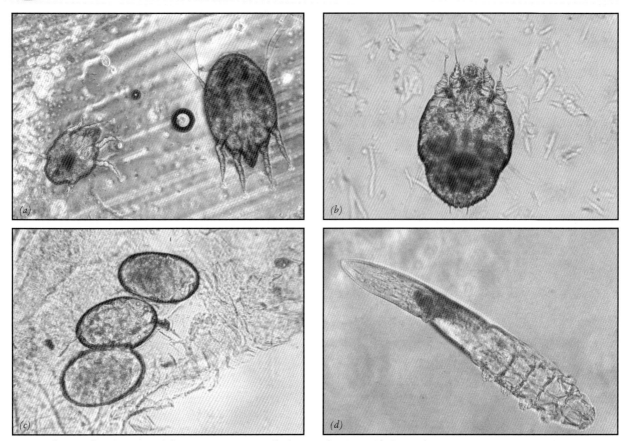

(a) Otodectes; (b) Sarcoptes *adult*; (c) Sarcoptes *eggs (high magnification)*; (d) Demodex.
© A. Foster/S. Shaw, University of Bristol

5.48 Life cycle and risk of zoonotic and cross-species infection for the common external parasites

Parasite	Zoonotic	Host specific	Life cycle
Ctenocephalides (flea)	Yes	No	Majority of cycle is off host. Eggs, larvae and adults present in environment
Dipteron (fly)	No	No	Eggs and larvae present on animal
Lignognathus (louse)	Yes	Yes	Permanently resides on animal. Transmitted from animal to animal by close contact
Trichodectes (louse)	Yes	Yes	Permanently resides on animal. Transmitted from animal to animal by close contact
Cheyletiella (mite)	Yes	No	Permanently resides on animal. Transmitted from animal to animal by close contact
Ixodes (tick)	Yes	No	Feeds on animal. Animals infected from environment
Sarcoptes scabiei (canine scabies)	Yes	No (rarely)	Permanently resides on animal. Transmitted from animal to animal by close contact
Otodectes (ear mite)	Occasionally	No	Permanently resides on animal. Transmitted from animal to animal by close contact
Notoedres cati (feline scabies)	Yes	No	Permanently resides on animal. Transmitted from animal to animal by close contact
Demodex (mite)	No	Yes	Found in small numbers in normal animals. Becomes significant when the animal's immune response is inadequate

5.49 Method of performing a Gram stain

1. Prepare a heat-fixed smear: pass the dry slide through a Bunsen flame several times until hot to the touch. Allow to cool
2. Flood the slide with crystal violet and leave for 1 minute
3. Wash off stain with Lugol's iodine, holding the slide at an angle
4. Flood the slide with Lugol's iodine and leave for 1 minute
5. Pour off the iodine and rinse with distilled water
6. Hold the slide at a slight angle and pour on 95% alcohol until the stain no longer discolours the alcohol
7. Immediately rinse the slide under running tap water to prevent excessive decolorization
8. Flood with carbol fucin (which acts as a counter stain) for 1 minute
9. Rinse the slide and gently blot dry

5.50 Inoculating a culture plate

Inoculating an agar plate using the streaking method. The loop should be flamed and cooled between each 'streaking'.

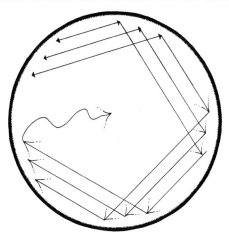

Bacteriology

Bacteriology smears

Smears can be prepared from fluid samples, from bacteriology swabs or from bacterial colonies grown on culture plates. The shape and staining characteristics will identify the type of bacteria. Appropriate antibiotics can often be selected on the basis of shape and their appearance on a Gram stain (Figure 5.49). Specific stains are used to identify specific families of bacteria. For example, Ziehl-Neelson stain is used to identify acid-fast bacteria such as the mycobacteria responsible for tuberculosis.

Bacterial culture

Many bacteria can be grown on blood-agar plates at 37°C. The plate is inoculated using a heat-sterilized metal loop to spread the sample across the plate. It is important to ensure that the loop has cooled before allowing it to contact the sample, since heat may destroy the bacteria within the sample.

Streaking is used to ensure that the concentration of bacterial colonies is low enough in some areas of the plate to allow single colony identification (Figure 5.50). Some bacteria produce distinct colonies, which can be identified by their appearance on an agar plate.

Virology samples

Virus detection is now commonly performed in veterinary practice. Desktop kits are available for detecting feline leukaemia virus, feline immunodeficiency virus and canine parvovirus. External laboratories can perform tests for many other viral diseases. The tests available for commonly encountered viruses are listed in Figure 5.51.

Histopathological samples

Samples of body tissue can be submitted for histopathological examination, but must be preserved immediately to be suitable for

5.51 Tests available for the common viral diseases of the dog and cat

Virus	In-house tests available	Samples required for external testing
Feline leukaemia virus (FeLV) FeLV antigen	Desk-top kits available for testing whole blood or saliva for antigen	Whole blood in heparin
Feline immunodeficiency virus (FIV) FIV antibodies	Desk-top kits available for testing whole blood for antibodies	Whole blood in heparin
Feline infectious peritonitis (FIP)	None	Serum and/or abdominal fluid for corona virus antibody titres
Feline calicivirus (FCV)	None	Oropharyngeal swab (in viral transport medium)
Feline herpes virus (FHV)	None	Oropharyngeal swab (in viral transport medium)
Feline infectious enteritis (FIE)	Canine parvovirus faecal antigen test may detect virus in some cases	Serum (two samples 4 weeks apart) and/or faeces
Canine parvovirus	Canine parvovirus faecal antigen test	Serum and faeces
Canine distemper virus (CDV)	None	Serum (two samples 4 weeks apart)

5.52 Preserving fluids for pathological specimens

Formol saline	40% formaldehyde solution	Used to preserve specimens which must be chilled
Buffered 10% formalin	10% solution of 40% formaldehyde and acid sodium phosphate monohydrate in distilled water	Used to preserve specimens which are kept at room temperature (must not be refrigerated as will cause artefacts)

examination. The available preservatives are listed in Figure 5.52.

Tissue samples should be small (< 1 cm^2) as poor cell preservation – resulting in cell death and destruction (necrosis) – will occur if larger samples are preserved by this method. Each tissue sample should be placed in at least 10 times the volume of formalin. For example: a 1 cm^2 piece of liver should be placed in a minimum of 10 ml of 10% formalin. 'Fixing' a sample with formalin often causes the sample to swell slightly and harden, and so the neck of the container needs to be wide enough to ensure that the sample can be removed with ease. Multiple samples should be submitted if possible.

Equipment

- Surgical kit
- Preservative – a minimum of 10 times the volume of the sample
- Bowl containing preservative (if the sample is to be fixed before being transferred to sealed container – a minimum of 24 hours to fix)
- Wide-necked container.

Cadavers for postmortem

Cadavers should be chilled not frozen and transported to the laboratory as soon as possible. Autolysis (postmortem decomposition) will occur if the temperature and humidity are not reduced and the cadaver is not examined quickly.

Toxicology

Each suspected toxin may require the collection of specific samples. It is vital that the external laboratory performing the tests is contacted to ensure that the correct samples are submitted. In general the following guidelines apply:

- Specimens must be collected fresh and free from environmental contamination
- Sample containers must be sterile and chemical-free
- Label with the usual details and the practice name and address
- Freeze all samples (except those for histopathology) and post on ice to the laboratory
- Accurate historical and clinical records must be sent with the samples.

Further reading

Bush BM (1975) *Veterinary Laboratory Manual*. William Heinemann Medical Books, London

Bush BM (1991) *Interpretation of Laboratory Results for Small Animal Clinicians*. Blackwell Science, Oxford

Davidson MG, Else RW and Lumsden JH (1998) *BSAVA Manual of Small Animal Clinical Pathology*. BSAVA, Cheltenham

Kerr MG (1989) *Veterinary Laboratory Medicine*. Blackwell, Oxford

Meyer D and Harvey J (1998) *Veterinary Laboratory Medicine. Interpretation and Diagnosis*, 2nd edn. WB Saunders, Philadelphia

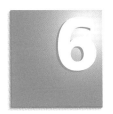

6 Surgical conditions and surgical nursing

Alasdair Hotston Moore and Cathy Garden

This chapter is designed to give information on:

- Preparation of small animals for surgery
- Providing the veterinary surgeon with general intraoperative assistance
- Postoperative care of small animals to promote a rapid recovery from surgery
- Problems in the pre-, peri- and postoperative periods
- Simple wound management under veterinary direction
- Common surgical conditions of small animals and the type of animal usually affected, the clinical signs of the disease and the basis for its treatment

Introduction

Diseases affecting small animals can be classified in a number of ways. An important distinction is between those requiring surgical treatment and those suitable for medical therapy.

This distinction is not absolute: many patients requiring surgery as part of their treatment also need medical therapy and some conditions can be treated by either medical or surgical methods. A common example of the latter is ear disease, when the veterinary surgeon may choose a medical or a surgical approach to the case. This decision will be constantly reviewed as the effect of treatment becomes apparent, and an initial medical treatment path may later be replaced by a surgical treatment.

In other instances, it is important that a condition requiring surgical treatment is recognized at the outset where surgery is an essential part of the case management. An obvious example is the fracture of a bone: early identification of the problem and appropriate surgical intervention will prove critical to a successful outcome.

Preoperative problems

The degree of preoperative care required in a particular case depends on the type of patient, the effect the surgical indication has had on the patient and the presence and effect of other diseases (Figure 6.1). Young, fit and healthy animals presented for elective surgery require the minimum of special care. Older animals are more likely to have concurrent disease; before surgery there is a need for closer assessment to identify such diseases and their effect. If necessary, preoperative treatment can then be arranged to minimize the potential morbidity and mortality associated with anaesthesia and surgery.

The impact of the indication for surgery must be considered during the assessment and preparation of the animal. For most elective surgeries (neutering, cosmetic procedures, chronic orthopaedic conditions), by definition, the indication has little effect on the patient's physiology. However, for emergency procedures, the animal can be severely affected by the disease (Figure 6.2).

Preparation of the patient

Patient preparation can vary greatly from case to case. Certain patients require longer periods to allow them to be optimally prepared for surgery. Some may require extended dietary control or medical treatment (e.g. diabetics) before they are ready for surgery. Other patients may need immediate surgical attention and preparation time may be limited.

This section will cover patient preparation for the more immediate preoperative period, starting with starvation through to the positioning of the patient on the table ready for the surgeon.

Starvation
Food is normally withheld for approximately 12 hours prior to surgery. This ensures an empty stomach and avoids vomiting in the perioperative period, which may be detrimental to the patient and the surgical incision. Surgery on certain parts of the alimentary tract may require dietary restriction for longer.

Bowel and bladder evacuation
Patients should be given the chance to urinate and defecate immediately prior to surgery. For most cases it is sufficient to allow them access to a litter tray or walk them before taking them into theatre. In some cases more extensive preparation is required.

6.1 Preoperative problems

Preoperative problem	Associated surgical complications	Steps in prevention
Advanced age	Exacerbation of pre-existing problems (e.g. organ failure)	Preoperative assessment and appropriate therapy
Obesity	Anaesthetic mortality Reduced surgical exposure	Normalize body condition prior to surgery
Emaciation	Delayed healing Reduced immunocompetence	Normalize body condition prior to surgery Modify surgical technique to allow for reduction in rate of healing Perioperative antibiotic use
Hypoproteinaemia	Delayed healing Reduced immunocompetence	Modify surgical technique to allow for reduction in rate of healing Perioperative antibiotic uses Plasma or blood transfusion
Therapeutic corticosteroids Cushing's disease (hyperadrenocorticism)	Delayed healing Reduced immunocompetence	Withdraw corticosteroid therapy prior to surgery Stabilize disease prior to surgery Modify surgical technique to allow for reduction in rate of healing Perioperative antibiotic use
Clotting or bleeding defects	Increased intra- and postoperative haemorrhage	Assess and treat before surgery Minimize bleeding during surgery by careful attention to haemostasis Fresh blood or plasma transfusion Postoperative monitoring
Organ failure	Exacerbation by hospitalization, anaesthesia and surgery	Assess and treat before surgery Tailor peri- and postoperative care appropriately
Skin infection Infections remote from surgical site (e.g. dental disease)	Infection of the surgical site	Assess and treat before surgery Perioperative antibiotic use

6.2 Factors to be considered and treated before, during and after emergency surgery

Complicating factor	Causes	Associated problems	Steps in prevention
Hypoventilation	Many, including: Respiratory tract obstruction Thoracic disease Abdominal distension Depression of the central nervous system	Hypoxia Hypercapnia Respiratory acidosis	Avoid worsening by stressing the patient or inappropriate use of drugs Oxygen supplementation before, during and after surgery if necessary
Dehydration	Inability or unwillingness to drink Increased fluid losses	Hypovolaemia Delayed recovery	Reverse before surgery if possible Use fluid therapy to expand blood volume (see Chapter 3)
Hypovolaemia	Dehydration Haemorrhage Septicaemia	Increased anaesthetic morbidity and mortality Surgical infection	Reverse before surgery if possible Use fluid therapy to expand blood volume (see Chapter 3)
Septicaemia	Trauma Organ rupture Migration of bacteria from gastrointestinal tract due to mucosal ischaemia	Increased anaesthetic morbidity and mortality Surgical infection	Aggressive pre- and intraoperative antibiotic and fluid therapy
Cardiovascular dysfunction	Many, including: Shock Septicaemia Toxaemia Gastric dilation volvulus (see later) Splenic diseases	Increased anaesthetic morbidity and mortality	Assess and treat underlying condition Specific treatment with drugs to suppress dysrhythmias (e.g. lignocaine) or increase force or rate of contraction (e.g. dopamine) may be required
Electrolyte or acid/base disturbances	Severe systemic disease of all types	Increased anaesthetic morbidity and mortality Delayed recovery	Reversal of hypovolaemia to allow homeostatic mechanisms to function Specific treatment may be needed, e.g. with potassium (for hypokalaemia), glucose and insulin (for hyperkalaemia) and bicarbonate or lactate (for acidosis)

Enemas

In cases of rectal or colonic surgery it may be necessary to be more certain that the patient has defecated. These cases will require an enema before surgery. A soap and warm water or phosphate (Fleet) enema is usually adequate for this. The patient may need bathing after administration of an enema. Enema administration is covered in more depth in Chapter 4.

Urinary catheterization

Other patients may need an empty bladder before surgery is undertaken. Gentle manual expression under general anaesthesia may be adequate or catheterization of the bladder may be required. An indwelling catheter can also be useful for measuring the production of urine during surgery and in the immediate postoperative period. Urinary catheterization is covered in more depth in Chapter 4.

Bathing

To remove loose hair and skin particles and so reduce the risk of contamination of the surgical site, it would be helpful to bath every patient prior to surgery. This is not always practical but it should be considered for patients that are excessively soiled or patients undergoing elective orthopaedic surgery with the use of implants (e.g. hip replacement). Enough time should be allowed to dry the patient thoroughly before surgery.

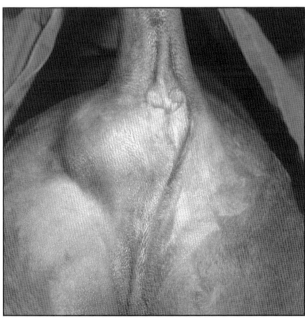

6.3 *Perineal area prepared for surgery by clipping, scrubbing and placement of a purse-string suture in the anus.*

6.4 Points to consider when clipping prior to surgery

- Clipping against the hair is the most effective, although it may be necessary to clip with the grain of the hair first to remove a thick coat
- Be neat: owners will not be impressed by untidy clipping
- Be gentle: avoid clipper rash and skin irritation
- Be thorough: clip a large enough area and consider the possibility of an extended incision if the surgery does not go as planned. The area clipped should extend 5–15 cm beyond the anticipated incision site
- If clipping near the eyes make sure they are appropriately protected before starting (e.g. by application of a bland ointment).

Clipping

There are advantages and disadvantages of clipping before or after the induction of anaesthesia and each patient should be considered individually – depending on the area to be clipped, the type of surgery and the temperament of the patient. For routine elective surgery the best time to remove the hair is after the induction of anaesthesia (Figure 6.3). This should be done in a preparation area outside the theatre. Loose hair and debris caused by clipping should be removed before the patient enters theatre, so reducing the risk of contamination.

To reduce the anaesthetic time, patients at greater anaesthetic risk may be clipped before induction if it can be done without causing distress, but this will increase the risk of postoperative wound infection. Clipping too soon before surgery, or clipping that causes damage to the skin, increases the skin bacterial numbers at the time of surgery and the incidence of incisional infection.

Points to consider when clipping prior to surgery are listed in Figure 6.4.

Skin preparation

Points to consider when preparing the patient's skin are listed in Figure 6.5. Once the initial preparation of the skin is complete the patient can be positioned on the operating table ready for surgery. Contamination of the skin is likely to occur during positioning and so a secondary scrub should be carried out in theatre immediately before surgery (Figure 6.5).

6.5 Preparation of the skin

Initial preparation

- Carried out in the preparation area, outside the theatre itself
- Wear gloves to prevent cross-contamination and protect the hands from sensitization to antiseptic solution
- Use either chlorhexidine or povidone–iodine. Do not change between the two during one procedure
- Mechanical scrubbing of the skin is important as it reduces the number of bacteria on the skin. Avoid abrading the skin surface
- Use lint-free swabs
- Start scrubbing at the incision site in the centre of the clipped area, work out towards the edges, discard the swab and start at the centre again with a clean swab. Be careful not to return a swab from the edges to the centre of the area to be scrubbed
- Include the hair at the edge of the clipped area to remove debris but be careful not to make the patient too wet
- Remove the soap with sterile water or alcohol and swabs, then repeat the scrubbing process.

Skin preparation in theatre

- Use sterile gloves and swabs for scrubbing
- Repeat the procedure described above for the initial preparation
- Mop up any pools of fluid caused by preparing the skin
- The final skin preparation should be performed in a sterile manner by a member of the surgical team. This usually consists of aseptic application of an alcoholic solution of skin disinfectant that is left to dry on the skin.

6.6 Points to consider during patient positioning

- Position the patient with the surgical site best presented to the surgeon
- Check that the positioning will not interfere with respiratory function or peripheral circulation, or cause muscular damage
- Use positioning aids to make the patient comfortable and avoid ischaemic damage
- If using some type of heat pad underneath the patient, remember that the patient will not be able to move away from the heat – make sure it is not too hot. Preferably use a thermostatically controlled electric heat pad or water blanket
- If monopolar diathermy is to be used, place the return electrode or patient plate against the skin under the patient. The plate should be in close contact with the skin in an area of good vascular supply. Some plates are used with contact provided by a saline-soaked cloth (check with the equipment manufacturer)
- Make sure everything is in place before the sterile preparation of the skin begins and the drapes are placed on the patient.

6.7 Points to consider during patient draping

- Drapes are applied by a scrubbed member of the surgical team once they are gowned and gloved and skin preparation is complete
- Drapes should cover the patient and the entire table, leaving only the surgical site exposed. The drapes *must* cover the area between the field of surgery and the instrument tray or trolley
- Water-resistant drapes are chosen for surgeries where irrigation or other fluids are likely to be present (for example, during exploration of a haemoabdomen). Another option is to use a sterile plastic drape under or over the cloth drapes to prevent strike-through
- Conventional drapes are secured to the skin with towel clips. If the tips of these penetrate the drapes, they are considered non-sterile and must be replaced
- Plastic drapes can be secured with sterile spray or may be self-adhesive; however, such drapes adhere unreliably in many situations
- Once in position, drapes should not be moved, since this would contaminate the surgical field. If placed incorrectly, they should be discarded and fresh drapes should be used
- Drapes can be made of either cloth or paper (advantages and disadvantages of different materials are discussed in Chapter 7)
- Some drapes have a pre-prepared opening for the surgical field (fenestration); for other surgeries the fenestration can be cut (if using paper drapes) or made to the required size using four plain drapes
- When applying individual drapes, the edges of each drape at the incision should be folded under before being placed on the patient.

Positioning of the patient

Although the initial positioning of the patient is usually a task for the veterinary nurse (Figure 6.6), it is wise to check on the final positioning with the surgeon or assistant before they begin to scrub up. Once surgery has started it is very difficult to alter the position of the patient without contaminating the sterile field.

Draping

Draping begins once the patient is correctly positioned and the final skin preparation is complete (Figure 6.7). Drapes are used to protect the exposed tissues from contamination from the surrounding skin (Figure 6.8). Figure 6.9 describes how to drape a patient.

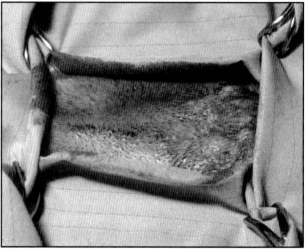

6.8 Prescrotal area draped for castration. Four plain drapes have been placed around the surgical site, leaving the area for incision open. Alternatively, a single fenestrated drape may be used.

Preparation of personnel for surgery

Scrubbing up

The aims of scrubbing the skin before putting on a surgical gown and gloves are to remove any gross dirt and to reduce as much as possible the number of microorganisms on the skin. Finally the scrub solution should have a prolonged effect in suppressing the levels of organisms on the skin once underneath surgical gloves.

There are variations in the methods for scrubbing up, mostly concerning the extent of the areas of the hands and arms that are scrubbed using a brush. Studies have shown that there is no difference between using reusable or disposable brushes, but frequent autoclaving of reusable brushes will eventually make them hard and harsh on the skin.

If the skin does become dry and damaged through repeated scrubbing procedures, there will be greater numbers of bacteria on the skin and the effectiveness of the scrubbing procedure will be greatly reduced.

Whichever variation in the method of scrubbing up is used (Figures 6.10 and 6.11), the basic principles remain the same:

- The procedure should be a routine
- It should not take up an excessive amount of time
- The antiseptic solution and technique should not be irritant to the skin.

6.9 How to drape a patient

Draping with four plain drapes
The order of draping is depicted in Figure 6.9a.

1. Pick up the first drape, still folded, from the trolley. Step back and unfold it away from the trolley and table so that it does not touch non-sterile areas.
2. One quarter of the drape is folded back underneath itself to produce a double layer at the edge of the draped area.
3. The drape is held along the folded edge, with the hands inside the drape so that they do not touch the patient as the drape is placed. Each subsequent drape is handled in the same way.
4. The first drape is placed on the side of the surgical field nearest the surgeon. This is so that the surgeon can later move close to the table and lean over to place the other drapes without contacting undraped areas.

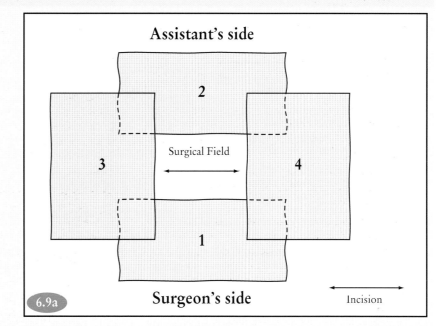

5. The second drape is placed on the opposite side of the surgical area (assistant's side) by the surgeon, who can approach the table, which is covered by the first drape, or by the assistant in the same way as the surgeon placed the first drape.
6. The third and fourth drapes are placed at either end of the surgical field (the order of these is not important).
7. Any remaining areas of the table or patient that remain exposed are covered by additional sterile drapes.
8. Drapes are secured with towel clips: one towel clip is used at each corner of the surgical field.
9. The clip is placed diagonally across the edges of the two drapes, with one tip on each. The tips are pushed down on to the skin and the clip is closed to pick up the drapes and a small fold of skin.
10. The clip is then placed under one drape at the corner.

Draping with one fenestrated drape

1. The drape is picked up, still folded, from the trolley and is unfolded away from the trolley and table (as in step 1 above).
2. The drape is held along the top edge, with the hands inside the drape so that they cannot touch non-sterile areas as the drape is placed.
3. Look through the fenestration and place the fenestration over the surgical field.
   - The size of the fenestration should approximate the area required – it is unsatisfactory to fold the drape to reduce the size of the fenestration if it is too large
   - The preferred alternative, if necessary, is to place further plain drapes over the fenestration to reduce its size.
4. Secure the drape with towel clips at each corner of the fenestration (see steps 8 and 9 above). The clips cannot be concealed beneath the drapes and are more likely to interfere with the instruments during surgery.

Other draping techniques

- Plastic drapes secured with adhesive spray or self-adhesive drapes can be usefully combined with conventional drapes to reduce strike-through in the presence of excessive fluids or as a form of subdraping (see below)
- Fenestrated and plain drapes can be used together to cover the patient and table effectively without leaving gaps where drapes overlap. For example, a large fenestrated drape with large fenestration can be placed as a second layer over a field surrounded by four plain drapes
- Some surgical sites require special techniques to drape effectively. For example:
   - On the limb, the foot may be covered by a sterile foot bag or surgical glove, or sterile cohesive bandage can be used to wrap the limb
   - Draping of the oral cavity requires additional towel clips or staples to secure the drapes to the lips
- *Subdraping* is the practice of placing additional drapes close to or against the incised skin edge to limit further the surgical field and reduce contamination from the surrounding skin. It is not routine in veterinary surgery but should be considered for procedures at particular risk of infection (placement of orthopaedic implants is one example)
   - Use of an adhesive plastic drape over the field that is incised with the skin is one such technique, but these types of drapes often peel away, particularly on concave surfaces and in the presence of fluids
   - Alternatively, small cloth drapes or towels can be secured to the skin edge with towel clips or skin clips (Michel clips), or disposable drapes can be sutured to the skin edges, following the initial skin incision.

6.10 How to scrub up

1. Remove any jewellery or watches.
2. Fingernails should be short and any varnish removed.
3. Stand at the sink with arms held forward away from the body and with hands higher than the elbows. This allows the water to run away from the scrubbed area and prevents possible recontamination (Figure 6.11).
4. The scrubbing procedure should take a minimum of 5 minutes, so allow at least 1 minute for each of the washing procedures.
5. Remove all organic matter from the skin by washing hands and arms (up to and including the elbows) with plain soap. Rinse, remembering to let the water flow down towards the elbows.
6. Repeat this procedure using surgical scrub solution and rinse in the same way.
7. Use a sterile brush to scrub the palm of each hand and each finger. Pay particular attention to the nail area. Either rinse the brush or discard it and use another one.
8. Repeat this procedure on the other hand. Always use the same system for this procedure to prevent missing out some areas. Rinse again.
9. Repeat the procedure in step 6. Wash hands and arms again using surgical scrub, but this time do not include the elbows, so that the hands do not touch areas that have not been scrubbed. Rinse.
10. Using a sterile hand towel, dry one hand in one quarter of the towel and one hand in another quarter. Dry the arms to the elbows on the two remaining quarters of the towel. Discard the towel.

This full routine should be used at the beginning of each surgical session. Between subsequent procedures, unless the hands have become grossly contaminated, an abbreviated 2-minute scrub, without the use of the brush, is adequate and helps to prevent trauma to the skin.

Gowning

Once the hands are dried the surgical gown can be put on (Figure 6.12). As described in Chapter 7, gowns are folded and wrapped for sterilization inside out so that the outside of the gown is not contaminated by being touched with ungloved hands. Although the surgical gown has been sterilized before use, when it is worn it is generally considered sterile on only the front, from the shoulder to the waist (including the sleeves.) This is to avoid accidental contamination of the surgical field.

Gloving

There are two main methods of gloving: open and closed. Both methods are widely used. Closed gloving is preferred – it minimizes the risk of contamination as the hands stay within the sleeves of the gown until they go straight into the glove. Only this method will be covered here (Figure 6.13). The methodology for open gloving may be found in publications listed under further reading.

The critical point to remember during gloving is to not touch the outside of the glove with an uncovered hand. During closed gloving the gloves are only handled through the sleeves of the gown and during open gloving only the inside of the gloves are touched by the scrubbed hands.

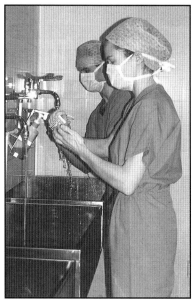

6.11 'Scrubbing-up' for surgery. The nurse is already dressed in theatre apparel (scrub suit, theatre clogs, hat and mask). The hands are kept above the elbows during scrubbing. A sterile brush has been collected from a wall dispenser (right of picture). The brush dispenser, taps and cleaning solution bottle are all elbow-operated.

6.12 How to put on a sterile gown

Gowning should be completed immediately after drying the hands. Even after the most rigorous of scrubbing procedures, hands can only be considered very clean – not sterile. The surgical gown is sterile and so to avoid possible contamination of the gown with the hands it should be handled by touching only the inside surface. Thus the gown is folded inside out, so that it can be handled without touching its outside surface.

1. Pick up the gown at the shoulders, hold it out in front of you and allow it to fall open.
2. Locate the sleeves, insert a hand into each sleeve opening, push your hands forward into the sleeves opening out your arms. Do not try to pull the gown up over your shoulders as this is a potential contamination risk.
3. An unscrubbed assistant should be available to adjust the gown as necessary, touching the inside of the gown only, and secure the gown at the back.
4. If the gown has front or side ties, these should be held out to the sides. The assistant should take the ties at the ends to avoid accidentally touching the gown and contaminating it. The ties should be secured at the back of the gown.

Like back-tying gowns, those that are tied at the side require an unscrubbed assistant:

1. The assistant makes the initial ties, touching the inside of the gown only.
2. The scrubbed person then passes one of the side ties, attached to a paper tape, to the assistant.
3. The assistant accepts the paper tape and takes it with the tie around the gown.
4. The scrubbed person can then pull the tie away, leaving the assistant holding the paper tape.
5. The scrubbed person can now tie the two ties together at the side of the gown.

How to put on sterile gloves – closed gloving method

1. Keep hands within the sleeves of the gown throughout.
2. Turn the open glove packet so that the fingers point towards the operator.
3. With the right hand, pick up the right glove (now positioned on the left of the packet) by the rim of the cuff.
4. Turn the hand over so that the fingers of the glove are now pointing down towards the elbow (see below).
5. With the left hand, pick up the other side of the rim of the cuff and pull it up and over the right hand.
6. Push the fingers of the right hand into the glove.
7. Keeping the left hand within the sleeve of the gown, the glove can be altered into a comfortable position.
8. With the left hand, pick up the left glove and repeat exactly the same process.
9. The cuffs of the gloves should entirely cover the wristlets of the gown.

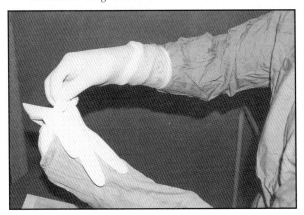

Intraoperative assistance

Nurses are often required to assist the veterinary surgeon during the surgical procedure. There are two main roles for the nurse in theatre: as a circulating nurse or as a scrubbed nurse.

Circulating nurse

A nurse present during the surgery who does not assist as a scrub nurse or a surgical assistant is described as a circulating nurse. This person should be in attendance at all times during the surgery and performs the following tasks:

- Helping in the preparation of the theatre
- Ensuring that the patient is correctly positioned on the operating table
- Assisting the surgical team with gowning
- Preparing the surgical site
- Assisting during the draping of the patient and the connection of any apparatus, such as diathermy or suction machines
- Fetching and unwrapping extra instruments or apparatus if they are needed during surgery
- Providing extra swabs or sutures and keeping account of used ones removed from the trolley
- Helping with anaesthesia if required
- Preparing and applying any dressing required at the end of surgery
- Clearing and cleaning theatre at the end of the procedure and preparing for the next procedure if appropriate.

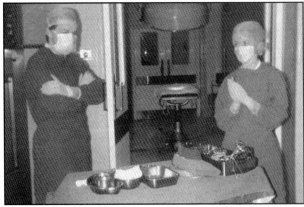

6.14   *Surgeon (left) and scrub nurse prepared for surgery. Both are gloved and gowned and the trolley is layed out for the operation.*

Scrub nurse or surgical assistant

The efficiency of the surgeon can be greatly increased with a competent surgical assistant. This is often the role of the veterinary nurse (Figure 6.14).

Duties of the scrub nurse include:

- Preparation of the instrument trolley for surgery (see Chapter 7)
  - To ensure easy use of the trolley, it should be set out in the same way each time, and instruments returned to the same place after use
  - Instrument handles should be placed towards the person in charge of the trolley
- Keeping instruments clean and orderly and wiped over when necessary
- Keeping the operating field neat and free of unnecessary instruments. Those instruments not currently being used by the surgeons should be returned to the trolley
- Anticipating the needs of the surgeon and having instruments at hand to pass as necessary
- Passing instruments, swabs, sutures and other equipment to the surgeon (Figures 6.15 and 6.16)
- Holding instruments or retracting tissues if necessary
- Removing soiled swabs from the surgical field
- Counting swabs, needles and sutures before surgery begins (the nurse should keep a close watch on the whereabouts of these items)
- Counting disposables again before the end of surgery to ensure that nothing is accidentally left in the wound.

6.15 How to handle and pass instruments

It is important for the scrub nurse to have some knowledge of the surgical procedure to be performed. This enables anticipation of the instruments that will be needed by the surgeon. Instruments should be:

- Passed to the surgeon in a positive manner: the surgeon should not have to look away from the site to take the instrument
- Passed firmly into the surgeon's hand, in a position that does not require the surgeon to reposition them before use (Figure 6.16)
- Ready for use when they are passed
- If curved, passed with the tip facing upwards
- Removed from the surgical site after use
- Cleaned with a swab if necessary and returned to the same place on the instrument trolley.

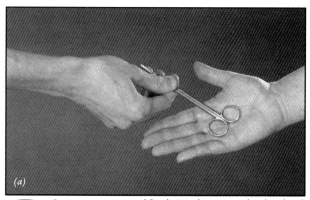

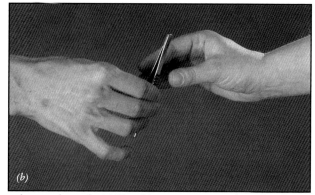

6.16 Instruments are pressed firmly into the surgeon's hand so that they may be grasped securely. (a) Ringed instruments are passed into the palm with the points outwards and curves upwards, ready for use. (b) The scalpel or dissecting forceps are passed into a finger grip, ready for use.

Intraoperative problems

There can be damaging results of surgery and anaesthesia in all cases. Some of these relate to particular procedures and these specific complications will not be considered. Others (such as respiratory and cardiac arrest) relate principally to anaesthesia, and are discussed in Chapter 8 and in the *BSAVA Manual of Advanced Veterinary Nursing*. General problems that occur include intraoperative contamination of tissues, haemorrhage and hypothermia.

Intraoperative contamination

Contamination of tissues may result from incisions into already infected tissues, spillage from incisions into the gastrointestinal, urogenital or respiratory tract or breaks in the aseptic technique (such as movement of drapes and other accidents). Such contamination is minimized by careful technique and the use of swabs or towels to isolate organs prior to incision.

If contamination occurs, irrigation of the area with isotonic fluids is recommended. If parenteral antibiotics have not been given, immediate administration is helpful in most cases with further doses of antibiotics given at the direction of the surgeon.

Haemorrhage

Blood loss is almost inevitable at the time of surgery. Careful technique combined with knowledge of anatomy will minimize the amount lost, as will control of bleeding points with instruments, ligatures, diathermy or pressure during surgery.

Catastrophic haemorrhage during surgery is not always readily controlled but in most cases even profuse arterial bleeding can be arrested by packing with swabs until definitive control can be established. After a measured 5 minutes of firm pressure, most sources of haemorrhage will be slowed enough for the surgeon to treat definitively.

Techniques for estimation of blood loss and decision making in blood replacement are covered in Chapter 8.

Hypothermia

Anaesthetized animals tend to cool because of their reduced metabolic rate and loss of homeostatic function. This can be exacerbated during surgery by exposure of viscera, with increased heat loss by convection and evaporation.

Warming of fluids used during surgery and preventing the animal becoming excessively wet will also help reduce unnecessary heat loss. Core temperature should be monitored periodically to assess the development of hypothermia and its response to corrective measures. Severe hypothermia is life threatening, in addition to prolonging recovery from anaesthesia.

Postoperative problems

Postoperative problems (complications) are often specific to certain procedures and these will not be discussed. Others relate to anaesthesia and are included elsewhere.

General postoperative problems include:

- Delayed wound healing (see Figure 6.38)
- Patient interference with the wound (Figures 6.17 and 6.18)
- Wound infection (see below)
- Prolonged recovery from anaesthesia (Figure 6.19)
- Pain
- Anorexia.

Postoperative monitoring

Post-operative care (Figure 6.20) begins when the last suture is placed, and anaesthesia is stopped. During this time the patient should not be left unattended until it is conscious.

6.17 Causes of patient interference with a wound

Cause	Prevention
Infection	Appropriate initial wound management and antibiotic therapy
Contamination or presence of a foreign body	Appropriate initial wound management
Tissue trauma during surgery	Careful surgical technique
Skin suture irritation	Place skin sutures loosely Use non-irritating suture material
Pain	Analgesia
Dermatitis (clipper rash)	Careful skin preparation with clean sharp clipper blades Avoid shaving the skin Avoid scrubbing the area with abrasive materials Treat pre-existing dermatitis prior to surgery

6.18 Prevention of patient interference

Prevention	Application
Attention to factors in Figure 6.17	All cases
Bandaging	All accessible sites (areas such as the perineum, groin and axilla are difficult to bandage without causing other difficulties)
Elizabethan collar (see Chapter 1)	All sites except the neck, distal limb and tail
Devices to prevent body flexion (stiff collars, body brace)	Wounds of the trunk and proximal limbs
Tranquillizers	Used with caution and often ineffective alone. Long-term use of questionable justification
Topical bitter substances	Sites prone to chewing rather than rubbing or scratching (e.g. not the head or perineum)

6.19 Causes of delayed recovery from anaesthesia

Cause	Prevention
Hypothermia	Take steps to prevent excessive heat loss during surgery and recovery
Anaesthetic overdose	Calculate anaesthetic dose carefully. Consider the impact of hypothermia on anaesthetic breakdown rates. Consider the impact of pre-existing disease on anaesthetic potency
Shock due to surgical complication	Avoid development of shock during anaesthesia. Treat with aggressive fluid therapy
Shock due to indication for surgery	Stabilize animal before anaesthesia whenever possible
Exacerbation of concurrent disease	Assess and treat concurrent disease prior to anaesthesia

The area where the patients recover after surgery should be kept warm: an ambient temperature of between 20 and 24°C should be adequate in most cases. Provision of a warmer area (for example, an incubator) is necessary for recovery of small patients in some instances.

In the recovery area there should be adequate space for any necessary equipment, and easy access to facilities and equipment such as suction and anaesthetic machines.

6.20 Points for consideration during the postoperative period

- The patient should be continuously observed until the swallowing reflex has returned and the endotracheal tube can be removed

- The animal is usually placed in lateral recumbency, with the head towards the front of the cage and the neck gently extended. The tongue is pulled forward from the mouth until the patient is swallowing freely

- Brachycephalic dogs require special care and are usually kept under constant observation until they are able to lift their heads. Prior to this, they are kept in sternal recumbency. These dogs often tolerate the endotracheal tube for longer periods than other breeds, particularly if local anaesthetic has been applied to the larynx and pharynx, and the tube should be retained for as long as possible

- The airway should be kept clear of any secretions. Suction equipment should be within easy access if required

- Temperature, pulse and respiration, mucous membrane colour and capillary refill time should be checked regularly. These are taken immediately the animal returns to the recovery area and then every 5 minutes. Following removal of the tube, every 10 or 15 minutes is suitable in most instances, but animals that recover more slowly require extra vigilance

- These parameters should be recorded to note any trends or changes that occur

- The patient's temperature should be maintained using blankets, heat pads or heat lamps. Overheating is a less common problem, but may be seen in giant breeds and in dogs with airway obstruction. Provision for cooling the environment, such as a fan, should be available

- To prevent hypostatic congestion of the lungs, the position of the patient should be changed periodically if longer recovery times are anticipated. Specifically, medium-sized and larger dogs should be turned over at least hourly

- Fluid therapy may need to be maintained. Fluids should be warmed before administration. The catheter must be checked for signs of blockage or extravasation of fluids

- The patient should be closely observed for signs of pain or discomfort. These include:
  - increased respiratory or heart rate
  - reluctance to move
  - chewing or biting at the surgical site.

  These signs should be reported to the veterinary surgeon so that further analgesia can be provided

- Urinary output may need to be observed for patients in longer periods of postoperative recovery. If necessary, a urethral catheter is placed, connected to a closed collection system. An output of 2 ml/kg body weight/hour indicates adequate kidney perfusion.

Shock as a complication of recovery

Shock can occur during recovery as a complication of surgery or be due to a pre-existing condition. The most common cause of postoperative shock is hypovolaemia. Other causes may be respiratory or cardiac insufficiency.

The signs of shock are:

- Tachycardia (rapid heart rate)
- Weak rapid pulse
- Shallow rapid respiration
- Pale or cyanotic mucous membranes
- Cold extremities
- Slow capillary refill time
- Delayed recovery from anaesthesia.

Haemorrhage from the wound can be an indication that hypovolaemia is developing but can be misleading: internal haemorrhage may not be evident at the incision and trivial wound haemorrhage is common. Internal haemorrhage after abdominal surgery may manifest as abdominal distension or abdominal pain. The production of large volumes of sanguinous wound fluid from drains also suggests that haemorrhage is occurring: measuring the volume and PCV of this fluid can be a useful guide to the severity of haemorrhage.

Types of surgical diseases and principles of treatment

This section is a general discussion of disease processes of surgical importance. It is followed by a section dealing with common surgical conditions for specific organ systems.

Inflammation

Inflammation is the way in which tissues react to injury, which may be chemical, thermal, infectious, or physical. The signs and processes of inflammation are covered in other texts (see Further reading).

Several types of inflammation can be distinguished (Figure 6.21). Inflammation is commonly classified as acute or chronic, reflecting the time course of the process and also the events occurring (Figure 6.22). Acute inflammation in particular is a dynamic process and several outcomes are possible, depending on the severity and type of the initial injury, the individual animal and the tissue affected (Figure 6.23).

The inflammatory process is in general beneficial to the individual, and results in an attempt to overcome the effects of the initial injury. For example, the inflammatory fluid contains cells of the immune system which help

6.21 Types of inflammation

Type	Characteristics	Examples
Catarrhal	Restricted to mucous membranes, where it is characterized by formation of excess mucous	Acute conjunctivitis
Purulent (suppurative)	Accumulation of fluid containing large numbers of neutrophils (pus)	Cat bite abscess
Serous	Fluid is watery in nature, consisting principally of serum leaking from local capillaries	Peritonitis
Haemorrhagic	Fluid contains large numbers of red blood cells	Cellulitis

6.22 Comparison of acute and chronic inflammation

Acute	Chronic
Short duration	Lasts more than a few days, sometimes months
Cardinal signs are all apparent	Cardinal signs usually less obvious
Nature of pathology changes rapidly (Figure 6.23)	Slow progression
Commonly systemic signs present	Usually signs are local in occurrence
Neutrophils are predominant cell type	Lymphocytes, monocytes and fibroblasts dominate

6.23 Outcome of acute inflammation

Outcome	Description
Resolution	Tissue returns to normal: long-term change
Repair of function	Tissue injury has occurred but healing and regeneration processes of tissue allow recovery
Degeneration	Tissue injury has occurred and affected cells do not repair
Necrosis	Cells within affected tissue die
Abscessation	Accumulation of polymorphonuclear white blood cells (PMNs) in a cavity within the tissue
Ulceration	Loss of surface epithelium
Sinus formation	Chronic inflammation of deeper tissues with discharging tract leading to skin surface
Fistulation	Loss of tissue between two epithelial surfaces, causing connection between them
Chronic inflammation	Inflammation is not resolved but degree reduces and types of cell responding change

overcome infection. However, the inflammatory processes can result in further tissue damage and unnecessary pain and so inflammation is often treated to overcome these adverse effects.

Ideally treatment should remove the inciting cause: for example, antibiotic therapy to eliminate infection or removal of a foreign body. Treatment to reduce the degree of inflammation is also used: for example, the veterinary surgeon may use drugs such non-steroidal anti-inflammatory drugs (NSAIDs) or corticosteroids which block some of the chemical pathways of inflammation. Another way in which acute inflammation can be reduced is the use of cold dressings applied soon after an injury has occurred.

Orthopaedic injuries

Fractures

Definition:
Fracture is disruption in the continuity of a bone.

Most fractures occur following trauma – for example, falls or road traffic accidents. Occasionally bones may fracture following trivial injuries, or even spontaneously. In the latter cases, this is usually because the bone strength is altered by an existing disease, such as a tumour. These are known as pathological fractures.

Fractures are classified in a number of ways (Figures 6.24 and 6.25). They can be treated in several ways, depending on the bone affected, the severity of the disruption, the age of the animal and its size (Figures 6.26–6.28). Bandaging techniques are described in Chapter 1.

Casts

Casts are still a common form of fracture repair in small animals; Chapter 1 describes how to apply, manage and remove a cast and gives details of the various casting materials that are available. Plaster of Paris is most commonly used and is the easiest to apply. The synthetics have the important advantage of higher strength-to-weight ratios but they conform less well to angular areas (e.g. the hock).

The cast is removed once the fracture is stabilized (clinical union). The healing period is variable and depends on the

6.24 Classification of fractures

Type	Description
Closed	Overlying skin is intact During first aid and initial management, care should be taken to prevent the fracture fragments pushing through the skin surface, resulting in an open fracture
Open (previously known as compound fractures)	Associated with a break in the nearby skin surface Infection of the fracture site is more likely and early treatment is important to a successful outcome
Simple	Containing a single fracture line and therefore only two fragments Simple fractures of a long bone may be transverse (break is across the shaft), spiral (break tends to run along the shaft) or oblique (break is in between these positions)
Incomplete (also known as greenstick fractures)	Does not completely disrupt the continuity of a long bone, i.e. one cortex is intact Usually seen in young animals
Comminuted	Containing more than one fracture line and several fragments
Avulsion	Resulting in the separation of the point of attachment of a muscle or tendon to a bone from the main part of the bone The pull of muscle tends to displace the fragment from its original site
Condylar	Fracture involving the condyles of a long bone (such as the distal femur or humerus) Needs accurate reduction and fixation to prevent interference with joint function

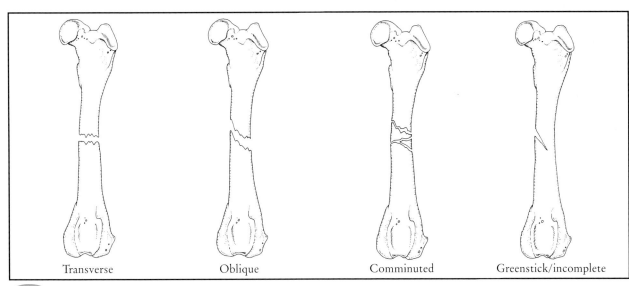

Transverse   Oblique   Comminuted   Greenstick/incomplete

6.25 *Classification of fractures.*

Methods of fracture treatment

Method	Application	Advantages	Disadvantages
First aid methods[a]			
Cage confinement	Recommended for fractures of the spine and of the limbs when the leg is fractured above the stifle or elbow	Effective in many cases	Less suitable for distal limb fractures
Splint	Fractures of the limbs below the stifle or elbow	Materials readily available	May be difficult in conscious patient
Robert Jones bandage	Fractures of the limbs below the stifle or elbow	Materials readily available available	If poorly applied, bulkiness of dressing may exacerbate injury
Definitive methods			
External coaption (splints, extension splints and casts) (Figure 6.27)	Suitable for fractures of the limbs below the elbow or stifle	Cheap to apply Technically simple	Limited application, poor healing of unstable fractures (comminuted, spiral) May result in pressure sores Immobilization of limb can cause fracture disease (joint stiffness, muscle wasting)
Internal fixation (IF)	Placement of metal implants to hold fragments rigidly in apposition during healing	Applicable to a wide variety of fractures Potentially allows rapid return to function Avoids fracture disease	Relatively expensive in terms of materials and instrumentation Time consuming Requires greater technical skill
Intramedullary pin (Steinmann pin)	Long straight pin placed within the medullary cavity across the fracture line to fix the fragments in alignment Placed at surgery (open pinning) or percutaneously (closed pinning) using a Jacob's chuck	Wide application for long bone fractures in cats and smaller dogs Little specialist equipment required Implant relatively inexpensive	Not suitable for fractures prone to collapse in length or rotation Less suitable for big dogs than other internal fixations
Rush pins	Less commonly used method of IF Used in pairs to stabilize supracondylar fractures		Limited application
Kirschner and arthrodesis wires	Similar to Steinmann pins and may be used in a similar way in small bones Used with other techniques to fix small bone fragments		Rarely suitable as sole method of fixation
Cerclage wires	Flexible surgical steel wire used to supplement other forms of IF Supplied in reels and cut to length as required Typically used to repair avulsion fractures, osteotomies and long bones		Rarely suitable as sole method of fixation
Bone plates and screws (Venables, Sherman, dynamic compression plates)	Plates are attached to bone across fracture sites and held in place with screws	Wide range of application Allow early limb use and avoid fracture disease	Relatively expensive and technically demanding method of fracture repair
External fixation (Kirschner–Ehmer apparatus or Ilazirov fixator)	Pins are placed through the skin into fracture fragments and the pins are linked together externally by a frame or bolts and rods	Suitable for complicated fractures, open fractures and for repair of limb deformities when other techniques are unsuitable	Relatively expensive and technically demanding method of fracture repair

[a] See also Chapter 9 in BSAVA Manual of Veterinary Care.

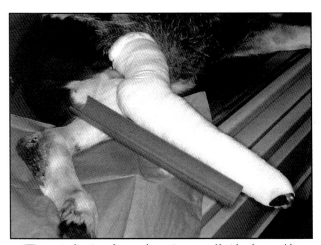

6.27 *Application of external coaption to a calf with a fractured lower limb. Incorporation of a gutter splint into a modified Robert Jones bandage is an effective and economical treatment.*

nature of the fracture, its site and the age of the animal. Radiographs may be used as a guide to the progress of healing.

Details of complex fracture repair will be found in *BSAVA Manual of Advanced Veterinary Nursing*.

Luxations

Definitions:

Luxation is displacement of joint surfaces from their normal articulation (synonym: dislocation).

Subluxation is incomplete luxation (i.e. some of the articular surface remains in contact).

Some luxations arise from congenital malformations of the joint structures. For example, small breeds of dog often have poorly developed articulations of the femur and patella, resulting in patellar luxation. Congenital luxations are treated by surgical procedures that aim to reproduce the joint architecture of the normal animal.

Other luxations arise as a result of trauma, causing separation of the joint surfaces, often with damage to the supporting structures of the joint (joint capsule and ligaments) and even fractures of the bones forming the joints. Traumatic luxations are treated by reduction of the joint surfaces (restoring to a normal position) and repair of the supporting structures if necessary. Often the joint is supported in a normal alignment after reduction by placement of a splint, bandage or cast (see Chapter 1).

Soft tissue injuries

Hernias and ruptures

Definitions:
Hernias and *ruptures* are defects in the body wall through which organs can protrude (prolapse).

Hernias are enlargements of existing anatomical holes.

Ruptures are tears that appear where there were previously sheets of tissue.

Reducible hernias are those where the protruding tissues can be returned to a normal position by pressure, without enlarging the hole.

Irreducible hernias are those where they cannot.

Incarceration is the reduction of blood supply to the contents of irreducible hernias so that the tissue is at risk of necrosis.

Hernia ring is the borders of the tissue in which a hernia is present.

Common sites of hernias in cats and dogs are:

- Umbilical – abdominal fat or organs protrude through the umbilical canal of the ventral abdominal wall
- Hiatal – abdominal organs (usually the stomach) protrude through the oesophageal hiatus of the diaphragm
- Inguinal – abdominal organs (such as the bladder) protrude through the inguinal canal of the groin.

Common types of rupture are:

- Diaphragm – tear in the diaphragm (Figure 6.29), usually as the result of trauma, allows abdominal organs (such as the liver) to enter the thorax
- Perineum – degeneration of the muscles of the pelvic floor allows pelvic structures (such as the rectum) to enter a subcutaneous position next to the anus
- Incisional – breakdown of a surgical repair of the abdominal wall allowing abdominal tissues to protrude into a subcutaneous position.

Ruptures and hernias are treated to prevent organ prolapse and incarceration. They are usually treated surgically by:

- Reduction of the herniated tissues (replacement into their normal position)

Factors in selection of a method of fracture treatment

Factor	Effect on bone healing	Suitable methods
Animal age	Delayed in older animals	Internal fixation preferred in older animals
Body size	Greater body weight destabilizes fracture sites	Internal fixation preferred in large dogs
Athleticism	Greater stress at fracture site	Internal fixation preferred
Bone affected	Distal limb fractures can be stabilized by external coaption	Internal fixation is preferred for proximal fractures
Severity of disruption	Presence of multiple fragments reduces stability and delays healing Presence of multiple fragments complicates placement of internal fixation	External fixator may reduce need for complete reconstruction
Stability of reconstructed fragments	Instability of fragments reduces stability, delays healing and can result in deformity	Unstable fractures require internal fixation or an external fixator

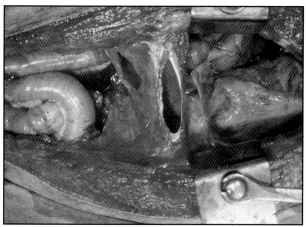

6.29 *Intraoperative photograph of a dog with a ruptured diaphragm. Part of the intestinal tract has entered the thoracic cavity (right) through a tear in the diaphragm.*

- Closure of the hernia ring (the ring can usually be closed by placing sutures across it)
- Occasionally, patching the hole instead with an implant of synthetic material such as plastic or steel mesh.

Abscesses

Definition:
An *abscess* is a discrete collection of purulent material (pus). It is often surrounded by a wall of inflamed and fibrous tissue, sometimes known as a *pyogenic membrane*.

Superficial abscesses usually develop after introduction of bacteria into tissue by sharp trauma, such as animal bites or infected surgical procedures.

Clinical signs of an abscess

- Local swelling (due to the presence of a pocket of pus and local oedema)
- Local pain
- Warmth and erythema of the overlying skin
- Systemic signs of toxaemia (e.g. pyrexia, depression, anorexia, tachycardia)
- Discharge of purulent fluid from the area if the overlying skin bursts (described as 'pointing').

Details of abscess management are in *BSAVA Manual of Advanced Veterinary Nursing*.

Ulcers

Definition:
An *ulcer* is a full thickness loss of epithelium at a tissue surface (skin or mucous membranes of other organs).
Decubitus ulcers occur over bony prominences as a result of skin trauma, reduced local circulation, local infection and poor tissue healing. They readily develop in animals that are recumbent and systemically ill.

Loss of epithelium can result from a number of processes, including:

- Trauma
- Local infection
- Neoplasia
- Drug therapy – notably the NSAID class of analgesics, which can cause ulceration of the gastrointestinal tract

- Foreign bodies – for example, corneal ulceration as a result of ocular foreign bodies.

Once ulceration has developed, further damage to underlying tissues is possible (for example, perforation of the stomach) and local infection is common.
Ulcers are treated by:

- Removing the underlying cause
- Local therapy to improve tissue healing (including wound dressing, see below)
- Surgical excision and closure of adjacent normal tissue if necessary.

Fistulae

Definition:
A *fistula* is a connection between two surfaces lined with mucous membrane.

Fistulae commonly develop after trauma to tissues. Once established, they require surgical repair. One example is the oronasal fistula (Figure 6.30 and below).
Occasionally congenital fistulae are encountered: for example, a connection between the vagina and rectum in bitches (rectovaginal fistula). Congenital clefts of the palate may be considered as oronasal fistulae.

Discharging sinus

Definition:
A *discharging sinus* is an opening in the skin lined by granulation tissue.

Discharging sinuses commonly arise as a result of chronic infection of deeper tissues, often due to the presence of a foreign body. The commonest example is anal furunculosis (see later).

Tumours

Definition:
Tumour is a non-specific term usually referring to uncontrolled growth of cells without physiological cause. This usually results in swellings which are more correctly termed *neoplasms*.

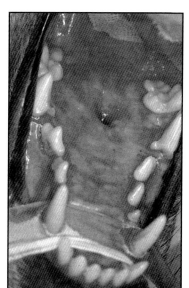

6.30 *Oronasal fistula in the hard palate of a dog following a dog bite. The dog also has marked stomatitis.*

Neoplasms can affect any tissue of the body and can be benign or malignant ('cancerous').

Benign neoplasms:

- Tend not to invade surrounding tissues
- Are often slow growing
- May be cured by surgical excision.

Malignant neoplasms:

- Invade surrounding tissues and/or spread (metastasize) via the lymphatics or blood to other tissues
- Often enlarge in size more rapidly than benign tumours
- Are more difficult to cure surgically or by other methods.

Tumours are named according to the tissue of origin and their tendency to malignancy:

- *-oma* refers to a benign tumour
- *-carcinoma* refers to a malignant tumour arising from glandular tissue
- *-sarcoma* refers to a malignant tumour arising from solid tissue.

Specific tumours will be mentioned in the sections on organ systems below.

Signs of neoplasia may be:

- Local:
  - signs caused by the presence of the tumour mass (such as obstruction of viscera, ulceration, impediment of movement)
- Systemic:
  - release of hormonally active substances, such as pseudoparathyroid hormone – this results in hypercalcaemia, a frequent finding in dogs with lymphoma

- cachexia – muscle wasting due to increased catabolism and often accompanied by anorexia
- histamine release – a feature of canine mast cell tumours (mastocytoma), resulting in anaphylaxis and gastric ulceration.

Determining the prognosis for tumours

Definition:
The *prognosis* for a disease is a statement of the way in which it is likely to progress and the way in which it may respond to treatment.

The prognosis for tumours of different types varies tremendously. It is important to determine the tumour type so that the correct treatment can be chosen and so that the owner can be informed of the likely outcome.

Information used in assessing prognosis in neoplasia includes:

- History – some tumours (rarely) affect typical breeds and ages of animal
- Appearance – some tumours (rarely) have a typical appearance
- Presence of attachment to deeper tissues – malignant tumours more frequently adhere to surrounding tissues
- Presence of ulceration – malignant superficial tumours often ulcerate
- Radiography or ultrasonography – to look for evidence of metastasis to other sites (such as the lungs)
- Biopsy – to determine the type of tumour and the prognosis.

A *biopsy* is removal of a piece of tissue from an animal for laboratory examination. This is usually the most reliable way in which a prognosis can be made (Figure 6.31).

Treatment of tumours is outlined in Figure 6.32.

6.31 Types of biopsy

Type	Application	Advantages/disadvantages
Fine needle aspirate biopsy (FNAB)	Any swelling, also bone marrow and solid organs (liver, etc.)	Quick and easy, rarely requires anaesthesia and no special apparatus Cytological processing also rapid Limited information on tissue type and prognosis in most cases
Needle core biopsy (Trucut, Jamshidi)	Any swelling or organ which can be reached at surgery or percutaneously	Relatively fast Often percutaneous biopsies can be taken without general anaesthesia Gives more tissue information than above but still limited by small sample size Requires specialized needle
Incisional (wedge) biopsy	Skin masses or organs/masses that can be reached surgically	Usually requires general anaesthesia No special instruments required A surgical procedure Greater tissue mass acquired increases information, particularly on invasiveness
Trephine	Bone lesions	Necessary to obtain good samples from calcified tissue
Excisional biopsy	Any mass that can be excised completely Reserved for cases when surgical excision requires no special planning or cure by excision is thought likely	Usually requires general anaesthesia No special instruments required A surgical procedure Greater tissue mass acquired increases information, particularly on invasiveness Possibly curative

6.32 Principles of treatment of neoplasms

Type of treatment	Application	Specific examples of use
Surgical excision (the extensiveness of surgery should be tailored to the tumour type)	Widely available Commonest form of treatment Limited use for locally invasive and metastatic tumours	Mammary tumours Solitary lung tumours
Chemotherapy	Less widely used Commonest use is for tumours of the white blood cells Occasionally used to prolong the survival of animals with malignant tumours, particularly after excision	Lymphosarcoma Mast cell tumour
Radiation therapy	Very restricted availability	Intranasal tumours

Wounds (including surgical incisions)

Definition:

A *wound* is any injury to a body tissue, although it usually refers to injuries to the skin and deeper layers caused by external trauma (including surgery).

Common causes of wounds are cuts (including surgical incisions), crushing and abrasions. Often these occur together: for example, during an animal bite the skin may be cut and the underlying tissues subjected to crushing.

Wound classification is given in Figures 6.33–6.34.

Wound healing

Following injury, biological processes to heal the damaged tissue begin (Figure 6.37). Details of these processes can be found in the further reading section.

Factors affecting wound healing

Wound healing occurs most rapidly in animals in a good general state of health, receiving adequate nutrition and in the absence of infection. Beyond ensuring that these factors are present, little can be done to accelerate the process. However, a number of factors decrease the rate of wound healing (Figure 6.38).

6.33 Classification of wounds

Type	Description	Common examples
Puncture (Figure 6.35)	Small skin penetration Often larger area of affected deeper tissue	Animal bite Stick injury
Avulsion	Flap of skin partially separated from surrounding area	Road traffic injury
Incised	Sharply incised skin edges Little trauma to surrounding tissues	Surgical incision Glass cut
Lacerated (Figure 6.36)	Torn skin edges Often concurrent contamination and trauma to underlying tissues	Road traffic injury Barbed-wire
Abrasion	Surface layers worn off Often contamination of underlying tissues	Road traffic injury
Shear	Extreme example of abrasion with deeper layers (muscle, ligaments, bone) also eroded	Road traffic injury to distal limb

6.34 Wound classification by degree of contamination

Type	Definition	Example
Clean	Created under aseptic conditions Not involving the urogenital, gastrointestinal or respiratory tracts	Simple surgical skin incision
Clean–contaminated	Created under aseptic conditions Entering one of the organs above, without gross spillage	Enterotomy
Contaminated	Wounds with contamination but not active infection	Fresh traumatic wounds Surgical wounds with break in aseptic technique or involving inflamed tissue
Dirty	Wounds with active infection already present	Traumatic wounds of more than 6 hours duration Surgical incisions encountering pus

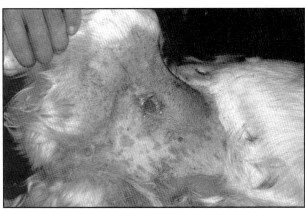

6.35 *Puncture wound in the groin of a bitch, probably caused by a stick penetration.*

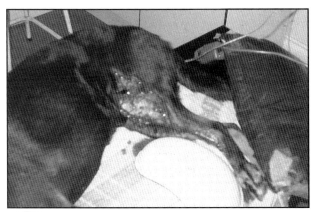

6.36 *Lacerated wound on a hindlimb, due to barbed-wire.*

6.37 Phases of wound healing

- *Inflammatory stage* – begins within a few minutes with the activation of inflammatory mediators
- *Repair stage* – removal of damaged tissue and debris
- *Fibroblastic phase* – deposition of collagen and new blood vessels (granulation tissue)
- *Epithelialization phase* – regeneration of epithelium over the wound surface
- *Contraction phase* – reduction of wound area by inward movement of surrounding skin
- *Remodelling phase* – replacement of initial repair tissue with more normal collagen.

6.38 Factors causing delayed wound healing

Local factors	Systemic factors
Infection	Cachexia (state of generalized tissue breakdown)
Excessive moisture	
Inappropriate topical therapy	Uraemia
Patient interference	Starvation/malnutrition
Presence of foreign material	Cytotoxic drugs
Tissue dehydration	Hormonal imbalance (hyperadrenocorticism, hypothyroidism)
Tissue movement	Corticosteroid therapy
Poor operative technique	Prolonged hospitalization

Open wound management

When wounds are not closed primarily (see Figure 6.40) they are managed as open wounds. The aims of this period of management are to:

- Reduce tissue contamination
- Remove devitalized tissue
- Promote the formation of granulation tissue
- Encourage wound contraction
- Encourage epithelialization.

These aims are met in several ways.

Debridement

Debridement is the removal of devitalized and necrotic tissue. This is usually done by sharp excision, but some dressings (such as wet to dry gauze dressing) and some topical treatments help in sloughing unhealthy tissue from the wound. Debridement is repeated as necessary during wound management. Repeated debridement is particularly useful when the presence of vital structures or a deficiency of tissue precludes initial aggressive debridement.

Lavage

Lavage is the flushing of the wound to remove foreign material, wound exudate and contamination. Gentle pressure is used, such as that from squirting fluid through a 20 G needle from a syringe. Commercial systems such as aerosols of sterile saline or water pumps are available, but excessive pressure must be avoided. The lavage solution must be non-toxic to tissues. Sterile saline or Hartmann's solution are both useful. Antiseptic solutions (chlorhexidine or povidone–iodine) offer little advantage, but if used must be isotonic and at low concentrations since they tend to be tissue toxic. Commercial preparations can also be used and are intended to promote the separation of necrotic and healthy tissue.

Wound dressing

Covering the wound prevents further tissue contamination and can promote tissue repair. Dressings and bandages are discussed in detail in Chapter 1.

The first layer of dressing (contact layer) is usually non-adherent, to reduce damage to the healing wound when it is changed, but sometimes gauze dressings are used that are soaked in saline initially and then removed after 12–24 hours. These 'wet-to-dry' dressings help to debride the wound in the early stages of management. The contact layer may be semi-occlusive, which tends to keep the surface moist and promote epithelialization, or non-occlusive, which is more useful when there is a heavy wound exudate. The type of contact layer chosen will vary as wound healing progresses (Figure 6.39).

The next layer is the absorbent layer, which soaks up the wound exudate. Finally a tertiary layer is used to protect the dressing and hold it in place.

The frequency of dressing change will be dictated by the degree of exudation: the dressing must not be allowed to become soaked with exudate. Initially this may require changes daily or more often. Once granulation is progressing, changes every few days may be appropriate. At each dressing change, the wound is inspected and lavaged or debrided as necessary. Wound dressing should be considered an aseptic procedure.

Surgical conditions and surgical nursing | **143**

Type	Description	Example	Application
Dry-to-wet dressings	Soak up wound exudate and adhere to necrotic tissues	Sterile surgical gauze	Open wounds with contamination and necrotic tissue and watery exudate
Wet-to-dry dressings	Soak up wound exudate and adhere to necrotic tissues	Sterile surgical gauze soaked in sterile saline	Open wounds with contamination and necrotic tissue and viscous exudate
Non-adherent semi-occlusive (pad type)	Retain some moisture within wound to promote epithelialization but allow exudate to pass through in addition	• Perforated plastic with absorbent backing • Petroleum impregnated gauze	Closed wounds Wounds undergoing healing
Non-adherent semi-occlusive (sponge type)	Sponge absorbs exudate whilst absorbing excess fluid Keeps wound hydrated	Commercially available	Contaminated wounds Healing wounds
Hydrocolloid	Occlusive non-adherent dressing of hydrocolloid with plastic backing	Commercially available	Healing wound undergoing epithelialization and contraction
Hydrogel	Thin layer of gel supported on plastic sheet Also available as gel for direct application and coverage by a semi-occlusive dressing	Commercially available	Healing wound undergoing epithelialization and contraction
Calcium alginate dressing	Felt-like pad of fibre derived from seaweed	Commercially available	Exudative wounds

Topical treatments

Substances can be applied to the wound surface to promote healing. They include antiseptics, antibiotics and debriding creams. In all cases, they are potentially tissue toxic and must be used with care. Once granulation is established, the wound is resistant to infection, and antibacterial treatment is often of little benefit.

Wound closure

Wounds can be closed at four times during treatment (Figures 6.40 and 6.41). The choice is made considering the degree of tissue contamination and devitalization and the area affected. Small wounds can be managed economically by second intention healing but in most cases wound closure makes the treatment course shorter and more economic.

Wound closure is undertaken once tissue contamination has been reduced or eliminated. Clean and clean–contaminated wounds should be closed as soon as possible to avoid further contamination or devitalization. Wounds with greater degrees of contamination or infection require treatment as open wounds before closure, or alternatively can be excised as a whole and the fresh larger incision created treated as a clean wound. This is only practical where further tissue loss is possible without interfering with closure.

The objectives at the time of wound closure are:

- Removal of devitalized tissue and contamination (by lavage and debridement)
- Removal of granulation tissue and areas of re-epithelialization (wounds closed after a delay of a few days or more)
- Elimination of dead space, defined as a pocket within tissue in which fluids (serum, blood or pus) may accumulate.

6.40 **Wound closure**

Time of closure	Application	Definition
Primary closure	Clean or cleaned wounds No skin tension	Immediate closure of skin edges (usually with sutures)
Delayed primary closure	Contaminated wounds Unknown tissue viability Skin tension present	Wound debrided and lavaged Closed after 2–5 days treatment
Secondary closure	Contaminated or dirty wounds	Closure delayed until 5 days or more after injury Granulation tissue and skin edges excised at time of closure
Second intention healing	Large skin defects with extensive tissue devitalization Used when closure is not possible	Healing by granulation, contraction and epithelialization

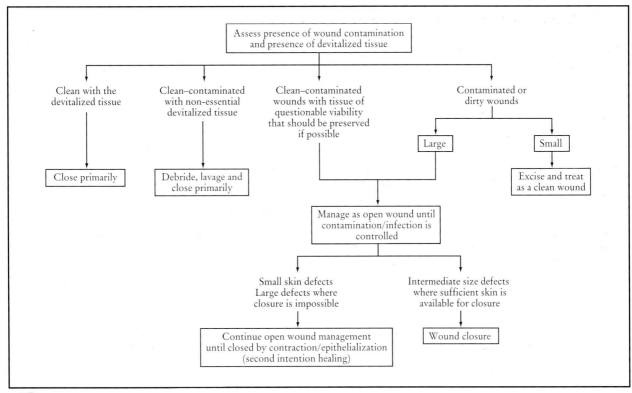

6.41 *Wound closure.*

- potentially present in all large wounds and those where there has been loss of subcutaneous tissue or extensive dissection has been undertaken
- potentiates the development of infection
- eliminated by apposition of deeper tissues by suturing, placement of drains within the wound to allow the evacuation of fluid as it accumulates, and application of pressure dressings following wound closure
- Apposition of skin edges – skin wounds heal most rapidly when the edges are closely aligned, without a step in height across the wound (Figure 6.42).

Following skin closure, wounds are often left uncovered but a dressing is applied in the following circumstances:

- Presence of exudation (indicates presence of contamination, infection or necrotic tissue and may require further treatment)

- Patient interference (often indicates presence of contamination or infection, dermatitis or tissue trauma during closure)
- Wounds on exposed areas (wounds on limbs may be covered to prevent external damage during healing)
- Pressure bandage (wounds under pressure bandages are usually covered with a non-adherent dressing; pressure bandages are often used on the limbs to prevent postoperative swelling, restrict movement or control postoperative haemorrhage).

If patient interference with a wound occurs, these possible causes and the prophylactic measures in Figure 6.43 should be considered.

6.42 Methods of skin apposition

Method	Comments
Suturing	Commonest method Widely applicable
Skin staples	Faster closure of very large wounds but more expensive than suturing
Adhesive strips	Commonly used for this purpose in people but not successful in animals due to poor adhesion
Surgical adhesives (cyanoacrylate glues)	Occasionally used, particularly for small wounds, but must be applied carefully to avoid interfering with healing

6.43 Prevention of patience interference

Cause	Prevention
Infection	Appropriate initial wound management and antibiotic therapy
Contamination or presence of foreign body	Appropriate initial wound management
Tissue trauma during surgery	Careful surgical technique
Skin suture irritation	Place skin sutures loosely Use non-irritating suture material
Pain	Analgesia
Dermatitis (clipper rash)	Careful skin preparation with clean sharp clipper blades Avoid shaving the skin Avoid scrubbing the area with abrasive materials Treat pre-existing dermatitis prior to surgery

Surgical drains

Definition:
Surgical drains are implanted devices to remove fluids or gases from a surgical site, body cavity or wound.

Drains in common use are plastic or rubber tubes or sheets. Gauze is also occasionally used as a seton drain, but there is undesirable tissue reaction to this material.

Drains can be considered in two groups (Figure 6.44):

- *Passive drains* – where exudate passes along or through the drain by gravity and capillary action (Figure 6.45)
- *Active drains* – where a source of negative pressure is used to pull fluid (or air) out through the lumen of a tube (Figure 6.46).

Applications

- Surgical wound with large dead spaces – Penrose or active wound drain usually chosen
- Localized peritonitis (e.g. associated with pancreatitis) – Penrose usually chosen
- Contaminated or infected wounds that have been closed
- Abscesses
- Thoracic surgery or trauma – thoracic drain used.

Care of drains

- Cover with a sterile dressing if possible, to prevent ascending infection. Dressing should be changed as necessary to prevent 'strikethrough' of wound fluid to the outer dressing layer

6.44 Types of surgical drain

Type	Description	Advantages	Disadvantages
Passive	Tube drains by gravity and capillary action	Simply managed	Effectiveness limited by action of gravity Open to ascending infection
Penrose (Figure 6.45)	Flat tube of soft rubber	Cheap Low tissue irritation	May become folded or displaced, limiting effectiveness
Corrugated	Length of stiff ridged plastic	Resistant to folding	Greater tissue irritation
Sump drain	Double lumen tube drain Commonly made by modifying a Foley catheter	Greater efficiency due to ingress of air	Stiffer than Penrose: greater tissue reaction because of this
Active	Tube connnected to source of vacuum	Wide variety of applications Less open to ascending infection	Greater cost and more nursing time required
Thoracic (chest) drain	Tube placed intercostally Drained intermittently with syringe or drained continuously by connecting to water tap or Heimlich valve	Suitable for draining pleural effusions or pneumothorax (see *BSAVA Manual of Advanced Veterinary Nursing* for more details)	Greater cost and more nursing time required
Active wound drain (Figure 6.46)	Tube placed within wound and attached to collapsible plastic reservoir	Action not limited by gravity	Greater cost than passive drain

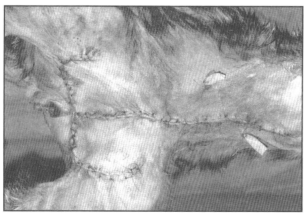

6.45 *Two Penrose drains have been placed after extensive reconstructive surgery using the skin of the ventral abdomen of this cat.*

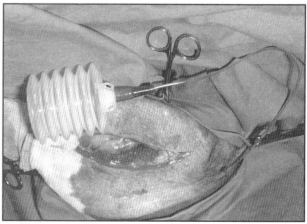

6.46 *A suction drain is placed after removal of a large tumour from the hindlimb of this cat.*

- Prevent the patient from interfering with the drain
- Empty the reservoir of active drains as necessary, in an aseptic fashion
- Keep in place as long as necessary, i.e. until drainage has practically ceased (the drain itself will provoke some exudate formation)
- Typically drains are maintained for 3–5 days, but this is highly variable depending on the circumstances
- Drains should not be used for longer than necessary because of the risk of ascending infection and the requirement for increased patient care (often animals are hospitalized whilst drains are in place).

Removal of skin sutures

Skin sutures are removed once the strength of the wound is sufficient to prevent it reopening in normal activity.

- Typically the sutures are removed after 10 days if wound healing has progressed normally, but they may be removed earlier (7 days)
- Delayed wound healing requires sutures to be left in place longer, but rarely beyond 14 days
- Sutures left in place too long tend to produce more scarring and irritation to the patient
- Sutures are usually removed in the conscious animal but sedation or anaesthesia is used in some cases – very nervous or aggressive animals, perineal surgery (especially urethrostomy, when it is important that all sutures are removed), ear surgery (because the area is very sensitive), eye surgery
- Sutures are removed with suture scissors or with a stitch-cutting blade. In both cases, one end is held up so that the blade can be passed under the knot and one piece of the suture is cut so that as little material as possible is pulled through the skin as it is removed
- Ensure that all sutures are removed. This may necessitate bathing off any scabs or exudate that are present and may obscure the sutures
- Skin staples are removed with staple removers (supplied with the stapler). In other ways, the same considerations as those for skin sutures apply
- Wounds closed with surgical adhesive do not require suture removal – the glue is sloughed once healing is complete

- Wounds closed with a subcuticular (buried) suture pattern do not usually require suture removal, since an absorbable (dissolving) suture material is commonly used
- Even when techniques are used that do not require suture removal, the wound is inspected at around 10 days to ensure healing is progressing normally.

Complications of wound healing

Wound healing complications (Figure 6.47) are caused by the same factors as those resulting in poor wound healing (above). Management of wound complications (Chapter 1) will be directed by the veterinary surgeon.

Wound dehiscence requires immediate first aid attention in some cases, particularly if there is concern about exposure of vital structures (this is always the case with laparotomy incisions):

- Cover with a clean, preferably sterile and non-adherent dressing
- Prevent the patient from interfering with the incision
- If evisceration occurs, there is a real risk of the animal damaging the prolapsed tissues. They should be wrapped in clean or sterile sheet and the animal treated as an emergency. The patient will usually be shocked and require aggressive treatment.

Common surgical conditions

The respiratory system

The upper respiratory tract comprises the nostrils, nasal chambers, nasal sinuses, pharynx and larynx. Figures 6.48–6.51 list common surgical conditions of these organs.

The following points concerning patient care should be considered:

- Immature patients with congenital defects require nursing until they are old enough for surgery. The tissues do not heal readily after surgery until the animal is 12 weeks old and so surgery is delayed until that time. Affected animals have difficulty feeding naturally and require tube feeding, by nasogastric or orogastric intubation. Episodes of rhinitis may need antibiotic treatment

6.47 Complications of wound healing

Complication	Definition	Predisposing factors	Consequences
Dehiscence	Opening of the wound along all or part of its length	Same factors associated with poor wound healing Poor operative technique Incorrect suture selection	Further wound contamination Exposure and damage to deeper structures (potentially catastrophic if all layers of abdominal or thoracic closure dehisce)
Seroma	Collection of tissue fluid under a wound	Poor wound healing Infection Patient interference	Potential for infection
Sinus	(See under inflammation)	Foreign material in wound (including buried sutures) Infection	Delayed healing Patient interference
Incisional	Dehiscence of abdominal wall with skin closure remaining intact	Poor operative technique Incorrect suture selection Patient debility	Strangulation of herniated contents Evisceration

6.48 Diseases of the nostrils (nares)

Condition	Description	Treatment
Congenital conditions		
Stenotic nares	Common in brachycephalic dogs – part of the brachycephalic obstructive syndrome (BOS)	Surgical widening, with good prognosis
Cleft lip (harelip)	Less common than clefts of the hard or soft palate, which often occur together with this disease Obvious at birth and may interfere with nursing	Surgical repair can be undertaken, but is delayed until the animal is at least 8 weeks old, when the tissues are more mature (may require tube feeding until that time)
Acquired conditions		
Neoplasia	Not uncommon, particularly in older cats with non-pigmented tissue Squamous cell carcinoma is the commonest type These tumours have a tendency to recur locally but rarely spread elsewhere	Cryosurgery, radiotherapy and excision of the nasal planum
Trauma	Can result in obstruction to the nostrils	Early wound management is necessary to avoid scarring

6.49 Diseases of the nasal cavities and sinuses

Condition	Description	Treatment
Chronic rhinitis	Common in cats, rarer in dogs May be associated with chronic viral infections in cats Nasal sinuses are also commonly involved	Response to medical or surgical treatments can be disappointing
Foreign bodies	Important cause of acute sneezing and nasal discharge in dogs	Some dislodge naturally May require removal by vigorous flushing under anaesthesia, forceps retrieval using endoscopy Occasionally open surgery (rhinotomy) is indicated
Fungal rhinitis	Uncommon in cats Important cause of nasal disease in dogs Infection with *Aspergillus*, causing sneezing, nasal discharge, nasal pain and nose bleeds (epistaxis)	Oral antifungal drugs and topical treatments Placement of indwelling catheters via the frontal sinuses and twice daily administration of enilconazole is an effective treatment but requires hospitalization and intensive nursing
Neoplasia	Important causes of chronic nasal disease (discharge, obstruction and epistaxis) in elderly dogs and cats	Surgery alone is not a helpful treatment Radiation therapy with surgery in dogs Chemotherapy in cats

6.50 Diseases of the palate

Condition	Description	Treatment
Congenital conditions		
Cleft palate	Not uncommon in kittens and puppies Results in difficulty in feeding and nasal discharge	Surgery is delayed until the animal is 12 weeks of age, when the tissues are more mature Nursing care and tube feeding are required until then Many breeders elect to have such animals euthanased if the defects are recognized soon after birth
Overlong soft palate	Part of BOS Causes dyspnoea and stertorous respiration (snoring)	Shortening by excision of the tip of the palate if other components of BOS are not severe
Acquired conditions		
Traumatic cleft palate	Often follows road traffic accidents or falls in cats	Many will heal eventually Assessment and treatment of concurrent injuries is important
Oronasal fistula	Usually follows trauma or tooth removal Removal of the upper canine teeth is a common cause Results in food entering the nose and chronic infection	Closed by creation of a flap of mucosa from a nearby area which is sutured to patch the hole

6.51 Diseases of the larynx

Condition	Description	Treatment
Laryngeal paralysis	Paralysis of the muscles of the larynx, most importantly those allowing the vocal cords to be opened Common in dogs, occasionally seen in cats Elderly, medium–large breed dogs, particularly Labrador and Golden Retriever, Irish Setter and Afghan Hound Results in coughing, rasping respiratory noise (stridor), altered bark and dyspnoea	Various surgical procedures that increase the size of the laryngeal opening, most commonly a 'tie-back' surgery, effective even in elderly patients
Laryngeal collapse	Component of BOS in which structures of larynx become distorted and collapse Results in laryngeal obstruction Usually severely dyspnoeic	Excision of the obstructing structures from within the airway Guarded prognosis
Neoplasia	Occasionally seen in cats and dogs	Most are lymphosarcomas in cats, and chemotherapy may produce a period of remission Usually malignant in dogs and treatment is not successful
Laryngospasm	Spasm of the muscles of the larynx, producing marked obstruction of the airway Most often seen in cats after endotracheal intubation	Usually resolves after treatment with corticosteroids or local anaesthetics

- Otherwise no special preparation for these surgeries is required. Cats are often anorexic after nasal surgery of any type and need to be tempted to eat, since the sense of smell may be lost and cats tolerate nasal obstruction poorly. Nasogastric feeding is contraindicated after nasal or pharyngeal surgery, however. Alternative routes of assisted feeding (pharyngostomy or gastrostomy tubes) are available, but in practice are usually not necessary
- After oral surgeries of these types, voluntary feeding is often resumed within a few hours. Soft food is given, but bones and biscuits are avoided for at least 2 weeks. Occasionally oral intake of food or fluids is contraindicated and tube feeding is necessary

- Antibiotic treatment for a few days is usually prescribed
- Flushing of the mouth with an oral antiseptic solution is sometimes advised, but is often unnecessary.

The lower respiratory tract comprises the trachea, bronchi, bronchioles and lungs. Figures 6.52 and 6.53 list common surgical conditions of these organs.

Care of the respiratory patient
In dealing with the respiratory patient each case should be monitored and have nursing care adapted to suit the individual patient following the particular surgery (Figure 6.54).

6.52 Diseases of the trachea

Condition	Description	Treatment
Tracheal collapse	Yorkshire Terriers commonly affected Results in characteristic honking cough	Results of surgical correction often no better than medical treatment
Trauma	Following external trauma (RTA, dog fight, stick penetration) or intubation injuries	Severe injuries require surgical repair Mild cases may heal without surgery
Foreign bodies	Usually inhaled grass seeds, occasionally pebbles and others Cause cough and sometimes dyspnoea	Endoscopic retrieval

6.53 Diseases of the lungs

Condition	Description	Treatment
Primary lung tumours	Solitary masses, often occupying an entire lung lobe Important cause of chronic coughing in elderly dogs	Usually malignant but surgery improves quality of life
Lung abscess	Usually due to a chronic inhaled foreign body	Lobectomy often required
Metastatic lung tumours	Arise from spread of distant tumours	Surgery rarely indicated

6.54 Points to consider in caring for the respiratory patient

- Make sure you are prepared during the final stages of the surgery of any respiratory case
- Have suction and sterile saline ready
- Consider keeping the endotracheal tube in for as long as possible. It may be useful to remove it with the cuff inflated to avoid debris passing into the trachea. Even after the endotracheal tube has been removed there should be a clean appropriate sized tube and a laryngoscope to hand
- Have oxygen on standby, with a suitable method of administration (face mask or nasal catheter)
- Handle respiratory cases carefully; avoid causing the patient unnecessary distress
- Regular monitoring is important:
  - Watch carefully for any changes in respiratory pattern or colour of mucous membranes
  - Watch to ensure that the volume of air movement is adequate
  - Check the patient's temperature regularly, as hyperthermia can develop in animals with respiratory obstruction
  - Conversely, hypothermia often occurs in patients after open thoracic surgery
- Have a suitable tracheotomy tube and small surgical kit ready in case of emergencies
- A patient that has been in lateral recumbency during a lengthy surgical procedure should not be turned on to the other side in recovery. The 'down lung' during surgery will be congested and underventilated and may interfere with respiratory function if it is placed uppermost. As soon as possible the patient should be placed in sternal recumbency
- Chest bandages can be used post surgery to protect the surgical incision or to hold a chest drain in place. Bandages should be checked regularly so that they are not so tight that they interfere with respiratory function. Two fingers should be held underneath the bandage during inspiration, when the chest is at maximum capacity
- Chest drains are usually placed at the time of surgery and a secure system is vital for the safety of the patient:
  - They should be sutured in place and held securely with a body bandage
  - Elizabethan collars may also be used
  - Any tubing used for chest drainage should be sterile
  - Patients connected to a drainage system should never be left unattended
  - Further details of chest drainage are in *BSAVA Manual of Advanced Veterinary Nursing*.

The alimentary tract

Oral cavity
Figure 6.55 describes common surgical oral diseases. Patient care is similar to that outlined for surgery of the upper respiratory tract.

Dental disease
Figure 6.56 describes common dental diseases. Patient care is similar to that outlined for surgery of the upper respiratory tract. After dental treatment, soft food should be given for 4–5 days, before gradually returning to a normal diet.

Oesophagus
Figure 6.57 describes common surgical conditions of the oesophagus. Oesophageal surgery is covered in *BSAVA Manual of Advanced Veterinary Nursing*. Following oesophagitis or removal of oesophageal foreign bodies, tube feeding should be considered for 5–10 days to allow the oesophagus to heal.

Stomach
Figure 6.58 describes common surgical conditions of the stomach.

6.55 Diseases of the oral cavity (see also Figures 6.48–6.51 and 6.56)

Condition	Description	Treatment
Fractured mandible	Common after RTA, especially in the cat Often open and comminuted	Internal or external fixation or by muzzle support May require tube feeding during healing
Separated mandibular symphysis	Common after RTA, especially in the cat	Cerclage wiring
Ulceration	Oral ulceration may be caused by ingested irritants, uraemia, liver failure, allergy and viral infections (cats)	Biopsy may be necessary to distinguish it from an ulcerating neoplasm
Epulis neoplasia	Non-specific term applied to benign masses arising from the gums Various benign and malignant tumours are reported Prognosis depends on site, size and tissue type Squamous cell carcinoma most common, particularly in cats	Local excision or more radical surgery Prognosis is poor after traditional surgery but fair after radical surgery

6.56 Dental diseases

Condition	Description	Treatment
Gingivitis	Inflammation of the gums, usually around the teeth Commonest tooth-related disease and usually associated with accumulation of plaque and tartar on the teeth and associated infection Also associated with causes of oral ulceration (Figure 6.55)	Removal of accumulated tartar and improved oral hygiene (oral antiseptics, short-term antibiotics, dietary change, tooth brushing) Prevented by attention to dietary hygiene
Periodontitis	Progression of gingivitis resulting in regression of gum-line and pocket formation around the teeth	Early cases may be reversed by treatment of gingivitis Other cases require gum surgery or tooth extraction
Caries	Demineralization and destruction of the tooth substance induced by bacteria Results in defect in enamel and deeper tissue Rare in animals cf. humans	Extraction or filling
Fractures of crown	Usually traumatic in origin Canines commonly affected	Often managed conservatively but may be capped or extracted
Feline neck lesions	Also known as subgingival resorptive lesions Seen exclusively in cats, cause unknown Causes cavities in the tooth substance at the gingival margin Painful	Filling or extraction
Retained deciduous teeth	Retention of deciduous canines is most significant Deciduous teeth should be shed by the time the permanent teeth are beginning to erupt Retention of teeth after this will lead to misplacement of permanent teeth and malocclusion	Retained teeth should be extracted, with care to prevent damage to the emerging permanent teeth

6.57 Oesophageal diseases

Condition	Description	Treatment
Megaoesophagus	(See Chapter 4)	
Oesophageal stricture	Stricture (narrowing due to scarring) usually follows an episode of oesophagitis Commonly develops within a few days of general anaesthesia if stomach contents have refluxed into the oesophagus Animals present with dysphagia and regurgitation	Managed by treatment of oesophagitis and repeated dilation of the stricture (bougienage) Prognosis guarded
Oesophageal foreign body	Various ingested objects may become lodged in the oesophagus Most commonly pieces of bone Fish-hooks are also encountered occasionally Terrier dogs are predisposed	Removal by forceps, endoscopy or surgery Complications of oesophageal perforation and aspiration pneumonia may develop
Vascular ring anomaly (persistent right aortic arch)	Congenital malformation resulting in obstruction of the oesophagus Animals present soon after weaning with regurgitation of solid food	Division of obstructive band at thoracotomy

Condition	Description	Treatment
Foreign bodies	Indigestible material of various types can lodge in the stomach Signs vary from none to severe vomiting	Induction of vomiting (if small and smooth), endoscopic retrieval or surgery (gastrotomy)
Neoplasia	Not uncommon in older animals Signs: vomiting, weight loss, haematemesis Diagnosed by radiography or endoscopy and biopsy	Most are large and malignant but surgery can be helpful occasionally Poor prognosis
Pylorospasm/pyloric stenosis	Narrowing of the outflow of the stomach Causes food retention and vomiting	Surgery to widen the outflow (pyloroplasty or pyloromyotomy)
Gastric dilation/volvulus syndrome (GDV, bloat)	Concurrent twisting of the stomach Seen in large and giant dogs with deep chests (Labrador, Irish Setter, Dobermann, Great Dane, etc.) Causes severe shock and can be fatal if not treated rapidly	Requires emergency treatment (see text)
Hiatal hernia	Prolapse of part of the stomach into the thorax through an enlarged oesophageal hiatus Results in oesophageal reflux, dysphasia and regurgitation	Managed medically, or occasionally by surgery

Treatment of gastric dilation/volvulus syndrome (GDV)

This is covered here in more depth since the veterinary nurse may have to assist with emergency treatment of the condition.

For treatment of GDV:

- Aggressive intravenous fluid therapy (100 ml/kg/hour initially, for rapid restoration of circulating blood volume)
- Gastric decompression, carried out concurrently with fluid therapy. Several methods are in use:
  - orogastric intubation (stomach tube) – possible without sedation in many cases, but may be difficult to enter the stomach if grossly distended or volvulus is present
  - nasogastric intubation – smaller diameter tube may be easier to pass in some cases
  - trocharization – passage of large gauge needles through the most distended flank into the stomach; advised in cases where intubation is not possible
  - flank gastrotomy – when decompression is not possible by other means, a limited surgical approach to the stomach under local anaesthesia may be used, but is rarely required
- Gastric lavage – flushing of the stomach with warm saline is often recommended
- Treatment of shock – continuation of fluid therapy and correction of acid/base and electrolyte disturbances until patient is stabilized
- Treatment of dysrhythmias – cardiac dysrhythmias are common in affected dogs and should be monitored by electrocardiography and treated if necessary; lignocaine by intravenous bolus or infusion is the treatment of choice
- Additional drug therapy – antibiotics are indicated because of the danger of septicaemia, and corticosteroids may be used in the treatment of shock
- Radiography may be used to confirm the diagnosis and assess the position of the stomach
- Surgical exploration of the abdomen under anaesthesia is recommended, once the patient is stable, to allow repositioning of the stomach and spleen if displaced, inspection of tissue viability and resection if necessary (the spleen and stomach may be partially necrotic) and surgical fixation of the stomach (gastropexy) to prevent future volvulus (twisting).

Advice to owners to reduce likelihood of recurrence

Owners of breeds prone to GDV, and in particular owners of dogs previously treated for the condition, should be advised on the recognition of the disease and steps that they may use to reduce the risk of recurrence. Owners should watch for:

- Restlessness and discomfort up to 3 hours after eating
- The animal retching but unable to vomit
- Abdominal distension
- Respiration that is rapid and laboured
- A pulse that is rapid and weak.

GDV can occur in any breed but is more common in large deep-chested dogs such as Irish Setter or St Bernard. To reduce the risk of recurrence:

- Avoid feeding large meals
- Avoid exercise immediately before or after eating
- The type of diet fed is now thought not to be an important factor in the development of the condition, but ingestion of air during feeding may be important. This may be reduced by postural feeding and discouraging the dog from gulping its food.

Care of patients after gastric surgery

Patient care following gastric surgery will be adapted according to the reason for surgery and the type of surgery performed. As with the care of any patient that has undergone surgery on the alimentary tract, fluid therapy, electrolyte balance and nutritional support are very important during the return to normal function.

- Offer very small amounts of water on recovery from anaesthesia
- If water is retained by the patient and no problems are encountered for 12 hours post surgery, small amounts of a bland diet can be offered
- Feed little and often and gradually increase over several days
- Return to a normal diet over approximately 3–5 days.

Small intestine, large intestine (colon), rectum and anus

Figures 6.59 and 6.60 describe common surgical conditions of these organs.

6.59 Diseases of the small and large intestine

Condition	Description	Treatment
Simple foreign body	Compact foreign bodies that are ingested can cause varying degrees of intestinal obstruction Commonest in younger animals Severity of signs greatest when obstruction is complete and in the proximal intestine Typical signs include vomiting, shock, abdominal pain, but in less severe cases include weight loss and diarrhoea	Can be managed conservatively if incomplete obstruction and carefully monitored More commonly surgery required: removal at enterotomy if intestinal wall viable, else resection and anastomosis (enterectomy)
Linear foreign body	Elongated foreign bodies (string, tape, etc.) cause more severe signs Typically the proximal end lodges at the pylorus or the base of the tongue Intestine becomes plicated along the foreign body Severe obstruction and often perforation as the foreign body saws through the intestinal wall	Removed at surgery: often requires several enterotomies and repair of perforations Prognosis cautious
Neoplasia	Intestinal neoplasia can be focal or diffuse Focal neoplasms produce obstruction and similar signs to simple foreign bodies (above) Diffuse neoplasms may cause obstruction or malabsorption, weight loss and diarrhoea	Majority are malignant but surgery can be helpful for focal neoplasms
Strangulation	Intestine can be strangulated/incarcerated by entrapment in a hernia or rupture Signs of obstruction are severe and intestinal compromise also causes pain, toxaemia and shock	Enterectomy
Intussusception	Invagination of part of the intestine into an adjacent part Commonest in younger animals, often after enteritis Results in partial or complete obstruction Ileocaecal is commonest site	Early cases may be reduced at surgery, but formation of adhesions requires resection and anastomosis
Megacolon	Loss of contractility of colon Commonest in older cats Results in constipation	Repeated evacuation and stool softeners or by surgery (subtotal colectomy)

6.60 Diseases of the rectum and anus

Condition	Description	Treatment
Neoplasia	Not uncommon in older animals Signs include tenesmus, haematochezia and constipation May be malignant or benign	Variety of surgical techniques are available to manage Prognosis is poor for malignant types
Polyps	Benign superficial lesions of the lining of the rectum or anus Signs as neoplasia	Prognosis is good after local excision if discrete Management is more difficult if diffuse
Anal furunculosis	Inflammatory disease of the skin around the anus Results in formation of discharging sinuses and local fibrosis Results in pain, dyschezia and incontinence Typically a disease of German Shepherd Dogs	By surgical excision of the affected area or cryosurgery Prognosis is guarded because of recurrence or postoperative incontinence
Anal sac disease (sacculitis, abscessation or impaction)	Results from obstruction of the anal sac canal and/or infection Causes pain and 'scooting'	Manual evacuation and antibiotics if necessary Sometimes flushing under sedation is helpful Occasionally excision of the sacs is used (anal sacculectomy)
Perineal rupture/hernia	Seen in older entire male dogs Loss of muscular support to the rectum results in dilation or deviation of the rectum and dyschezia Other signs occasionally seen if other organs pass into the rupture (small intestine, prostate, bladder)	Managed conservatively by stool softeners and manual evacuation or by surgical repair Significant risk of recurrence after surgery, though this is reduced by castration

Preparation of animals for intestinal surgery

The time required for preparation of the patient for intestinal surgery will vary according to the area of surgery (small or large intestine) and if the patient is presented as an elective or emergency case. Points to consider for a patient undergoing elective large intestinal surgery are listed in Figure 6.61.

Preparation of animals for anorectal and perineal surgery

The considerations given above also apply in these cases. For surgery carried out in the terminal rectum via the anus, the surgeon may wish to pack the descending rectum with swabs or bandage to keep intestinal contents away from the surgical site. During perineal surgery, a purse-string suture is usually placed in the anus for the same purpose.

6.61 Points to consider for patient undergoing elective large intestinal surgery

- Starvation of patients undergoing large bowel surgery may need to be longer than the normal 12 hours to ensure that the gut is as empty as possible at the time of surgery
- A low residue diet fed for 3–5 days before surgery may reduce the volume of large intestinal contents
- The day before surgery, withhold food and give an enema
- On the day of surgery, another (non-irritant) enema can be given if necessary
- Recovery after surgery will be improved if the patient is not lacking in nutritional requirements at the time of surgery. Prolonged pre- or postoperative starvation should be avoided
- The technique of giving oral antibiotics before surgery to reduce intestinal bacterial load is no longer considered good practice
- In some cases, the surgeon may prefer enemas not to be given, since liquefied intestinal contents may be more difficult to deal with at surgery than firm faecal material.

6.62 Points to consider for patients after intestinal surgery

- Offer very small amounts of water within hours after surgery, as this may stimulate gut activity
- When water is taken successfully by the patient, and if no vomiting occurs, small amounts of a bland food can be offered; this will gradually be increased if no problems occur
- Tube feeding may be necessary in patients that refuse food
- Total parenteral nutrition (nutritional support via an intravenous catheter) could be considered in vomiting patients, but it is expensive and technically difficult to do in a safe and effective manner
- Early signs of ileus (lack of significant peristaltic activity) are difficult for the nurse to observe but may be signified by abdominal distension due to the retention of gas, abdominal pain, vomiting and anorexia
- Watch when faeces are passed: observe for consistency, colour, signs of blood and whether any straining is present.

Care of patients after intestinal surgery

Following surgery on the intestinal tract, consider:

- Fluid and electrolyte balance
- Nutritional support
- Return to normal function of the alimentary tract.

Immediate postoperative monitoring should include all the basic parameters such as temperature, pulse, respiration and colour of mucous membranes. Specific points to consider for patients after intestinal surgery are listed in Figure 6.62.

Liver and spleen

Figure 6.63 describes common surgical conditions of these organs.

Liver biopsy

Biopsy is occasionally required for diagnosis of liver disease. Available methods include:

- Fine needle aspirate
- Needle core biopsy (e.g. Trucut)
- Surgical biopsy (wedge biopsy).

A clotting profile should be carried out before liver biopsy, since animals with liver disease are at risk of clotting defects. Following biopsy by any technique there is a risk of severe haemorrhage and the animal must be observed closely for signs of developing shock – poor recovery from anaesthesia, tachycardia, cool periphery, pale mucous membranes, etc.

Urinary tract (kidneys, ureters, bladder and urethra)

Figure 6.64 describes common surgical diseases of these organs.

Management of urinary obstruction

This condition usually occurs in males, because of the relatively long and narrow urethra in this sex. There are various causes but feline lower urinary tract disease and urolithiasis are most important (see Chapter 4). Affected animals strain unsuccessfully to urinate and later become systemically affected (shocked, uraemia, vomiting, collapse).

Important steps in management are:

- Fluid therapy, to correct fluid deficits and electrolyte imbalances (typically affected animals are hypovolaemic, acidotic and hyperkalaemic)
- Emptying of bladder, by cystocentesis or passage of a urethral catheter
- Establishment of diagnosis and specific treatment
- Urethral stones can often be flushed back into the bladder and removed by cystotomy
- Recurrent cases may require urethrostomy to bypass an area of obstruction or to bypass the penile urethra (narrowest part).

Care of patients undergoing surgery of the urinary tract

Following urinary tract surgery it is important to maintain a good fluid and electrolyte balance. Fluid therapy is covered in detail elsewhere but adequate fluid administration can be maintained by intravenous and/or oral fluid therapy. Initially a high rate of infusion may be used for the administration of intravenous fluids to encourage the production of urine. Oral

6.63 Diseases of the liver and spleen

Condition	Description	Treatment
Hepatic tumours	Relatively common in older dogs Signs are usually non-specific (weight loss, anorexia, vomiting)	May be surgically treatable if discrete although they are usually malignant
Portosystemic shunts	Abnormal blood vessels joining the portal vein to the systemic circulation Result in signs of liver failure, particularly neurological signs	Medical management often helpful Surgical ligation of the anomalous vessel possible in some cases (an advanced surgical technique)
Trauma to liver or spleen	May result in severe haemorrhage Falls, crush injuries and car accidents are common causes	Usually haemorrhage will stop if animal is supported with fluids/blood transfusion Surgical treatment is rarely required
Splenic tumours	Haemangiosarcoma most frequent Common in older large breed dogs Results in vague signs or collapse due to intra-abdominal haemorrhage	Splenectomy, but poor prognosis since malignant
Splenic haematoma	Similar presentation to splenic tumours Prognosis better Histopathology necessary to differentiate the diseases	Splenectomy

6.64 Diseases of the kidneys, ureters, urethra and bladder

Condition	Description	Treatment
Kidney tumours	Uncommon diseases Signs include haematuria and abdominal mass	Nephrectomy if no gross metastasis
Kidney trauma	Follows blunt abdominal trauma	Kidneys usually recover without surgery Less commonly surgical repair or nephrectomy is required
Ureteral trauma	Occasional consequence of abdominal trauma or surgical misadventure Results in accumulation of urine within the abdomen or in the retroperitoneum, or hydronephrosis	Repair or ureteronephrectomy
Ureteral ectopia	Congenital condition in which the ureters insert into the urethra or vagina Causes incontinence	Ureteral repositioning or ureteronephrectomy
Bladder tumours	Cause urinary frequency, urgency and haematuria in older bitches Usually extensive at the time of diagnosis	Rarely amenable to surgical treatment
Urolithiasis (stones)	Most commonly affect the bladder but all parts of the urinary tract may be affected In males, usually cause dysuria due to urethral obstruction In females, usually cause signs of cystitis (urgency, frequency) Several chemical types occur: may be associated with infection	Depends on stone type; includes elimination of infection, surgical removal and dietary manipulation
Feline lower urinary tract disease (FLUTD, FUS)	Syndrome of signs associated with the bladder and urethra May cause frequency, urgency and haematuria in females and males Commoner presentation in males is obstruction of the urethra by stones or mucus	Dietary and drug treatment often helpful Males with recurrent obstruction may require urethrostomy to prevent further difficulties
Urinary incontinence	Wide variety of causes	Depends on specific diagnosis Some cases respond to medical treatment, others benefit from surgical intervention

intake of fluids should be encouraged as soon as possible. Water may also be added to the patient's normal diet to increase fluid intake.

Monitoring of urine output

Cystitis occasionally occurs following surgery of the urinary tract.

- Observe the patient for frequency of urination and the amount passed each time
- Observe for signs of difficulty or discomfort in passing urine
- Check the colour of the urine passed
- Watch for the presence of blood
- Check the smell of the urine and note any changes.

Indwelling urinary catheters

To reduce bacteria tracking up the catheter, a closed drainage system is preferable. This also enables the nurse to monitor urine production, take samples if necessary and watch for any changes in the type or volume of urine produced.

Flushing of the urinary catheter may be required to remove blood clots from the urethra or bladder. If necessary, this should be performed using sterile saline.

The patient must be prevented from interfering with indwelling urinary catheters: Elizabethan collars are usually used.

Management of urethrotomy/urethrostomy

Prevention of self-mutilation is vital to the success of these cases. Elizabethan collars, and possibly sedation in the initial postoperative period, may be required. Patients should be given plenty of opportunity to urinate. The area around the wound should be kept clean and petroleum jelly may be applied to surrounding skin to prevent scalding initially. Cat litter trays should be filled with shredded newspaper or something of a similar consistency for 4–5 days post surgery, since particles of litter may irritate the site.

Reproductive system

Testes, prepuce, scrotum, penis and prostate gland

Figures 6.65 and 6.66 describe common surgical diseases of these organs.

Castration

This is the commonest surgical procedure of this system in the male and is defined as removal of the testes (orchidectomy, gonadectomy).

6.65 Diseases of the testes, scrotum and penis

Condition	Description	Treatment
Cryptorchidism	Failure of one or both testicles to descend to scrotal position by usual time (typically birth) Usually unilateral Most are abdominally retained in the dog, but in the cat many are inguinal or subcutaneous The condition has a heritable component	Abnormally located testicles have increased incidence of torsion and of neoplasia, justifying their removal prophylactically Bilateral castration is recommended
Testicular neoplasia	Represent 5% of canine neoplasms Most are benign, but some are oestrogen secreting and related signs may be seen Remainder present with testicular enlargement and/or distortion	Castration
Testicular torsion	Uncommon, but occurs principally to retained testicles Especially those having undergone neoplastic transformation Presenting signs are those of abdominal pain and/or an abdominal mass	Castration
Orchitis	Not uncommon in the dog Acute onset of pain, swelling and local oedema, may be systemic signs (fever, listlessness) Prostatitis may be present concurrently	Castration is usually the most appropriate treatment Antibiotics, analgesics and hypothermia may be attempted
Scrotal haematoma	Commonest complication of castration due to patient interference, haemorrhage (from scrotal tissue, septum or testicular vessels) and trauma at surgery or preparation Particularly a problem in larger mature dogs, for which routine scrotal ablation should be considered at the time of castration	Prevention of patient interference and/or scrotal ablation in susceptible animals
Balanitis (infection of the penis and prepuce)	Slight purulent preputial discharge is common in normal mature dogs, and does not represent disease Infections of the penis and prepuce do occur occasionally, resulting in irritation, copious purulent to serosanguineous discharge and occasionally adhesions	Careful search should be made for underlying diseases (foreign bodies, trauma, neoplasia) before treatment with local irrigation and antibiotic therapy is started Condition tends to recur

6.66 Diseases of the prostate gland

Condition	Description	Treatment
Benign prostatic hyperplasia (BPH)	Common in older entire male dogs Usually causes dyschezia without systemic signs	Treated hormonally or by castration
Prostatitis	Bacterial infection of the parenchyma of the gland Often causes systemic signs of pyrexia, lethergy, etc. Also dyschezia, dysuria, tenesmus and purulent penile discharge	Systemic antibiotics and hormonal therapy or castration
Prostatic abscessation	Often concurrent with prostatitis Similar signs but mass can also cause pelvic obstruction	Drainage percutaneously or at surgery as well as treatment for prostatitis Cautious prognosis
Prostatic cysts	Usually accompany BPH	Drainage at surgery or percutaneously as well as treatment for BPH
Prostatic neoplasia	Carcinoma commonest type Unlike other prostatic diseases, occurs frequently in castrates Painful enlargement of the gland with marked tenesmus and dysuria/dyschezia Malignant and locally invasive	Not usually attempted Grave prognosis

Indications include:

- Social (undesirable sexual behaviour, dominance, prevention of pregnancy)
- Scrotal/testicular neoplasia
- Hormonally responsive conditions (perianal adenoma, perineal rupture, benign prostatic disease, stud tail)
- Prophylaxis of above diseases
- Cryptorchidism (prophylaxis of testicular neoplasia or torsion)
- Testicular or scrotal trauma
- Inguinal herniation

Preparation of the cat for castration

- Pluck or clip the hair from over the testicles
- Give the area a gentle surgical scrub, wiping the fur away from the area of incision.

Preparation of the dog for castration
Careful preparation is important as hurried preparation may lead to scrotal dermatitis which will interfere with postoperative healing.

- Clip under anaesthesia to try to avoid damage to the skin of the scrotum with the clippers
- Skin that is wet or damp is more difficult to clip and damage to the skin is more likely
- Povidone–iodine is generally more irritant to the skin, so use chlorhexidine surgical scrub to avoid skin irritation after clipping
- To avoid dermatitis, some surgeons prefer to minimize preparation of the scrotal skin; instead, they exclude the scrotum from the surgical field.

Patient care after castration
Interference with the wound by the patient post surgery may cause wound breakdown or worsen the formation of scrotal haematoma. If some degree of scrotal dermatitis is present after surgery, the patient will be more inclined to lick the area.

Elizabethan collars are useful to prevent patient interference. Owners should be advised to look for:

- Signs of redness, swelling or bruising at the surgical site
- Discharge from the wound
- Discomfort in the patient.

Ovaries, uterus, vagina and mammary glands
Figure 6.67 describes common surgical diseases of the ovaries, uterus and vagina.

Ovariohysterectomy (OHE) (spay) in the bitch and queen
Spaying is the commonest surgical procedure of this organ system in the female. It is common practice to remove the ovaries and uterus together, though in many cases ovariectomy alone would produce similar benefits.
Indications include:

- Prevention/termination of pregnancy
- Social (elimination of oestrus)
- Management of medical disorders (diabetes mellitus, epilepsy)
- Prevention of mammary tumours (see below)
- Ovarian disease (neoplasia, irregular cycles)
- Uterine disease (pyometritis, complications of pregnancy)
- Vaginal disease (hormonally responsive conditions).

Timing of OHE

- Technically feasible from a few weeks old (preferred by some rehoming organizations)
- Leaving surgery until after first oestrus in the bitch may reduce the incidence of incontinence, vaginitis, infantile vulva
- Avoid surgery during oestrus (increased vascularity) or false pregnancy (may be prolonged)
- Ovariectomy early in life reduces the incidence of mammary neoplasia (see below)
- Kittens are typically neutered at 4–6 months, bitches during anoestrus after the first season.

6.67

Condition	Description	Treatment
Ovarian tumours	Uncommon in bitches (1% of canine neoplasms), rare in cats	OHE Prognosis is limited by potential for metastasis
Pyometra (synonym: pyometritis, 'pyo')	Disease of the mature bitch, most commonly in bitches over 6 years old Hormonally mediated cystic uterine change accompanied by a bacterial infection Usually in entire females Occasionally seen in the uterine remnants of spayed females ('stump pyometra') under the influence of exogenous progestagen treatment or those with ovarian remnants Disease occurs during metoestrus, typically 5–80 days after oestrus Association exists between the incidence of the disease and irregular oestrous patterns and also with the use of oestrogens (for example, for misalliance) and progestagens Less common in cats and has a less distinct relationship with oestrous Clinical signs of pyometra: • depression, lethergy, anorexia • vomiting and diarrhoea • polydipsia and polyuria • purulent vaginal discharge • abdominal distension • pyrexia	Ovariohysterectomy is the treatment of choice in the majority of cases following supportive care
Vaginal neoplasia	Usually present as perineal swelling, in entire bitches of around 10 years, and show oestral-related growth Usually benign	Episiotomy and submucosal dissection OHE is essential to prevent recurrence
Vaginal hypertrophy	Excessive hypertrophy of the vaginal mucosa occuring in oestrus Can cause perineal or vulval swelling, or vaginal prolapse Most cases occur at the first oestrus and regress in dioestrus Affected breeds include Boxer, Bullmastiff, Bulldog and Sharpei	Tissue should be lubricated and replaced if not devitalized, and OHE performed at next oestrus
Vaginal prolapse	Occurs postpartum or associated with vaginal hypertrophy (q.v.)	Submucosal resection is indicated if mucosa is devitalized Otherwise reduction and placement of a purse-string retaining suture

Caesarean section

This is the removal of term foetuses by hysterotomy. Obstetrical intervention in bitches and queens is restricted to drug intervention, limited vaginal manipulation and Caesarean section. Around 60% of canine dystocias are managed by Caesarean section.

Fundamental to successful use of this surgical technique are careful preparation of the dam, selection of anaesthetic technique and care of the neonate. These are covered in more detail elsewhere. The dam must be handled quietly and as much preparation be made prior to anaesthetic induction as possible. Adequate assistance must be available for preparation, surgery and care of the neonates.

Care of the dam after Caesarean section

• Gently clean the surgical area before the neonates begin to suckle
• The dam should be put back with her litter as soon as possible, but should not be left unattended until she has recovered sufficiently from the anaesthesia as she may inadvertently cause damage to the neonates when moving or trying to stand
• Following surgery, place the dam in a large kennel with clean bedding. Ideally there should a bed or enclosed area where the dam can lie with her litter and an area where she can move away to avoid their attentions

- Environmental conditions are important. The area should be draughtfree, the atmosphere should be warm but not so warm that the dam will become too hot. The dam should be free to move away to a cooler area if she wishes.

Care of the neonates after Caesarean section

- Check the mouth for any debris or mucus that may be blocking the airway
- If necessary, remove debris from the mouth or nostrils with swabs or gentle suction. Swinging a neonate to remove fluid from the airways is less satisfactory, since it may damage the delicate brain
- Wrap the neonate in a warm towel and gently rub to dry it and stimulate respiration
- Have oxygen and a respiratory stimulant to hand in case they are needed
- Make a quick check for any congenital abnormalities, such as cleft palate or imperforate anus
- Keep the neonate warm until it can be returned to the dam at the earliest opportunity
- Once the neonates have been returned to the dam they should be watched to avoid accidental damage by the dam while she is recovering from anaesthesia
- Suckling should be encouraged at the earliest opportunity.

Diseases of the mammary glands

Three pathological processes are encountered:

- Hypertrophy – a physiological process during late pregnancy but pathological during false pregnancy or following exogenous progesterone treatment
- Inflammation (mastitis) – usually associated with bacterial infection around the time of parturition
- Neoplasia – the most important surgical disease of this organ.

Mammary tumours in the bitch

Mammary tumours (Figure 6.68) represent around 25% of canine neoplasia with around half of those neoplasms occurring in the bitch. There is an obvious age distribution, with a peak incidence at 10 years; mammary neoplasia is rare below 5 years of age.

Ovariectomy significantly reduces the incidence of mammary tumours if it is performed early in the bitch's life. However, after 2–3 years an ovariohysterectomy has no effect on the incidence of later mammary neoplasia, and there is no evidence at present that ovariohysterectomy at the time of mastectomy improves the survival times.

Prognosis depends heavily on the histopathological type. Thus histopathology should be carried out so that owners can be offered an accurate prognosis. The prognosis is excellent for simple and benign mixed tumours, or for malignant tumours where the tumour is small (less than 5 cm diameter) and local invasion or distant metastasis has not occurred. As with all neoplasia, clinical appearance and examination are not reliable guides to prognosis.

Mammary tumours in the cat

The relative and absolute incidence of mammary tumours in the cat is lower than in the bitch, but they do represent the second most common solid neoplasm of this species after skin neoplasia.

The prognosis in the cat is poorer than that in the dog since 85–90% of tumours are malignant (commonly adenocarcinomata). Intact females are at greater risk than spayed females, and Siamese cats may be overrepresented.

Eye

Figure 6.69 describes common surgical diseases of the globe, eyelids and conjunctiva.

6.68 **Mammary tumours in the bitch**

Tumour types

A variety of histopathological types occur:

- Benign (represent 52% of the total)
- Carcinomata (represent 40% of the total)
- Sarcomata (represent 4% of the total)
- Malignant mixed tumours (represent 4% of the total).

Surgical treatment

The surgical approach will remain the primary treatment of mammary neoplasia in the bitch. Non-surgical management with chemotherapy and radiotherapy is occasionally of value but is principally indicated for palliation if local recurrent disease occurs.

Surgical techniques include:

- *Local excision* (lumpectomy)
- *Simple mastectomy* – removal of tumour and associated glands
- *Partial radical mastectomy* – removal of tumour complete with glands associated with it, by lymphatic drainage with or without the nodes
- *Radical mastectomy* – removal of tumour with all glands of that side, with or without the nodes
- *Bilateral radical mastectomy* – removal of all mammary tissue.

The value of each of these techniques remains equivocal and most surgeons would opt for simple excision with small nodules but a more radical procedure for larger nodules, particularly if there was any clinical evidence of malignancy. Overall it is wiser to perform a radical excision at the outset to prevent local recurrence and the need for repeated surgeries.

Diseases of the globe, eyelids and conjunctiva

Condition	Description	Treatment
Perforation	Caused by trauma or uncontrolled infection	Enucleation when a non-functional eye is painful or shrunken
Prolapse of the eyeball	Follows head trauma, particularly in brachycephalic dogs with protruding globes Priority is to prevent further trauma to the eye and prevent desiccation	Moisten and lubricate eye with saline and aqueous gel Replacement is urgent: usually requires general anaesthesia Restrain animal to prevent self-inflicted trauma
Cataracts	Opacification of the lens resulting in loss of vision when severe May be inherited in some breed, idiopathic or associated with diabetes mellitus	Intraocular surgery to remove the lens is indicated if retina is believed to be functional
Corneal ulceration	Many causes, including: trauma, foreign bodies, infection (especially feline upper respiratory tract viruses), keratoconjunctivitis sicca (dry eye) Risk of perforation of globe if severe	Treat underlying cause if possible Surgery to promote healing and protect the globe may be indicated (third eyelid flap or conjunctival flap)
Eyelid tumours	Relatively common Particular tumour types are adenoma (benign, usually wart-like in appearance) and squamous cell carcinoma (SCC, locally malignant) SCC are most common in unpigmented skin	Adenoma respond well to local excision SCC require more radical surgery or radiation treatment
Distichiasis	Aberrant lashes growing at the margin of the eyelids	Often insignificant If symptomatic, treated by plucking, diathermy or excision of the follicles
Entropion/ectropion	Rolling in or out of the eyelid margin Cause irritation to the cornea or conjunctiva Often associated with the conformation of certain breeds (Sharpei in particular, but also others with droopy faces)	Variety of plastic surgical techniques to improve the architecture of the lids is available
Conjunctival foreign bodies	Cause of severe or chronic conjunctivitis Grass seeds a common type Careful ocular examination under local or general anaesthesia Important to eliminate in such cases	Removal of the FB

Diseases of the pinna, ear canal and middle ear

Condition	Description	Treatment
Squamous cell carcinoma (SCC) of the pinna	Commonly affects tips of ears of white cats (or those with white ears) Pre-cancerous change of actinic keratosis found prior to SCC Presents as alopecia and crusting of ear tip progressing to ulceration and distortion Often bilateral	Early cases may respond to reducing exposure to sunlight (confinement and sun block) SCC requires surgical amputation of pinna
Trauma to pinna	Can result in marked haemorrhage	Usually heal well following wound management and bandaging First aid includes head bandage to control haemorrhage and reduce effects of head shaking
Aural haematoma	Haematoma formation between skin and cartilage of pinna Usually a canine disease May indicate ear canal disease (check for this)	Managed by drainage and various surgical procedures May respond to drainage and corticosteroid administration Left untreated, distortion of pinna will result
Foreign body within ear canal	Typically grass seeds in summer (usually dogs) Hair accumulations can also cause irritation Results in head shaking and discomfort	Removed with forceps under sedation/general anaesthesia
Acute otitis externa (OE)	Various causes (yeast infection, bacteria, foreign bodies, ear mites) and underlying conditions (atopy, conformation, hypothyroidism, etc.)	Usually respond well to medical treatment Further investigation and surgery may be indicated for resistant or recurrent cases

Figure 6.70 continues ▶

Condition	Description	Treatment
Chronic otitis externa	Usually a result of unresolved acute OE Ear canal tumours, middle ear infection and anatomical abnormalities are also causes	May respond to intensive medical treatment, including ear flushing Surgery indicated in resistant cases
Middle ear infection	In dogs, usually follows otitis externa and managed concurrently In cats, seen as primary disease in young cats	May respond to medical management or require drainage at surgery (ventral bulla osteotomy)
Middle ear polyps (nasopharyngeal polyps)	Almost exclusively cats, usually young Cause signs of middle ear diseases (head tilt, Horner's syndrome, loss of balance), otitis externa (if extending into ear canal) or pharyngeal obstruction (if extending through Eustachian tube into nasopharynx)	Traction and/or middle ear exploration (ventral bulla osteotomy)

Care of patients after ocular surgery

- Where possible, house patients that have undergone ocular surgery in cages without bars, as the patient may cause damage to the eye by putting its nose through the bars
- Manual restraint of patients following intraocular surgery should be gentle so as not to cause an increase in intraocular pressure
- Analgesia for patients following ocular surgery is important as pain or discomfort may cause the animal to rub at the surgical site
- Foot bandages can be used to prevent damage to the surgical site with the front feet
- Elizabethan collars can be used to prevent self-mutilation. Some patients may cause more damage by wearing or trying to remove the collar, so careful patient selection is required.

Ear

Figure 6.70 describes common surgical diseases of the pinna, ear canal and middle ear.

The two commonest types of surgical procedure are treatment of aural haematoma and ear canal surgery for otitis externa.

Treatment of aural haematoma

Most cases of aural haematoma are treated by surgical drainage. Several techniques are described. In all cases an incision is made through the skin on the hairless (concave) surface of the pinna to evacuate the haematoma. Continued postoperative drainage is achieved by placing a drain (Penrose or teat cannula) into the cavity or by excising an ellipse of skin. A series of large mattress sutures may be placed through the pinna to eliminate the dead space. The ear is usually bandaged postoperatively, to prevent patient interference, protect the drain or wound, reduce dead space and prevent the adverse effects of head shaking.

Some cases of aural haematoma are treated by surgical drainage with subsequent infusion of corticosteroid suspension. Commonly, a bandage is applied after such treatment.

Care of patients after ear canal surgery

In the care of patients following ear canal surgery it is important to prevent self-trauma by the patient, as this will lead to breakdown of the surgical site. The way in which each case is treated may vary due to the response of the patient following surgical intervention.

Further reading

Hickman J and Walker RG (1980) *An Atlas of Veterinary Surgery*, 2nd edn. Lippincott, Philadelphia

Slatter D (1993) *Textbook of Small Animal Surgery*, 2nd edn. Saunders, Philadelphia

Swaim SF and Henderson RA (1997) *Small Animal Wound Management*, 2nd edn. Williams and Wilkins, Baltimore

Williams J, McHugh D and White RAS (1992) Use of drains in small animal surgery. *In Practice* 14, 73–81

7 The surgical environment and instrumentation

Cathy Garden

This chapter is designed to give information on:

- The preparation routine required in the operating room before surgery
- The reasons for specialized theatre clothing, the use of drapes during surgery and the different varieties of drapes
- Asepsis and methods of sterilization, including methods of packing for sterilization
- Instrument cleaning and care, including functional checks and methods of identification

Introduction

The care and maintenance of the surgical environment and the instruments and equipment within it is vitally important for the smooth running of all the procedures performed within the operating room. Whether there is a purpose-built theatre with all the latest equipment, or rooms converted into an operating theatre with minimal equipment, there are basic rules that should be followed. The previous chapter covered preparation of the patient; this chapter is concerned with the preparation of the operating theatre, the instruments and the surgical team. General care and maintenance of instruments will also be covered.

The surgical environment

In order to achieve an aseptic technique within the operating theatre, the surgical environment itself must be maintained to a high standard of cleanliness. All efforts to practise aseptic techniques will be wasted if the environment itself is not clean.

It is advisable to have a routine preparation for surgery that is followed strictly whenever surgery is performed. Work schedules may be set out for daily and weekly cleaning routines; this helps to maintain the operating theatre at the appropriate standard.

The following is a guide – some of the points may not be appropriate for all situations but they can be adapted to particular circumstances in order to achieve the best results of cleanliness.

Theatre design and layout

Very few nurses will be able to design their own operating facilities but an awareness of the ideal requirements will assist in the adaptation of existing facilities if appropriate. Consider the following points in the design and layout of the patient preparation and surgery areas.

All areas of the surgical suite should be clearly marked, ideally with coloured floor tape and door signs. This marks areas of restricted access to all members of staff and warns that the appropriate theatre clothing should be worn before proceeding into these areas. The theatre suite can be made up of several rooms, including the preparation room and the theatre.

Preparation room

This is where the induction of anaesthesia takes place and where any preoperative procedures such as clipping, bathing or catheterization are performed before the patient is moved into the operating room. The preparation room should lead into the operating room.

Chapter 1 describes the functional and hygiene standards of the preparation room (such as surfaces, storage facilities, anaesthetic induction and clipping-up equipment, lighting, ventilation and sound insulation) and the necessary cleaning and equipment preparation procedures.

- It is sensible to have an anaesthetic emergency box or crash kit in the preparation room
- The clippers (with surgical blades) and vacuum cleaner to remove loose hair after clipping should be positioned by the table
- Preparation tables incorporating sinks are ideal for cleaning the patient or emptying its bladder prior to surgery
- There should be a sink for cleaning anaesthetic equipment.

Theatre

If facilities permit, there may be more than one room for operating, so that each theatre may be designated for a specific type of surgery – for example, orthopaedic surgery, soft tissue surgery and dirty procedures such as dentistry.

- Ideally, the operating room should have only one doorway so that it does not become an area for through traffic. This doorway must be large enough to allow trolleys or pieces of large equipment into or out of the theatre
- The room should have good natural lighting with additional ceiling lighting, preferably flush mounted
  - Operating lights, usually ceiling mounted, should have maximum manoeuvrability
  - Two lights pointed at the surgical site from different angles give ideal lighting
- The room should be easy to clean, and if possible constructed of impervious materials, with no seams where dust could collect and make cleaning difficult
- There should be minimal furniture and shelving, as these will also collect dust
  - Areas of storage should be located in the preparation or scrub areas
  - If storage cupboards are necessary they should be recessed in the wall or built from floor to ceiling to prevent dust collection. Trolleys are preferred.
- Room temperature is important to maintain the patient's body temperature under anaesthesia and create a pleasant working environment
  - A room temperature of 15–20°C is acceptable
  - Methods of heating vary but fan heaters create dust movement and so should be avoided
- Ideally ventilation should be achieved by using air conditioning; it should not be provided by open windows
- The room should have plenty of splash-proof electrical sockets in appropriate places
- An X-ray viewer, preferably flush mounted, should be available in the theatre
- Near to the theatre there should be a room where patients can recover after surgery, with all the necessary equipment to deal with any post-surgical emergencies (see Chapter 1)
- Scrub sinks should not be located in the theatre itself; ideally they should be in a separate room or in the preparation room.

Preparation of the operating theatre

Cleaning

Daily damp dusting
All surfaces and equipment should be wiped with a suitable disinfectant that is bactericidal, fungicidal, sporicidal and viricidal. The disinfectant should be diluted according to the manufacturer's instructions.

Cleaning between operative procedures
As soon as the patient is removed from theatre and before the next one arrives in the anaesthetic room:

- Remove dirty instruments for cleaning and resterilization
- Wipe over all flat surfaces, anaesthetic equipment, operating table and other equipment that may have become dirty, using a suitable disinfectant as described above for damp dusting
- Clean the floor only if necessary (usually this applies only to the soiled areas around the operating table)
- Reposition the table, heating pad and diathermy plate
- Restock if necessary
- Prepare the instruments and equipment for the next surgery.

Cleaning at the end of the day
Immediately after surgery finishes, the operating room should be thoroughly cleaned. This is best done at the end of the day when no operations are scheduled. This gives any airborne particles, disturbed during cleaning, time to settle before the next procedure begins. At the end of the day the operating room should be ready for use again, either for the following day or in case of any emergencies.

- Clean and resterilize all instruments that have been used during the day, ready for use again when needed
- Thoroughly clean all surfaces, equipment and the floor within theatre, including the scrub sink area
- Restock and refill supplies and drugs as necessary
- Empty and clean all bins and vacuum cleaners
- Wash all drapes and theatre clothing, including boots and shoes worn in theatre.

Weekly cleaning
Weekly cleaning is important to maintain the standards of cleanliness and reach all areas not cleaned in the daily routine. Where possible, this cleaning should include the preparation rooms and changing rooms associated with the theatre.

- The operating room should be emptied of movable equipment, which should be cleaned (including the castors, where appropriate) before it is returned to theatre
- Working from ceiling to floor, all fixed structures should be cleaned – including walls, floors, scrub sinks and drains – using a disinfectant as described above for damp dusting
- Although cupboards are not recommended in theatre, they are necessary in the preparation and scrub areas; all of them should be emptied, cleaned and restocked during the weekly clean.

Preparation of the operating table
After cleaning, the table should be put into position for surgery. Any heat pads, supports and other equipment should be put in place. The operating table is very important to the procedures taking place within the surgery and the positioning of it may be crucial to the success of the surgery.

There are many different types of operating table and they can vary hugely, so it is impossible to describe how to set out a table for each procedure. However, the following points should be considered when setting out the table for surgery:

- The table should be adapted for the correct position of the patient according to the surgical procedure that is to be used
- The table should be of a suitable size for the size of patient
- The height of the table should be easy to adjust to enable it to be positioned correctly for the height of the surgeon
- To make the table more comfortable there should be some sort of padding (preferably anti-static) available for the area where the patient will be recumbent. This will reduce the risk of muscle damage through ischaemia and reduce heat loss from the patient
- Theatre lighting should always be checked prior to the start of surgery.

Preparation of diathermy and anaesthetic equipment
There are two types of diathermy: bipolar and monopolar. If monopolar diathermy is to be used during surgery, the patient must be 'earthed'. This is done by means of a contact plate,

which should be placed in a suitable position, and contact gel should be placed on the plate. Bipolar diathermy requires no contact plate. Figure 7.1 shows how a diathermy unit would be set up for use.

Anaesthetic equipment is discussed in Chapter 8.

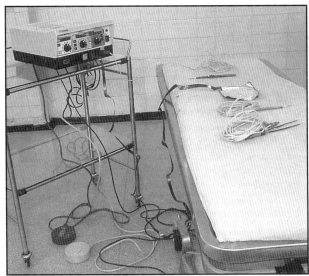

7.1 *Diathermy unit set up for use.*
Courtesy of A. Hotston Moore.

Preparation of other equipment

- Have ready scrub solutions, brushes, towels, gowns and gloves suitable for the surgical team
- Set out skin preparation materials for the patient
- Lay out the instrument trolley and put ready any spare instruments, drapes, swabs and sutures that may be required during the surgery. It is always better to have them close at hand in case of an emergency.

Instrument trolley

The preparation of the instruments (Figures 7.2 and 7.3) is one of the duties performed by the nurse in the immediate preparation for surgery. It should be done in an area of the operating room that is away from the preparation of the surgeon and the patient, and it should be performed in a sterile manner, using a pair of cheatle forceps.

7.2 How to lay out an instrument trolley

1. Use an instrument trolley that is an appropriate size
2. Make sure that it is clean (it should have been damp dusted in the daily preparation for surgery)
3. Cover the base of the trolley with a sterile water-resistant layer such as paper wrap to prevent bacterial strike if the trolley should become wet
4. On top of this put a double layer of sterile linen drapes. (The water-resistant and linen layers may already be wrapped around the surgical kit in such a way that they cover the trolley top when unwrapped.)
5. The trolley is now ready for the instruments. It is most logical to place these from left to right in the order in which they are most likely to be used
6. Sterile extras may be added if necessary, such as swabs, sutures and bowls
7. A sterile cover should be placed over the top of the instrument trolley until it is ready for use (Figure 7.3).

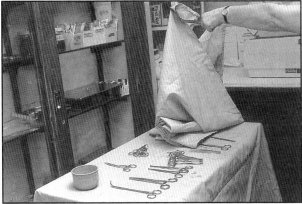

7.3 *Instrument trolley set up and with a sterile cover to protect it until ready for use.*
Courtesy of A. Hotston Moore.

Theatre clothing

Theatre clothing cannot be considered as sterile, but as a permeable barrier to microorganisms. The material should be lint-free, hard wearing and comfortable.

Scrub suits

Most scrub suits consist of top and trousers. Ideally, to reduce the shedding of microorganisms from the skin into the environment, the top should be worn tucked inside the trousers, which should have cuffed legs or be worn inside surgical boots.

To reduce the risk of contamination of the surgical site by organisms on the scrub suit, all scrub suits (particularly those of the surgeon) should be:

- Worn only within the operating room
  - Those worn outside the operating room should be covered
  - They should not be worn outside with the intention of returning to the operating room in the same scrub suit
- Changed at least daily, or more frequently if soiled
- Periodically autoclaved (in a steam autoclave with a drying cycle).

Footwear

Theatre footwear should only be worn within the operating room. Areas of access should be clearly marked with coloured floor tape and appropriate signs, as described earlier. This helps to prevent theatre shoes being worn outside the restricted area and also helps to make others aware that outside shoes should not be worn within the operating room

- Shoes or boots should be anti-static, comfortable and easily cleaned
- Shoe covers can also be used; they should be lightweight, waterproof and durable.

Theatre hats

It is recommended that head covers are worn by all personnel in theatre, as hair sheds particles that may contain bacteria. There are several different types of head cover that can be worn in theatre.

Theatre hats are made of many different materials. They should be lint-free, durable and comfortable and should cover all hair easily.

Face masks

Face masks only cover the nose and mouth. Although studies have shown that the wearing of face masks does not significantly affect the levels of environmental bacteria, they still have a role in the prevention of contamination in the surgical wound.

Most masks give effective filtration of organisms shed from the nose and oropharynx, but it should be noted that these organisms can reach the surgical environment via the sides and bottom of the mask. This can be prevented by wearing a hood-type theatre hat with the sides of the mask incorporated under the edges of the hat.

Face masks can be made of cloth or, more commonly, disposable materials. Disposable masks are made of synthetic and natural materials; they usually have, across the nose, a section that can be shaped for comfort and they have pleats that give greater efficacy.

Surgical gowns

The aim of a surgical gown is to provide a barrier to the transmission of microorganisms. Studies have shown that the use of disposable non-woven materials during surgery dramatically reduces the number of microorganisms isolated from the surgical environment compared with the use of cloth materials (Figure 7.4).

There are basically two types of gown available: those that are tied at the back and those that are wrapped around and tied at the side. The wrap-around gowns are usually made of a disposable material.

Ideally all gowns should:

- Have an overlapping back, to ensure complete sterility
- Have wide sleeves, to allow comfortable movement during surgery
- Be available in a range of sizes to fit all.

Long-sleeved gowns with knitted cuffs or wristlets are preferred. The cuffed part of the sleeves of any gown can act as a wick, so these should be covered by the surgical gloves.

After use, reusable gowns need to be folded ready for sterilization. There are several variations in the method for folding, one of which is described in Figure 7.5. The most important point is that the gown is folded with its outside surface on the inside, to ensure that only the inside surface will be touched when the gown is being put on. (Gowning is described in Chapter 6.)

Disposable non-woven gowns are pre-packed, sterile and folded. Although these gowns are considered sterile, areas that are subjected to more friction, such as the elbows, may become more permeable. It should also be remembered that, during particularly lengthy surgical procedures, the gown will be subjected to more pressure and stretching and will have an increased risk of contamination through moisture strike. To repeat the warning given in Chapter 6: any surgical gown should only be considered as sterile from the surgeon's shoulder to waist, including the sleeves.

Surgical gloves

Surgical gloves are worn as a barrier between the surgeon's hands and the tissues of the patient. They come pre-packed in specific sizes with sterility guaranteed, unless the packet is damaged. They should be chosen to fit snugly but not too tightly. Sterile gloves should be worn for all operative procedures.

Some gloves are lubricated with a fine starch powder that is put on to assist the wearer in the gloving procedure. However, the powder can cause a foreign body inflammatory response which may interfere with wound healing and possibly cause adhesions during the healing process. When using these gloves it is advisable to wash off the powder with sterile water and wipe over with a sterile towel before commencing surgery.

7.4 Reusable and disposable gowns: advantages and disadvantages

	Advantages	Disadvantages
Reusable cloth gowns	Can be washed and resterilized many times, so have long-term use Conforming and comfortable Cheaper to purchase as only initial cost	Not resistant to body fluids so are not considered sterile once wet Time-consuming to wash, fold and resterilize Each time the gown is washed the pore size is slightly increased, further reducing the properties of the material as an aseptic barrier
Disposable non-woven gowns	Lint-free material Resistant to body fluids and water Save time and resources as do not require washing, folding and resterilizing	Less conforming than reusable gowns More expensive as must be continually kept in stock

7.5 How to pack a gown for sterilization

1. Lay the gown on a flat surface with the outside facing up
2. Position the sleeves and ties so that they will be folded within the gown
3. Fold one edge to the middle
4. Fold the remaining edge right over to the other side
5. Concertina the gown from the bottom upwards, leaving the collar on the top.

The folded gown is ready to be packed for sterilization. For convenience, a hand towel is often packed with the gown.

Gowns are usually sterilized by autoclaving, as this is the most practical method. It is also possible to sterilize gowns with ethylene oxide. Autoclaves used for sterilizing gowns or other materials must include a drying cycle in the sterilization process. Items that are wet at the end of the sterilization cycle and then left to dry cannot be considered sterile.

Alternatively, gloves without the addition of powder can be used and should be considered as the gloves of choice particularly when surgery involves delicate tissues, such as ophthalmic procedures.

Even the most rigorous hand scrubbing procedure does not remove all the bacteria. Therefore, if a glove is punctured during a surgical procedure, it should be changed as soon as possible, or another glove should be applied over the top of the first one.

When changing gloves during a surgical procedure, the contaminated glove can be removed by the wearer and replaced by the open gloving method or removed by an assistant and replaced by the closed gloving method described in Chapter 6.

Drapes

The aim of using drapes is to maintain an aseptic technique by reducing the risk of contamination to the wound from the hair of the patient and the immediate surrounding area. Most drapes are made of cloth (reusable) or are paper-based (disposable). Figure 7.6 gives some of the advantages and disadvantages of each type. Some drapes are self-adhesive or have adhesive areas around the incision site.

Drapes should be:

- Readily available, conforming, water-resistant and lint-free
- Cover the whole of the patient
- Have a suitably sized fenestration for the surgery being performed.

Types of drapes

There are basically two different types of drapes, but as these are available in different forms the final choice is more extensive. The two main types are plain and fenestrated.

- Plain: rectangular drapes, placed one at a time at right angles around the surgical site. Four drapes are used to create a 'window' around the incision site
- Fenestrated: a single drape that already has a 'window' prepared in it.

The exact method of draping a patient depends on the available materials, the type of surgery to be performed and the size of the patient. Details of how to drape a patient are given in Chapter 6.

Asepsis

Asepsis is described as freedom from infection. Therefore 'aseptic technique' is the term used to describe all precautions taken to prevent infection arising from contamination of the wound during surgery, which would cause a delay in postoperative wound healing.

The rules of an aseptic technique are that:

- Only scrubbed personnel should touch sterile items
- Non-scrubbed personnel should touch only non-sterile items
- Only sterile items should touch patient tissue
- Only sterile items should touch other sterile items
- Any sterile item touching anything non-sterile becomes non-sterile itself
- If the sterility of any item is in doubt, it should be considered non-sterile.

Sterilization

- *Disinfection* is defined as the destruction of vegetative forms of bacteria, but not necessarily spores
- *Sterilization* is the process of destroying all microorganisms, including spores.

Sterilization can be achieved by several different methods, usually divided into:

- Cold or chemical sterilization
- Heat sterilization.

Heat sterilization can be further divided into wet or dry heat: the addition of moisture destroys the bacteria at a lower temperature and in a shorter time. Hence the most common method of sterilization is the autoclave, which provides moist heat in the form of saturated steam under pressure.

Boiling water does not reach high enough temperatures to destroy bacteria and should therefore only be considered as disinfection.

Methods of sterilization

Heat sterilization

Hot air oven
Sterilization is achieved by exposure to a very high temperature for a long period of time. This is a slow method of sterilization but is useful for items that cannot tolerate moist heat, such as glass, perishable rubber, oils and powders.

7.6 Reusable and disposable drapes: advantages and disadvantages

	Advantages	Disadvantages
Disposable drapes	Water-resistant Impermeable to microorganisms Pre-packed and folded Guaranteed sterility Lint-free	More expensive Often less conforming Large stock needed Less adaptable to size of fenestration
Reusable drapes	Conforming and soft Readily available Fenestration can be easily adapted Cheaper	Not water-resistant Become poor quality with repeated use Time spent washing and folding Sterility not guaranteed after autoclaving in a benchtop model with no drying cycle

It is also suggested that sharp cutting instruments may also be sterilized by this method so as not to damage the cutting edge, with the possibility of rusting; however, a long cooling period is needed before use and the very high temperatures may cause damage to the metal.

Autoclave

This method is commonly used in veterinary practice. The destruction of microorganisms is achieved through applying a higher temperature, by producing steam under pressure. The steam comes into direct contact with the items to be sterilized, penetrating or heating each one to the desired temperature. Figure 7.7 gives temperature, time and pressure combinations.

7.7 Autoclave temperature, time and pressure combinations

Pressure (psi)	Temperature °C	Time (minutes)
0	100	360
15	121	9–15
20	125	6.5
25	130	2.5
35	133	1

Cold sterilization

Ethylene oxide (EO)

Items to be sterilized are exposed to ethylene oxide gas in adequate concentrations at an appropriate temperature and humidity for a sufficient time. The gas diffuses and penetrates items rapidly; after sterilization it diffuses away; therefore objects sterilized with this method should have a suitable time for 'airing' before use.

- It is a very efficient method of sterilization but the gas is highly flammable, explosive and toxic to body tissues
- It can be used for the sterilization of objects that would be damaged by heat sterilization, such as reusable plastic items
- It should always be used with the correct equipment (a plastic container with an attached ventilation system) provided by the manufacturers and with strict adherence to their instructions, so as to comply with COSHH regulations
- Items sterilized by this method must be aired after exposure to the gas, as suggested by the manufacturer.

Radiation

This method is used for items that cannot be sterilized by heat or chemicals. It is not a method used within veterinary practice, although many items used will have been sterilized by this method prior to their supply, such as some suture materials.

7.8 Sterilization and packing methods

Packing materials	Advantage	Disadvantage	Type of sterilization method
Linen drapes	Readily available Conforming Can be used to pack difficult items	Porous Liable to wear Time spent laundering and folding	Autoclave with a drying cycle, or ethylene oxide if not too tightly packed
Paper drapes	Water-resistant so useful as an outer layer to package surgical kits	Non-conforming Can be easily torn	Autoclave with a drying cycle or ethylene oxide
Self-seal sterilization bags	Easy to pack Clear front so able to see contents	Heavier or sharp instruments may puncture the bag (to prevent punctures double packing may be necessary, which increases cost)	Autoclave, ethylene oxide
Nylon film	Cheap Long-lasting Readily available	Punctures easily — punctures are not easily seen so may be missed	Autoclave
Metal tins	Easy to pack Very long-lasting after initial expense Cannot be punctured by sharp or heavy instruments	Expensive to buy Bulky to store Need a large autoclave with a drying cycle	Autoclave, hot air oven
Special polythene bags supplied by the manufacturers of ethylene oxide	Easy to use, strong bags	Must use specific polythene bags with correct equipment Can overpack so gas cannot circulate	Ethylene oxide
Cardboard cartons	Sturdy and not easily punctured by sharp objects Regular shape makes them neat to store	Expensive to buy Can be bulky to store	Autoclave with drying cycle

Method	Comments	Use with
Chemical indicator strips	Show a colour change when exposed to the correct conditions. Should be placed in the centre of a pack before sterilization	
	• Chemical indicator strips: paper strips that change colour when exposed to the correct conditions of temperature, pressure and time. Also available for ethylene oxide	Autoclave Ethylene oxide
	• Brownes tube: small glass tube filled with an orange liquid that changes colour to green when the correct temperature is reached and maintained for the correct length of time. Available for different temperatures	Autoclave Hot air oven
Indicator tape	Tapes are often used as a method of securing other packing methods. Both of these tapes only indicate exposure, not that the correct time or pressure has been achieved. Therefore they cannot be considered as a reliable method for checking sterilization methods	
	• Bowie Dick tape: a beige tape with a series of lines on it that change to black after exposure to a temperature of 121°C	Autoclave
	• Ethylene oxide tape: green tape with a series of lines that change to red after exposure to EO gas	Ethylene oxide
Spore strips	Paper strips that contain a controlled-count spore population. After sterilization the strips are cultured for 72 hours to see if all the spores have been destroyed. The main disadvantage of this system is the delay in obtaining the results	Autoclave Hot air oven Ethylene oxide

Chemical solutions

This refers to the soaking of items to be sterilized in a liquid to kill the bacteria. It should really only be regarded as a method of disinfection rather than sterilization. It is commonly used for cleaning endoscopes. The type of solutions that may be used are based on glutaraldehyde or chlorhexidine.

Methods of packing for sterilization

Many different methods are available for packing instruments and equipment ready for sterilization. Choice will be affected by a variety of factors, the most important of which is probably the method of sterilization to be used. For example, some packing materials suitable for use with an autoclave may not be suitable for use with gas sterilization. Figure 7.8 gives some examples of different packing materials with an appropriate method of sterilization.

Whatever the method used for packing, each pack should be labelled with the following information before sterilization:

- Contents of the pack (e.g. 'large gown', 'general kit')
- Full date on which the pack was sterilized (e.g. '30.5.99')
- Name of the person who prepared the pack for sterilization.

Efficacy of sterilization methods

It is advisable to check the method of sterilization regularly, to ensure that the correct conditions for sterilization have been met. Different types of indicator are available for this purpose (Figure 7.9).

Storage after sterilization

- If possible, sterile packs should be stored in closed cabinets rather than on open shelves: in closed cabinets, storage times are generally longer and there is less chance that the packs will come into contact with water

- The packing method may also affect the length of time the pack can be safely stored before resterilization should be considered
- Any pack that is damaged or becomes wet during storage should be considered non-sterile
- If there is any doubt regarding the sterility of a pack it is safer to consider it non-sterile and to resterilize it before use
- As a general rule, any item not used 3 months after the sterilization date should be resterilized before use.

Instruments

Surgical instruments may be made of either chromium-plated carbon steel or stainless steel.

- Chromium-plated carbon steel instruments are lower in price and are commonly used in practice. However, the surface is susceptible to attack by solutions with a low pH. This makes the instruments prone to pitting, rusting and blistering and they may need replacing more frequently
- Stainless steel instruments are of better quality and are usually more durable, with better resistance to corrosion.

Some stainless steel instruments, such as scissors or needle holders, have tungsten carbide inserts added to the tips of cutting or gripping surfaces. This makes the instruments tougher, with better resistance to wear, but they are more expensive. Such instruments can usually be identified by their gold-coloured handles.

There are many different types of surgical instruments available. It is not necessary to know every different one; it is more important to know the commonly used instruments (Figure 7.10) and it is useful to know instruments used in the practice.

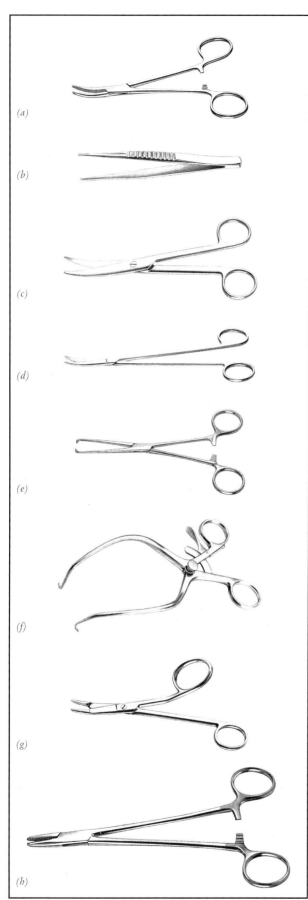

7.10 Examples of commonly used instruments: (a) Spencer Wells artery forceps; (b) Treves rat-tooth dissecting forceps; (c) Mayo scissors; (d) Metzenbaum scissors; (e) Allis tissue forceps; (f) Gelpi self-retaining retractors; (g) Gillies needleholders; (h) Mayo needleholders.
Courtesy of Veterinary Instrumentation.

7.11 Surgical function and instrument examples

Function	Example
Cutting	Scalpel handle and blade
Dissection	Dissecting forceps, Mayo or Metzenbaum scissors
Haemostasis	Artery forceps
Tissue-holding	Allis forceps
Retraction	Gelpi or Langenback retractors
Suturing	Needle holders and suture scissors

7.12 Examples of instrument kits

General surgical kit	Scalpel handle (No. 3)
	Dissecting forceps –
	  rat-toothed fine and plain fine
	Scissors
	  Mayo – straight
	  Metzenbaum
	Artery forceps x 8
	Allis tissue forceps x 2
	Retractors
	  Gelpi
	  Langenbeck
	Probe
	Backhaus towel clips x 6
	Needle holders
	Suture scissors

General eye kit	Eyelid speculum Small scalpel handle (beaver handle) + blade Fine dissecting forceps Fine scissors Corneal scissors Capsular forceps Irrigating cannula Vectis Iris repositor Castroviejo needle-holders
Abdominal kit	**General set +** Self-retaining retractors Long-handled artery forceps x 6 Long dissecting forceps x 2 Bowel clamps x 4
Thoracic kit	**General set +** Periosteal elevator Rib cutters Rib retractors Long-handled artery forceps x 6 Long dissecting forceps x 2 Lobectomy clamps
Orthopaedic set	Periosteal elevator Osteotome Chisel Mallet Curette Hohmann retractor x 2 Rongeurs Bone-cutting forceps

Surgical kits

It is often helpful to have some surgical kits made up ready for use. The contents of these will vary, depending on the type of surgery they are intended to be used with and personal preference.

When making up surgical kits, it is important to remember the size of the animal that the kit will be used with and then assemble instruments for each function (Figure 7.11).

The addition of swabs, bowls of a suitable size and drapes may also be appropriate.

In some circumstances it will be necessary to make up more specialized kits. Figure 7.12 gives examples of a general surgical kit and some more specialized ones.

Instrument care and maintenance

Routine maintenance

There are three stages in the cleaning of a surgical instrument:

- Manual cleaning
- Ultrasonic cleaning
- Lubrication.

Manual cleaning

- Gross visible debris should be removed immediately so that blood and tissue debris does not have a chance to dry in joints and serrations
- The instruments may then be soaked for a short time in warm water (preferably deionized) containing a mild, non-corrosive instrument-cleaning agent
- Next, each instrument should be carefully scrubbed with a small hand brush, paying particular attention to the areas where debris may become trapped
- Finally, the instruments should be rinsed in water – preferably distilled or deionized as this gives a neutral pH and will not leave deposits on the surface of the instrument that might promote corrosion.

Ultrasonic cleaning

Ultrasonic cleaners are very efficient and remove debris from areas that are not accessible to manual cleaning. They work by a process called cavitation, in which minute bubbles form on the surface of the instruments. The bubbles expand until they implode (burst inwards), releasing energy which dislodges debris from the surface of the instrument. After being cleaned in the ultrasonic cleaner, the instruments should be rinsed thoroughly.

Lubrication

Lubrication is essential to maintain the working life of the instruments. Without proper lubrication, all instruments (especially those with box joints) will become stiff and difficult to use. However, unsuitable types of lubricant (such as mineral oil) can leave a film coating on the surface of the instrument, which may prevent adequate contact between steam and the organisms during sterilization.

There are many different types of instrument lubricants available and these are special preparations that do not interfere with steam sterilization. Many also contain anti-rusting agents and antimicrobial agents to inhibit the growth of organisms.

Instrument identification

The marking of instruments is often used as a method of identification for a specific surgical pack. The most suitable method is to use thin strips of a coloured plastic autoclave tape. Engraving the surface of the instrument should be avoided as this causes damage and predisposes the instrument to corrosion.

Routine instrument checking

After cleaning and before sterilizing, all instruments should be inspected to ensure that they are functioning properly. A few simple tests to ascertain condition and function may save time during surgery.

- Check hinged joints for stiffness
- Check the alignment of jaws and teeth
- Check sharp instruments carefully for nicks or burrs
- Check instruments with screws or pins for tightness of the screw or pin
- Check forceps by lightly closing the jaws to see that the tips meet and that there is no overlap
- Check that needle holders will hold a needle without it rotating easily
- Check that ratchets do not easily spring when lightly tapped against a solid object
- Check the tips of towel clips for damage. If the tips are bent out of position they will not hold the drapes in place.

Specialized instrument care

Compressed air machines

These machines should never be immersed in water or cleaned in an ultrasonic bath.

- The machine and air hose should be wiped carefully as soon as possible after use, then dried
- The machine should be oiled before sterilization – the oil recommended by the manufacturer of the machine should be used
- Several drops of oil should be put down the air coupling and around the quick coupling and the triggers
- The machine should then be reconnected to the air supply and run for approximately 30 seconds
- Any excess oil should be wiped off before packing the machine for sterilization.

Motorized equipment

The care of these machines is very similar to that of the compressed air machines. Special attention should be paid to the manufacturer's instructions, as these machines may seize up after repeated autoclaving.

Dental instruments

A good standard of dentistry work relies on good quality, well maintained instruments and equipment. There are two types of dental instruments: hand-held and mechanical.

- Hand-held instruments (such as scalers, picks, luxators and curettes) may have delicate points or tips and should be very carefully washed and dried. Many of these instruments then require sharpening with an Arkansas stone and oil. Autoclaving may then be carried out as normal, although care should be taken to protect delicate tips and points
- Mechanical instruments (such as ultrasonic cleaners and polishers) need regular maintenance. The manufacturer's instructions will give the best guidance for each specific

type of equipment but the following points may be useful:

- Oil the handpiece after each use and before cleaning, by putting two drops in the inlet port
- Regularly remove the turbine from the high-speed handpiece and clean with an aerosol lubricant
- Check filters according to the manufacturer's instructions
- Check compressor and air line for leaks

Suction equipment

- The containers on the suction unit (usually plastic or glass jars) should be emptied, cleaned, disinfected and dried as soon as possible after use, or replaced if the units are designed to be disposable
- An anti-foaming agent is available to put in the jars to prevent foam getting into the mechanics of the machine
- The filters should be changed regularly; the frequency

depends on usage, but monthly (at least) is recommended
- Regular servicing by the manufacturing company is also recommended.

Sutures

There are two main categories of suture materials: absorbable and non-absorbable. These two categories can be further divided into:

- Natural or synthetic
- Monofilament or mutifilament
- Coated or uncoated.

Figures 7.13 and 7.14 give details of some of the commonly used suture materials.

7.13 **Non-absorbable suture materials**

Suture material	Trade name	Mono/multifilament	Synthetic/natural	Coated	Knot security	Duration	Comments
Polyamide (nylon)	Ethilon (Ethicon)	Monofilament	Synthetic	Not	Fair	Permanent	Causes minimal tissue reaction and has little tissue drag
Polybulester	Novafil (Davis & Geck)	Monofilament	Synthetic	Not	Fair	Permanent	Very similar to Ethilon, with similar properties
Polypropylene	Prolene (Ethicon)	Monofilament	Synthetic	Not	Fair, can produce bulky knots that untie easily	Permanent	Very inert, produces only a minimal tissue reaction. Very strong but also very springy. Little tissue drag
Braided silk	Mersilk (Ethicon)	Multifilament	Natural	Wax coat	Excellent	Eventually may fragment and breakdown	A natural material with good handling properties but high tissue reactivity and should not be used in infected sites
Braided polyamide	Supramid or Nurolon (Ethicon)	Multifilament	Synthetic	Encased in outer sheath	Good	Outer sheath can be broken	Better handling characteristics than the monofilament polyamide. Can be used in the skin but should not be used as a buried suture
Surgical stainless steel wire		Available as either monofilament or multifilament	Synthetic	Not	Excellent although knots may be difficult to tie	Permanent	Not commonly used now, but can be useful in bone or tendon. Difficult to handle, may break

7.14 Absorbable suture materials

Suture material	Trade name	Mono/multifilament	Synthetic/natural	Coated	Duration of strength	Absorption	Comments/uses
Polyglactin 910	Vicryl (Ethicon)	Multifilament (braided)	Synthetic	Yes (calcium stearate)	Retains 50% of tensile strength at 14 days, 20% at 21 days	Absorption 60–90 days by hydrolysis	Dyed or undyed Low tissue reactivity Uses: subcutis, muscle, eyes, hollow viscera
Polyglactin 910	Vicryl *rapide* (Ethicon)	Multifilament (braided)	Synthetic	Yes (calcium stearate)	Retains only 50% of tensile strength at 5 days. Provides wound support for 10 days	Absorption is complete by approximately 42 days. Absorbed by hydrolysis	Although this material is the same as Vicryl, changes in the way the material is manufactured make it lose tensile strength and be fully absorbed much faster
Polydioxanone	PDS II (Ethicon)	Monofilament	Synthetic	No	Retains 70 % tensile strength at 14 days, 14% at 56 days	Only minimal absorption by 90 days, absorbed by 180 days. Absorbed by hydrolysis	Good for infected sites as monofilament. Very strong but springy. Minimal tissue reaction. Uses: subcutis, muscle, sometimes eyes
Polyglycolic acid	Dexon (Davis & Geck)	Multifilament	Synthetic	Can be coated with polasamer	Retains 20% at 14 days	Complete absorption by 100–120 days. Absorbed by hydrolysis	Similar to polyglactin, but has considerable tissue drag. Uses: as for polyglactin
Poliglecaprone 25	Monocryl (Ethicon)	Monofilament	Synthetic	No	Retains approximately 60% at 7 days, 30% at 14 days. Wound support maintained for 20 days	Complete absorption between 90–120 days. Absorbed by hydrolysis	A new synthetic suture material. Less springy than other monofilament absorbables with minimal tissue reaction and drag. Available dyed or undyed
Polyglyconate	Maxon (Davis & Geck)	Monofilament	Synthetic	No	Retains 70% at 14 days	Complete absorption by 60 days Absorbed by hydrolysis	Similar to polydioxanone but easier to handle. Uses: also similar to polydioxanone
Chromic catgut		Essentially monofilament	Natural Made from purified animal intestines	Coated with chrominum salts	Retains tensile strength for approximately 28 days	Absorbed by enzymatic degradation and phagocytosis	Always causes a moderate inflammatory response
Plain catgut		Essentially monofilament	Natural Made from purified animal intestines	No	Retains tensile strength for approximately 14 days	Absorbed by enzymatic degradation and phagocytosis	Also causes an inflammatory response and rapidly loses tensile strength

Suture materials

The choice of suture materials will depend on:

- Personal preference
- Type of tissue in which the material is to be used
- Risk of contamination
- Length of time the sutured tissues will require support.

As a general rule:

- Absorbable sutures are used to close internal layers where initial strength is required while tissue healing takes place
- Non-absorbable sutures are used in the skin when they can be removed once sufficient healing of the wound has occurred. They are also used in areas where tissues may be slow to heal and so long-term support of the tissues is required.

Alternatives to sutures

There is an increasing number of alternatives to suture materials that are becoming used more routinely, including staples, glue and adhesive tape.

Staples

There are several different types of metal staples designed for use in different situations. Packed in a gun-type applicator, they are quick to insert. Skin staples are commonly used and are easily removed with the correct staple-removing forceps. Specialized staples can also be used for procedures such as intestinal anastomosis and ligation.

Tissue glue (cyanoacrylate)

These glues, used for skin closure, are designed to give rapid healing. They are usually applied to small superficial wounds.

Adhesive tapes

These are designed for skin closure in humans. The tapes do not adhere well to animal skin and are therefore of limited use in veterinary practice.

Suture needles

Needles vary in design and shape (Figures 7.15 and 7.16). They are available with eyes, through which suture materials are threaded, or with the suture material already swaged on (Figure 7.17). Choice of needle is dependent on:

- type of wound to be sutured
- tissue to be sutured
- characteristics of available needles.

7.15 Shape of needle

Fully curved	• Entire length of needle is curved into an arc • Various degrees of curvature are available • Half circle is most common
Curved on straight/half curved	Sharp end of needle is curved but eye end is straight
Straight	Entire needle is straight

7.16 Design of point and shaft

	Features	Suggested uses
Cutting	• Point and sides of needle are sharp • Triangular in cross section with apex on inside of curve	Skin (other dense tissues)
Reverse cutting	• Point and sides of needle are sharp • Triangular in cross section with apex on outside of curve • Design used with small needles	Skin (other dense tissues)
Round bodied	• Needle is round in cross section with no sharp edges	Delicate tissues e.g. fat; thin walled viscera
Taper out	• Needle is similar to cutting needle at tip • As needle widens, becomes round bodied in design	Dense tissues other than skin e.g. fascia; thick walled viscera; mucous membranes

7.17 Attachment of needle to suture

Swaged-on	• Length of suture is bonded by the manufacturer to a disposable needle • Passes through tissue with less drag than eyed needle • Since a new needle is used each time, it is sharp • Suture is secured to needle • Relatively expensive • Useful for delicate tissues as less traumatic
Eyed	• Surgeon threads the needle at the time of the surgery • Greater bulk of suture at eye increases drag (needle should not be double threaded since this worsens drag further) • Needles are commonly re-used and therefore cheaper • Care must be taken to keep needle joined to suture!

Further reading

Lane DR and Cooper B (1999) *Veterinary Nursing*, 2nd edn. Butterworth-Heinemann, Oxford

McCurnin D (1990) *Clinical Textbook for Veterinary Technicians*, 2nd edn. WB Saunders, Philadelphia

Pratt PW (1994) *Medical, Surgical and Anaesthetic Nursing for Veterinary Technicians*, 2nd edn. American Veterinary Publications Inc., Goleta, California

Slatter D (1993) *Textbook of Small Animal Surgery*, 2nd edn. WB Saunders, Philadelphia

8 Anaesthesia and analgesia

Garry Stanway and Annaliese Morgan

This chapter is designed to give information on:

- The anaesthetic machine – how it works, how to test it before an anaesthetic, how to look after the compressed gas cylinders and how the machine is used
- Anaesthetic circuits – how they work and which is the most suitable circuit for each case
- Vaporizers – how they work and how to use them correctly
- Anaesthetic techniques – premedication, induction and maintenance techniques, including the drugs used and their desirable and adverse effects
- Intubation – how to intubate a patient and how to check that it has been intubated correctly
- Monitoring anaesthesia – what should be monitored and how to assess the depth of anaesthesia
- Anaesthetic emergencies – the kind of emergencies seen in veterinary anaesthesia, how to spot a potential emergency and how to deal with emergencies when they occur
- Analgesia – which analgesic drugs to use and when to use them

Introduction

This chapter looks at the concept of anaesthesia and how it applies to veterinary medicine. The functions of the anaesthetic machine and its correct use are discussed. The different techniques used in anaesthesia and the drugs commonly used in practice are considered. An explanation of what to do in an anaesthetic emergency and the correct use of analgesics is also given.

What is general anaesthesia?

General anaesthesia is defined as reversible insensitivity to pain. The patient should be insensible to noxious stimuli and unable to recall them.

When was anaesthesia invented?

In 1799, Sir Humphrey Davey first noticed that nitrous oxide, when inhaled, produced analgesia and exhilaration. In 1844 an American dentist used nitrous oxide for a tooth extraction and in 1846 Thomas Green Morton used ether to anaesthetize a patient undergoing surgery to remove a jaw tumour. In 1853, chloroform was administered to Queen Victoria whilst she was giving birth to Prince Leopold.

When is general anaesthesia used?

General anaesthesia is used to perform surgery humanely and painlessly on animals. It is also commonly used to facilitate the humane handling of animals. The Protection of Animals Act, 1964 and its amendments makes the use of anaesthesia a legal requirement for almost all operations performed on animals.

How is anaesthesia produced?

The exact mechanism of most anaesthetic agents on the brain is poorly understood. However, there is a variety of drugs available which, when inhaled or injected, induce a state of anaesthesia. They also produce a variety of undesirable side effects. It is possible to use these drugs to produce the desired state of anaesthesia whilst minimizing their side effects. It is important to be aware that anaesthetic agents do have adverse effects and to be prepared to minimize them if they occur.

Anaesthetic equipment

In order to induce and maintain anaesthesia safely, a wide variety of special equipment has been developed (Figure 8.1).

The anaesthetic machine

Most inhalation anaesthetic agents are liquids at room temperature. They are highly volatile and the resulting vapour, when inhaled, has anaesthetic properties. The anaesthetic machine is used to produce the exact mixture of gas and vapour needed by the patient. It consists of:

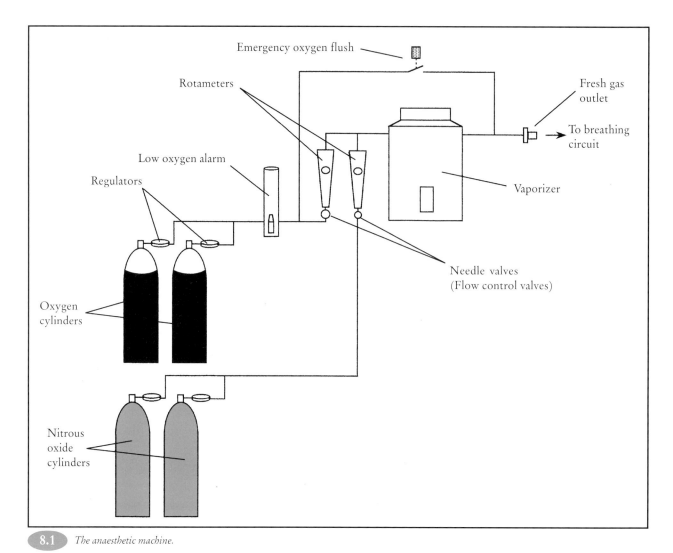

The anaesthetic machine.

- A supply of oxygen
- Regulators to control the pressure of the gas within the machine
- Needle valves and rotameters
- An emergency oxygen flush valve
- One or more vaporizers.

Some anaesthetic machines also include a supply of nitrous oxide and alarms which warn the anaesthetist that the oxygen supply is running low.

Gas supply

- Oxygen cylinders have a black cylinder body and white top
- Nitrous oxide cylinders are blue.

Figure 8.2 describes how to use a piped gas system. Figure 8.3 shows how to change a pin index cylinder; Figure 8.4 explains how to estimate the contents of a cylinder.

The machine
Figure 8.5 sets out how to check the anaesthetic machine and circuits.

Low oxygen warning devices
These devices give an audible warning (and in some cases a visual warning) when the oxygen pressure falls to a dangerously low level.

8.2 How to use a piped gas system

Many veterinary practices use a system of piped gas where the anaesthetic gases are stored in large cylinders and piped to the individual machines. There are a few points that need to be remembered when using such systems.

- The pressure gauges on the machines only show the pressure in the pipeline and not the pressure in the cylinders. In order to estimate the contents of the cylinders, the pressure gauges on top of the cylinders must be consulted
- At the end of the day the anaesthetic machine should be disconnected from the gas supply. This is usually achieved by twisting the metal collar on the supply coupling
- When disconnecting the gas supply, the nitrous oxide should be disconnected first, followed by the oxygen supply
- When connecting the piped gas supply, the oxygen should be connected first, followed by the nitrous oxide.

- Most are driven by the oxygen remaining in the cylinder
- Older alarms are driven by nitrous oxide. With these, it is important to ensure that there is a supply of nitrous oxide to run the alarm. If the nitrous oxide supply fails, the low oxygen alarms will not sound.

8.3 How to change a pin index cylinder

1. Make sure that the cylinder valve is fully closed
2. Undo the screw that holds the cylinder to the yoke and lift up the connecting bar
3. Pull the cylinder off the index pins (be prepared to take the weight of the cylinder)
4. Make sure that the Bodok washer has not come away with the old cylinder
5. Remove the plastic seal that protects the new cylinder
6. In order to make sure that there is no dust in the cylinder valve, open the valve momentarily to release a little gas before fitting it to the machine. (Because of the pollution hazard of nitrous oxide, do this in the open air.)
7. Offer the cylinder up to the yoke and engage it on to the index pins. Use your foot to help to support the weight of the cylinder
8. Close the connecting bar and tighten up the retaining screw
9. Open up the cylinder valve and listen for any leaks. If there is a leak, try tightening the cylinder retaining screw. If this does not work, the leak is most commonly due to a missing Bodok washer or dirt on the washer. Remove the cylinder, check the washer and refit the cylinder. Sometimes turning the washer around can cure the problem
10. Once the cylinder is fitted, open the valve fully and then back it off half a turn. This reduces wear on the valve
11. Check the cylinder pressure gauge to ensure that the cylinder is full
12. Label the cylinder with either a FULL or IN USE label, as appropriate.

8.4 How to estimate the contents of a cylinder

Oxygen

- The pressure in the oxygen cylinder falls proportionately as the gas is used up
- Use the pressure gauge to estimate the amount of oxygen left
- A full oxygen cylinder is at a pressure of 137 bar (13.7×10^3 kPa = 2000 psi)
- A half-full oxygen cylinder is at a pressure of 68 bar (6.8×10^3 kPa = 1000 psi).

Nitrous oxide

When nitrous oxide is compressed in the cylinder, it condenses into a liquid. The pressure above the liquid is constant until all of the liquid has evaporated.

To estimate the contents of a nitrous oxide cylinder:

1. Weigh the cylinder
2. Subtract the weight of the empty cylinder (which is stamped on the valve block)
3. This gives the weight of the liquid nitrous oxide inside
4. Multiply the weight (kg) of the liquid nitrous oxide by 534 to get the number of litres of nitrous oxide left in the cylinder.

8.5 How to check the anaesthetic machine and circuits

1. • If fitted, *turn on the spare oxygen cylinder* and check the pressure gauge. A full cylinder should read 137 bar (13.7×10^3 kPa = 2000 psi).
   • *Turn off the spare oxygen cylinder.* (If the spare cylinder is left turned on at the same time as the in-use cylinder, both cylinders will empty together.)

2. *Turn on the in-use oxygen cylinder* and note the pressure. If the pressure reading is in the red, change the cylinder

3. • If fitted, *turn on the spare nitrous oxide cylinder* and note the pressure reading. It should be 44 bar (4.4×10^3 kPa = 640 psi).
   • *Turn off the spare nitrous oxide cylinder*

4. *Turn on the in-use nitrous oxide cylinder* and note the reading on the pressure gauge. Again it should be 4.4×10^3 kPa. If it is lower than this, the cylinder is nearly empty and should be replaced

   • Note: Whilst checking the cylinders, listen for any leaking gas. Leaks are most commonly due to a faulty Bodok washer

5. • Check the low oxygen alarm: *turn off the in-use oxygen cylinder* and operate the oxygen flush valve. The alarm should sound once the pressure falls to a dangerously low level
   • *Turn on the in-use oxygen cylinder*

6. • Connect the scavenging receiver to the fresh gas outlet
   • Open each rotameter valve, starting with the nitrous oxide, and check that the bobbin or ball rises smoothly and rotates inside the tube
   • Ensure that a good fresh gas flow rate can be produced, by opening the rotameter valves until the rotameters are at their maximum reading

7. Operate the oxygen flush valve and check that you get a good flow of oxygen out of the common gas outlet

8. Check that the vaporizer is connected properly and that it is full. Check that the control valve will operate correctly. If there are several vaporizers on the machine, check each in turn, making sure that you never have more than one vaporizer switched on at one time

9. Check that the circuit you have selected fits your machine. Check the circuit for signs of damage. Pay particular attention to the inside tube in coaxial circuits. Check the reservoir bag for leaks and damage

10. Check that the endotracheal tube you have selected fits your circuit and that it is undamaged. If it is a cuffed tube, inflate the cuff and check for any leaks.

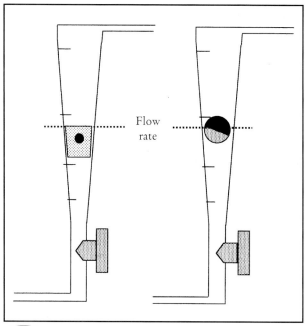

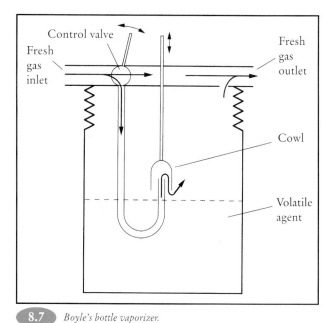

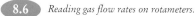
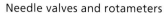

8.6 *Reading gas flow rates on rotameters.*

8.7 *Boyle's bottle vaporizer.*

Needle valves and rotameters

The flow rate is read off the top of the bobbin or through the centre line of the ball (Figure 8.6).

- Never overtighten the control knob, as the valve seat is easily damaged
- The bobbin or ball must rotate freely in the tube. If it does not, the reading will be inaccurate.

Emergency oxygen flush valve

This valve is used to deliver a high flow of pure oxygen to the breathing circuit, flushing the anaesthetic agents out of the circuit and providing the patient with 100% oxygen.

Vaporizers

Uncalibrated

Uncalibrated vaporizers include Boyle's bottle (Figure 8.7) and basic draw-over types

- The output of the vaporizer cannot be predicted. It can be varied, using the control, but it also varies with temperature and the flow of fresh gas through the vaporizer
- Draw-over vaporizers are included in some circle circuits (e.g. Goldman and Komazaroff vaporizers).

Calibrated

Calibrated vaporizers include the 'Tec' and 'Penlon' types (Figure 8.8).

- They are designed to produce a known concentration of anaesthetic vapour regardless of temperature and fresh gas flow
- To remain accurate, they must be serviced annually.

Anaesthetic circuits

The pipework that is used to connect the patient to the anaesthetic machine is called the anaesthetic circuit. Its function is to:

8.8 *Tec and Penlon type vaporizers.*

- Deliver oxygen-rich carrier gas (and anaesthetic vapour) to the patient
- Carry carbon dioxide-rich gas away from the patient
- Deliver potentially harmful waste anaesthetic agents to the scavenging system, which carries them away from the operating theatre.

Figure 8.9 defines some of the respiratory terms used in this section and gives some of the relevant values.

Adjustable pressure limiting (APL) or pop-off valve

The APL valve allows gas out of the circuit without letting air from the atmosphere back in. In order to carry out intermittent positive pressure ventilation (IPPV), it is sometimes necessary to use the control knob to increase the pressure at which the valve opens to let gas out.

Circuit classification

The older classification of anaesthetic circuits was confusing: the same circuit was classified differently, depending on the way it was used. The following simpler classification (taken from *Ward's Anaesthetic Equipment*, Baillière Tindall, with kind permission) is much more useful:

8.9 Definitions of some respiratory terms and their values

Term	Definition	Values
Tidal volume	The volume of gas an animal breathes in during a normal breath	Dog, cat: 10–15 ml/kg
Respiratory rate	The number of breaths an animal takes each minute	Dog: 10–30; cat: 20–30 breaths/min
Minute volume	The total volume of gas breathed in by an animal in 1 minute (= tidal volume x respiratory rate)	Dog, cat: 200 ml/kg/min
Oxygen consumption	The volume of oxygen metabolized by an animal in 1 minute	5–10 ml/kg/min
Dead space gas	Gas that has been breathed in by the animal but has not reached the alveoli and so has not been used in gas exchange. In anaesthesia, this is taken to include the gas in the endotracheal tube as well as any gas within the dead space of the breathing circuit	

8.10 Circuit classification and examples

Classification	Circuits fitting the classification
Non-rebreathing systems (use a valve to control gas flow)	'Ambu bags' (used for resuscitation in situations where a source of compressed gas is not available)
Systems where rebreathing is possible although not intended (with bidirectional flow within the system)	T-piece; Magill; Lack; Bain
Circuits containing soda lime	Circle; to-and-fro

- Non-rebreathing systems (with unidirectional flow of gas within the system)
- Systems where rebreathing is possible, although not intended, (with bidirectional flow of gas within the system)
- Non-rebreathing systems utilizing carbon dioxide absorption:
  - unidirectional (circle) systems
  - bidirectional (to-and-fro) systems.

Figure 8.10 gives examples of circuits that fit these classifications. Figure 8.11 compares some of the advantages and disadvantages of the rebreathing and carbon dioxide absorption systems. Figure 8.12 suggests how to choose a suitable circuit.

Systems where rebreathing is possible
These contain bidirectional flow within the system.

Jackson Rees modified T-piece
The absence of a pop-off valve means that this circuit (Figure 8.13) offers little resistance to breathing, making it especially suitable for small patients. It is difficult to scavenge from, because of the open-ended bag:

- Fresh gas flow rate should be 400 ml/kg body weight per minute (equal to twice the patient's minute volume)
- Suitable for continuous IPPV.

Magill, Lack and parallel Lack circuits
Magill and Lack circuits can be used at lower flow rates than the 200 ml/kg/min usually prescribed. This is because the first gas to be expired by the patient is dead space gas. Dead space gas can be rebreathed as it has not reached the alveoli and so does not contain carbon dioxide. This rebreathing will occur if the fresh gas flow rate is reduced to 170 ml/kg/min.

8.11 Advantages and disadvantages of circuits

Magill, Lack, T-piece, Bain	Circle, to-and-fro
Need high fresh gas flow rates and use relatively large amounts of volatile agent	Very efficient use of anaesthetic agent and oxygen
Very low resistance to breathing and so more suitable for small animals	Not suitable for animals weighing less than 10 kg
Cheap lightweight construction	Expensive to buy
The large volumes of cold dry anaesthetic gases used with these circuits will result in greater cooling of the patient, especially during long procedures	During long procedures, the patient loses less heat and moisture, as warm and moist exhaled gas is rebreathed
The concentration of anaesthetic vapour delivered to the patient is the same as the vaporizer setting	The concentration of anaesthetic vapour being delivered to the patient is not known
Changes to the vaporizer setting are almost immediately followed by changes in the concentration of anaesthetic vapour delivered to the patient	Changes to the vaporizer setting are only slowly reflected in changes in the concentration of anaesthetic vapour delivered to the patient
Can use: – trichloroethylene – carbon dioxide – nitrous oxide[a] with these circuits	Cannot use: – trichloroethylene – carbon dioxide – nitrous oxide[a] with these circuits

a Unless respiratory gas monitoring is available.

8.12 How to choose a circuit

Circuit	Suitable for patients weighing	Suitable for continuous IPPV	Can be used with N₂O	Short procedures
T-piece	< 8 kg	Yes	Yes	Yes
Bain	8–30 kg	Yes	Yes	Yes
Lack	10–60 kg	No	Yes	Yes
Magill	> 8 kg	No	Yes	Yes
Circle	> 20 kg	Yes	No^a	No
To-and-fro	>15 kg	Yes	No^a	No

a Unless respiratory gas monitoring is available

- When thinking about which circuit to use, consider the size of the patient's lungs as well as its weight. A fit young Whippet will have a larger lung capacity but weigh less than an overweight terrier
- Circuit choice for obese dogs should be based on their correct weight and not their actual weight
- Circle and to-and-fro circuits need high fresh gas flow rates in the first few minutes of use and take several minutes to achieve a stable anaesthetic. For this reason, these circuits are less suitable for use with very short procedures.

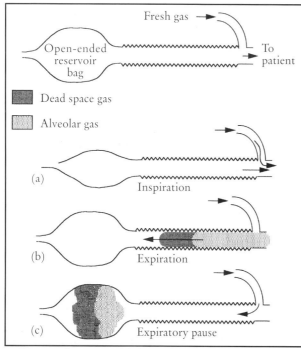

8.13 *Jackson Rees modified T-piece circuit. (a) When the patient breathes in, fresh gas is drawn partly from the fresh gas entering the circuit and partly from the gas within the corrugated tube. (b) During expiration, the exhaled gas is prevented from flowing back up the fresh gas supply tube because of the pressure of the high flow of fresh gas coming into the circuit. All of the expired gas passes into the relatively wide corrugated tube. The first gas to be exhaled is the patient's dead space gas. This is immediately followed by the carbon dioxide-rich alveolar gas. (c) If the expiratory gases were not flushed away by the fresh gas entering the circuit during the expiratory pause, the animal would inhale this stale alveolar gas. To ensure that this does not occur, the fresh gas flow rate needs to be 400 ml/kg/min (using a circuit factor of 2.5). The open-ended bag is used to give a visual indication of the patient's respiratory work and to facilitate intermittent positive pressure ventilation.*

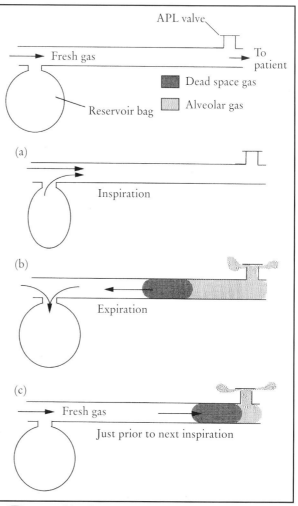

8.14 *Magill breathing circuit. (a) As the animal takes its first breath, it sucks gas out of the circuit. Some of this gas derives from the fresh gas coming in from the anaesthetic machine but, as the animal's peak inspiratory flow is greater than the flow of fresh gas entering the circuit, most of the gas comes out of the reservoir bag. This leaves the bag partially empty. (b) The animal then expires and gas flows back into the circuit. A small amount of pressure is required within the circuit before the APL valve opens. This does not occur straight away. Initially, expired gas travels back down the circuit, forcing fresh gas from within the connecting pipe back into the rebreathing bag. (Some fresh gas from the anaesthetic machine also flows into the rebreathing bag.) Once the bag is full, the pressure in the circuit rises sufficiently to open the APL valve. The remaining portion of the expiratory gas is expelled through this open APL valve. (c) During the expiratory pause, fresh gas from the anaesthetic machine pushes the rest of the expired gas out through the APL, leaving fresh gas in the circuit ready for the next breath. Fresh gas flow rate: 200 ml/kg/min (using a circuit factor of 1.0).*

The Magill circuit (Figure 8.14) is difficult to scavenge from, because of the position of the valve:

- Fresh gas flow rate should be 200 ml/kg/min (equal to the patient's minute volume)
- Not suitable for continuous IPPV.

The Lack circuit is similar to the Magill but the pop-off valve has been moved away from the patient connector and placed near the anaesthetic machine. The parallel Lack (Figure 8.15) and coaxial Lack (Figure 8.16) are identical in operation:

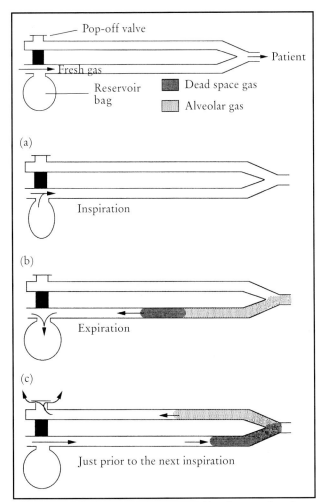

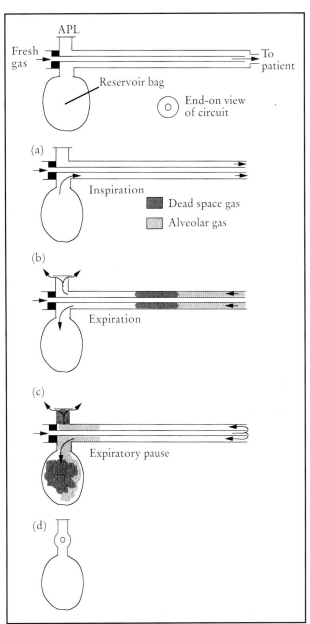

8.15 *Parallel Lack circuit. (a) The animal breathes gas in from the circuit, collapsing the bag. (b) The early portion of the expired gas from the patient flows back towards the rebreathing bag. (c) Once the bag is full, the later portion of the expired gas flows up towards the APL valve. During the expiratory pause, the remainder of the expiratory gas is driven towards the APL by incoming fresh gas. Fresh gas flow rate: 200 ml/kg/min.*

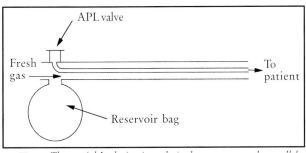

8.16 *The coaxial Lack circuit works in the same way as the parallel Lack circuit, except that the pipes are arranged one inside the other rather than being next to each other.*

- Fresh gas flow rate should be 200 ml/kg/min (equal to the patient's minute volume)
- Not suitable for continuous IPPV.

Bain and T-piece
In these circuits (Figure 8.17) the fresh gas flow rate must be 400 ml/kg/min to ensure that rebreathing of carbon dioxide-rich alveolar gas does not occur.

Non-rebreathing systems utilizing carbon dioxide absorption
For larger dogs and 'large animals', it is more efficient to absorb the carbon dioxide chemically, rather than relying on the fresh gas flow to remove the waste gas from the circuit.

8.17 *Bain circuit. (a) When the patient first inspires, the gas is drawn partly from the fresh gas coming into the circuit through the inner pipe and partly from the outer pipe, causing the rebreathing bag to collapse slightly. (b) During expiration, the first gas to be exhaled is the dead space gas, which is driven up the outer tube towards the APL, followed immediately by the alveolar gas. (c) During the expiratory pause, the exhaled gases are driven up the outer tube and either into the reservoir bag or out of the APL valve (using a circuit factor of 2.5). (d) Section through the reservoir bag and the APL showing how the bag and the valve are connected to the same pipe.*

Circuits containing soda lime
Two systems in which the carbon dioxide is removed chemically are:

- Circle circuit (Figures 8.18 and 8.19)
- To-and-fro circuit (Figure 8.20).

Both types contain soda lime (NaOH), which reacts with the carbon dioxide, removing it from the circuit:

$$CO_2 + 2NaOH = Na_2CO_3 + H_2O$$
$$Na_2CO_3 + Ca(OH)_2 = 2NaOH + CaCO_2$$

Soda lime also contains a chemical indicator which changes colour as the ability of the soda lime to absorb carbon dioxide

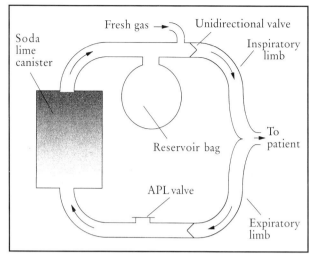

 8.18 *Circle circuit. When the patient breathes in, gas is drawn from the circuit, collapsing the reservoir bag. The one-way valves ensure that the inhaled gas only comes from the inspiratory limb. During expiration, the one-way valves direct the gas down the expiratory limb of the circuit, through the soda lime and back into the reservoir bag. As the gas passes through the soda lime, the carbon dioxide and the soda lime react and the carbon dioxide is effectively removed from the circuit.*

During the respiratory cycle, more gas will have entered the circuit through the fresh gas inlet. Because of this, there will be more gas in the circuit at the end of expiration than there was at the beginning of inspiration. The excess volume of gas leaves the circuit through the APL valve.

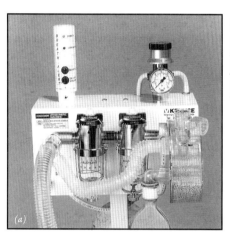

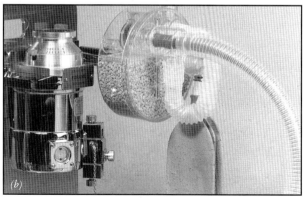

8.19

Circle circuit machines.
(a) With in-circuit vaporizer.
(b) With out-of-circuit vaporizer.

becomes exhausted (Figure 8.21). There are two indicators in common use:

- One in which pink soda lime changes to white
- One in which white soda lime changes to purple.

The expected colour change is indicated on the manufacturer's packaging.

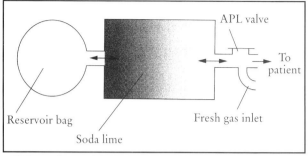

8.20 *The to-and-fro circuit incorporating a Waters' canister. During inspiration, gas is drawn mainly from the reservoir bag and partly from fresh gas coming in from the anaesthetic machine. During expiration, the carbon dioxide-rich exhaled gas is blown back through the soda lime (where the carbon dioxide is removed) and into the reservoir bag. During the respiratory cycle, more gas will have entered the circuit and so the excess gas is vented through the APL valve.*

The layer of soda lime closest to the patient is the first to come into contact with the exhaled gas and so is the first to lose its ability to absorb carbon dioxide. This means that at the end of expiration the very last portion of the exhaled gas does not come into contact with the soda lime. This carbon dioxide-rich gas is rebreathed by the patient with the next breath. Over time, the volume of exhausted soda lime increases, along with the volume of carbon dioxide-rich gas rebreathed. This steady increase in the amount of rebreathing is one of the to-and-fro circuit's major limitations.

8.21 Replacing the soda lime

Soda lime contains an indicator that changes colour as the soda lime's ability to absorb carbon dioxide becomes exhausted. This colour change is most pronounced immediately following use. If exhausted soda lime is allowed to stand for a few hours, its colour regenerates slightly.

Soda lime that appears to be exhausted at the end of anaesthesia should be replaced and not allowed to stand. This ensures that the next person who uses the circuit will not be fooled into thinking that the soda lime is fresh.

> ⚠ Remember that soda lime is caustic. Handle it with care.

Circle circuits

- The soda lime canister in circle circuits should be filled according to the manufacturer's instructions
- Do not partly fill a canister in order to save soda lime. The reaction between the expired gas and the soda lime is not instant. The gas must stay in contact with the granules for a short time. This occurs during the expiratory pause when the exhaled breath is held within the canister. If the canister is not filled, some of the expired gas may only pass through the granules and so have insufficient time to react with the soda lime.

To-and-fro circuits

- When filling the Waters' canister from a to-and-fro circuit it is important that the canister is packed tightly. If it is not, the exhaled gas may be able to pass over the top of the granules and bypass the soda lime
- It is possible to place a pan scourer in the end of the canister in order to hold the soda lime in place.

Figure 8.22 gives some hints on using circle and to-and-fro circuits. In comparing the two types, there are many disadvantages and no real advantages to the latter.

When using a circle or to-and-fro circuit, it is important to note that changes in the inspired vapour concentration only slowly follow changes in the vaporizer setting. The lower the oxygen flow rate, the more slowly the inspired concentration changes.

Therefore if the inspired concentration needs to be changed quickly, *the oxygen flow rate must be increased.*

Timing	Oxygen flow rate (l/min)	Vaporizer setting	Result (%)
Immediately post-induction	4–8	2–3	Washes nitrogen out of circuit and patient
Once anaesthesia is stable	1–2	0.7–2	Low oxygen flow rates produce stable anaesthetic because concentration of inspired anaesthetic vapour will only change very slowly
End of anaesthesia	4–8	0	Oxygen flow rate is increased to wash anaesthetic out of circuit and allow patient to recover

With a circle circuit:

- Unidirectional valves direct the gas around the circuit and through the soda lime
- The circuit's weight is supported by the anaesthetic machine
- There is a large resistance to breathing and so circles are generally not suitable for use with patients under 20 kg.

With a to-and-fro circuit incorporating a Waters' canister:

- Gas passes backwards and forwards through the soda lime as the patient breathes
- As the soda lime is exhausted, the active face moves away from the patient, resulting in an increase in circuit dead space. The patient will rebreathe ever larger volumes of carbon dioxide-rich gas until its own level of carbon dioxide reaches dangerous levels. The volume of dead space could eventually exceed the patient's own tidal volume
- The close proximity of the soda lime to the patient can result in irritant dust being inhaled by the patient.

Reservoir bags

The reservoir bag in a circuit containing soda lime should be of a greater volume than the tidal volume of the patient to which it is connected. In general, for dogs between 15 and 60 kg, a 2 l reservoir bag is suitable.

Circle circuits and vaporizers

It is possible to include a basic uncalibrated draw-over vaporizer within a circle circuit (see Figure 8.19a). This type of machine can be found in many veterinary practices.

Nitrous oxide and soda lime

 Nitrous oxide should not be used routinely with circuits that contain soda lime.

Unlike oxygen, nitrous oxide is not removed from the circuit. Its concentration will slowly increase as the circuit is used.

Consider a situation where nitrous oxide and oxygen are both being introduced into a circuit at a rate of 1 l/min. A 40 kg dog will use 200 ml oxygen/min. However, none of the nitrous oxide will be metabolized. This means that, at the end of one minute, the ratio of oxygen to nitrous oxide will be only 0.8:1 Eventually, the oxygen concentration can become dangerously low. Nitrous oxide can be used if respiratory gas monitoring is available.

Anaesthetic techniques and commonly used anaesthetic drugs

It is easiest to consider drugs in the order in which they are used during a typical anaesthetic. However, because some drugs (such as isoflurane and propofol) can be used as both induction and maintenance agents, drugs will be defined according to their most common usage. For example, isoflurane will be considered to be a maintenance anaesthetic agent and propofol will be classed as an induction agent.

Analgesics will also be considered in this section as they are used both as premedicants and for postsurgical analgesia.

Premedication

Drugs used for premedication are set out in Figure 8.23, and premedicant combinations for dogs and cats are shown in Figure 8.24.

Sedatives

Sedatives calm the induction of and the recovery from anaesthesia. (This is especially important when methohexitone is used as the induction agent.)

Sedatives are often classified according to their pharmacological grouping (Figure 8.25).

Analgesics

Analgesics provide relief from suffering and reduce distress and excitement during the recovery period.

Using analgesics routinely in premedication is a good habit. It should be remembered that the effects of some analgesics are fairly short lived (for example, pethidine only provides analgesia for 1–2 hours and morphine for only 4–5 hours in dogs). It is often necessary to give repeat doses of analgesic throughout the postsurgical period. Analgesics will be discussed more fully later in this chapter.

Neuroleptanalgesia

The combination of a phenothiazine or benzodiazepine sedative with a strong opioid analgesic is called neuroleptanalgesia (Figure 8.26). At low doses, they are useful for premedication. At higher doses, the central depression produced is sufficient to carry out minor surgical procedures.

8.23 Drugs used for premedication

Drug family	Typical use	Drug names
Anticholinergics	Drying agents Traditional use (required when ether is used as maintenance agent) No real justification for routine use with modern inhalation agents Used to treat bradycardias during anaesthetic emergencies	Atropine Glycopyrrolate
Sedatives	Used to calm patient prior to anaesthetic induction Synergistic effect with opiates (neuroleptanalgesia)	Acepromazine Diazepam Alpha-2 agonists
Analgesics	Use prior to surgery prevents spinal cord wind-up[a] and leads to enhanced postsurgical analgesia	Pethidine Morphine Methadone Buprenorphine Butorphanol Papaveretum Carprofen

a When pain is first perceived, the spinal cord pain pathways become overly sensitive to any further pain signals from the same area. With time, this increases the sensation of pain from that region.

8.24 Premedicant combinations

Species	Premedicant	Dose	Combined with	Dose
Dog	Acepromazine	0.03–0.05 mg/kg	Pethidine or morphine or methadone or papaveretum or buprenorphine	1–2 mg/kg 0.1–0.5 mg/kg 0.1–0.3 mg/kg 0.2–1.0 mg/kg 10 µg/kg
	Diazepam	0.1–0.25 mg/kg	Pethidine or morphine	1–2 mg/kg 0.1–0.5 mg/kg
	Medetomidine	10–40 µg/kg		
Cat	Acepromazine	0.03–0.05 mg/kg	Pethidine or morphine or buprenorphine	1–3 mg/kg 0.1 mg/kg 0.01 mg/kg
	Medetomidine	25–80 µg/kg		

8.25 Sedatives

Group/drug	Usage and effects	Contraindications and warnings
Phenothiazine derivatives: Acepromazine	Perhaps the most commonly used sedative premedicant in veterinary anaesthesia	Has been associated with causing seizures. Should be avoided in patients with epilepsy or undergoing anaesthesia for myelography. Boxers particularly sensitive to effects of acepromazine – should be used with caution and at greatly reduced dose in this breed
Benzodiazepines: Diazepam	Used as premedicant for sick patients and to treat seizures Most useful as premedicant when combined with morphine or pethidine	Does not always cause sedation in veterinary species; more likely to cause excitement than sedation in fit dogs, especially when used on its own

Figure 8.25 continues ▶

Group/drug	Usage and effects	Contraindications and warnings
Alpha-2 agonists: Xylazine and medetomidine	Newer sedatives used on their own or in combination with opiates for sedation for simple procedures or as premedicants Medetomidine has specifically licensed 'reversal agent' (atipamezole) which can be used to reverse its effects at end of a procedure, or during anaesthetic emergency	Alpha-2 agonist drugs have profound effects on cardio-vascular system of dogs and cats. Produce extreme bradycardia (heart rate in dogs may fall to below 40 beats/min). Useful but drugs should be used with caution, and avoided in sick or debilitated patients. Alpha-2 agonists reduce required dose of intravenous induction agents by *up to 80%*. (They also increase delay between intravenous injection of an anaesthetic induction agent and its effects being seen.) Great care should be taken when using alpha-2 agonists prior to induction of anaesthesia with intravenous induction agents

8.26 Neuroleptanalgesic combinations

Combination	Comments
Acepromazine and buprenorphine	Common premedicant combination
Acepromazine and morphine	Common premedicant combination
Acepromazine and pethidine	Common premedicant combination
Fluanisone and fentanyl	Commercial mixture used for sedation, used prior to diazepam for anaesthesia in rabbits
Acepromazine and etorphine	Commercial mixture that produces central depression and analgesia sufficient to perform major surgery Etorphine is a very potent drug and even small amounts can be fatal to humans

Routes of administration of premedication

Subcutaneous

- Slow uptake of drugs
- Not reliable in patients that are dehydrated or in physiological shock
- Easy to administer
- Not usually painful.

Intramuscular

- Can be painful
- More reliable uptake of drug
- Most failures due to inadvertent injection into fat
- Difficult in some dogs.

Intravenous

- Technically quite difficult
- Some drugs not suitable for intravenous injection.

Induction

The induction techniques of intravenous injection, intramuscular injection and mask induction are compared in Figure 8.27. Induction agents are listed in Figure 8.28 (intravenous anaesthetic agents) and Figure 8.29 (intravenous and intramuscular combinations for inducing anaesthesia in the cat and dog).

Induction is one of the most dangerous periods of anaesthesia. Cardiac arrest often occurs in the immediate postinduction period and Figure 8.30 describes how to check a patient at this stage, following the 'ABC' steps.

Steps in the intubation and extubation of dogs and cats are set out in Figure 8.31.

8.27 Induction techniques

Intravenous injection

- Produces a smooth induction of anaesthesia
- Dose of induction agent can be titrated so that patient gets just enough to induce anaesthesia and no more
- Most induction agents can only be given by intravenous injection
- Must have good patient restraint.

Intramuscular injection

- Technically easier than intravenous injection
- Must give the induction agents according to patient's weight
- Cannot easily dose to effect
- More suitable for very fractious patients where intravenous injection not possible.

Mask induction

- Can be very distressing for patient
- Significant pollution hazard (ventilate room well to reduce this)
- Induction in anaesthetic chamber useful for small mammals.

8.28 Intravenous anaesthetic agents

Group/drug	Usage and effects	Contraindications and warnings
Barbiturates:		
Pentobarbitone	A medium-acting barbiturate anaesthetic agent Slower onset of action and longer duration of anaesthesia when compared with more modern barbiturates Duration of surgical anaesthesia following single injection is very variable but, on average, lasts 30 min Only commonly used to control status epilepticus and, at a higher dose, for humane euthanasia	Use with caution in weak or toxaemic subjects Like thiopentone, extravascular injection will cause severe tissue reactions Can take between 6 and 18 h for dogs to make a complete recovery from this drug. Cats may take as long as 72 h to make a complete recovery There may be excitement on induction as the drug is slow to cross the blood–brain barrier
Thiopentone	Short acting. A single intravenous dose induces around 20 min anaesthesia in the dog Recovery from anaesthesia is mainly through redistribution of the drug into the patient's fat and not through metabolism Available in a number of concentrations: 2.5% (25 mg/ml) concentration should be used in small animals; 1.25% (12.5 mg/ml) is more suitable for use in very small dogs and cats	Can cause severe injury including skin slough if injected extravascularly Unstable in solution. Made up from crystalline form with sterile water. Made-up solutions should be kept refrigerated and any unused portion should be discarded after 24 h Prolonged recoveries seen in Greyhounds and other sight hounds; the drug should be avoided in these breeds Not suitable for use in puppies and kittens under 3 months of age Thiopentone is cumulative and so is not suitable for use as a maintenance agent
Methohexitone	Short acting. A single injection of methohexitone induces around 10 min anaesthesia Twice as potent as thiopentone Irritant if injected extravascularly Will often cause brief period of apnoea following induction of anaesthesia More rapidly metabolized and so not as cumulative as thiopentone. Further small doses can be given to prolong anaesthesia. Safe to administer a total maintenance dose equal to half the induction dose in small boluses as required	Quality of recovery is very dependent on the premedication used. Excitement seen in patients that have *not* been given a sedative premedicant Like thiopentone, unstable in solution and so any reconstituted methohexitone should be discarded after 24 h

Figure 8.28 continues ▷

Group/drug	Usage and effects	Contraindications and warnings
Steroids:		
Alphaxalone and alphadolone	A combination of these two steroids is marketed as 'Saffan'® When given intravenously it produces around 10 min anaesthesia Saffan can be administered by the intramuscular route but the volume needed can be very large. The combination is non-irritant if given extravascularly Saffan is licensed for the induction of anaesthesia in cats, ferrets and goats. It is suitable for use in a variety of exotic species	The two steroids are not soluble in water and the preparation contains the solvent, Cremophor EL, which causes severe anaphylaxis in dogs, making the drug *unsuitable* for use in this species Also results in histamine release in cats which can cause swelling of paws and ears. Laryngeal oedema may occur in some cats anaesthetized with Saffan
Dissociative anaesthetic agents	Produce light plane of anaesthesia along with profound analgesia. Animal appears dissociated from surroundings and procedure being carried out	
Ketamine	Used on its own, produces profound muscle rigidity. Used in combination with alpha-2 agonists, opioid analgesics and benzodiazepines to produce anaesthesia in dogs, cats and small exotics such as rabbits and small rodents Used with alpha-2 agonists for the induction of anaesthesia in horses	Not suitable for use in animals with impaired renal or hepatic function
Tiletamine	Similar to ketamine Available premixed with zolazepam (a benzodiazepine) in USA and Australia	
Substituted phenol		
Propofol	Marketed as milky-white emulsion in soya bean oil, egg phosphatide and glycerol Intravenous injection results in a rapid induction of anaesthesia which, if not maintained with inhalation agents or further increments of propofol, lasts about 15–20 min Rapidly metabolized in liver and elsewhere in body. Animals with impaired liver function less likely to experience prolonged recoveries when given propofol Because of rapid metabolism, it is non-cumulative and can be used as a maintenance agent	Some individuals develop severe muscle twitches after prolonged use Following intravenous injection, transient fall in blood pressure and brief period of apnoea Does not contain any preservative. Any part-used vials should be disposed of after use Does not produce prolonged anaesthesia in Greyhounds and other sight hounds

8.29 **Intravenous and intramuscular combinations for inducing anaesthesia in the cat and dog**

Species	Combination	Dose	Route
Cat	Medetomidine with ketamine and butorphanol	40 µg/kg 1.25–2.5mg/kg 0.1 mg/kg	Intravenous injection
	Medetomidine with ketamine and butorphanol	80 µg/kg 5 mg/kg 0.4 mg/kg	Intramuscular injection
	Medetomidine with ketamine	80 µg/kg 2.5–5 mg/kg	Intramuscular injection
	Diazepam with ketamine	0.1–0.25 mg/kg 5 mg/kg	Intramuscular injection
Dog	Xylazine followed 10 min later by ketamine	1–2 mg/kg 5 mg/kg	Intramuscular injection

8.30 How to check the patient following the induction of anaesthesia

Induction is one of the most dangerous periods of anaesthesia. Cardiac arrest often occurs in the immediate postinduction period. There is a lot going on in the theatre following the induction of anaesthesia and an arrest can easily be missed. By carrying out the following 'ABC', any problems will be quickly noticed.

Airway
Intubate the patient and check that the endotracheal tube is correctly positioned.

Breathing
Watch the patient's chest and the reservoir bag of the breathing circuit to see whether the patient is breathing or not. There is often a short period of apnoea following the induction of anaesthesia with thiopentone or propofol. If this occurs, ventilate the patient until spontaneous respiration returns.

Circulation
Check that the patient has a pulse. The femoral and lingual pulses are easy to check but remember to check more peripheral pulses such as the carpal or dorsal pedal artery. These give a much better idea of the adequacy of the peripheral perfusion.

Intubation
Before intubation is possible, the patient must be sufficiently deeply anaesthetized to abolish any gag reflex. Intubation should be possible if:
- The patient's jaw tone is relaxed

- The patient's tongue can be pulled out of the mouth without any resistance
- Attempts to introduce the endotracheal tube into the patient's oropharyngeal region do not result in swallowing or gagging movements.

8.31a How to intubate

Dogs

- The dog is positioned in ventral or lateral recumbency
- An assistant holds the dog's head, supporting it behind the ears with the left hand and pointing the dog's nose upwards
- The tongue should be gently pulled rostrally until it is fully extended and the larynx can be visualized (ensuring that the tongue lies between the two lower canine teeth) and the mouth opened by pulling down gently on the tongue
- Use a suitably sized and lubricated endotracheal tube to push the soft palate dorsally, away from the epiglottis. (This is not always necessary.) The epiglottis is then pushed down with the end of the tube, which is gently inserted between the vocal folds
- A laryngoscope is useful for brachycephalic dogs.

Cats

- The cat is positioned in ventral or lateral recumbency
- A laryngoscope makes intubation in cats much easier
- An assistant holds the cat's head, extending its neck and supporting it behind its ears
- The cat's tongue should be gently pulled rostrally until it is fully extended and the larynx can be visualized (ensuring that the tongue lies between the two lower canine teeth). Be very careful not to damage the delicate frenulum whilst doing this
- Hold the cat's tongue between the thumb and first finger and hold the laryngescope with the other fingers. This leaves the other hand free to manipulate the endotracheal tube
- The tip of the laryngoscope blade should be used to press down on the cat's tongue just rostral to the epiglottis. It should not be used to push down the epiglottis itself

- The larynx must be desensitized with a local anaesthetic spray and a few minutes allowed for the local anaesthetic to work
- A lubricated tube is gently passed between the laryngeal folds. This is made easier by observing the movement of the laryngeal folds as the cat breathes. The tube should be inserted during inspiration, whilst the vocal folds are open.

Checking the position of the tube and inflating the cuff

- Ventilate the patient with 100% oxygen, using the breathing circuit, whilst observing the chest wall. The chest wall should move as pressure is applied to the reservoir bag. If this is not visible, it may be necessary to palpate the chest to feel the movement
- If the tube is correctly positioned, the cuff can be inflated. Only inflate it sufficiently to prevent oxygen from escaping around the cuff. Overinflation can damage the tracheal mucosa or occlude the tube.

Tying the tube in place

- In order to reduce the risk of accidental extubation, the endotracheal tube can be tied in place with a piece of material such as a bandage
- The tie should be fastened around the end of the tube, over the plastic connector. The connector supports the wall of the tube and ensures that the tube does not collapse as the tie is pulled tight
- The material is then fastened behind the patient's head, muzzle or mandible to secure the tube in place
- Ensure that any knot used to fasten the tube in place is easily released in the event of an emergency. A simple bow is best, because people are familiar with it and know how to release it in an emergency.

8.31b How to extubate

- The cuff should be left inflated until just before the tube is removed
- During oral surgery some fluid may go around the endotracheal tube and down the trachea. In dogs, the endotracheal tube can be removed with the cuff partially inflated. This removes a lot of the debris from the proximal trachea
- Dogs should be extubated once their gag reflex has returned
- Cats should be extubated *before* their gag reflex returns (if a cat gags on an endotracheal tube, the trauma to the laryngeal mucosa can cause laryngeal oedema)
- The endotracheal tube should always be removed gently in a downward arc, so as to avoid damage to the larynx or trachea.

Maintenance

Most of the modern anaesthetic induction agents only produce a short period of anaesthesia. If the procedure is going to require a longer anaesthetic, a maintenance agent is used.

Most maintenance agents are inhalation anaesthetic agents (Figure 8.32) but some intravenous anaesthetic agents can be used for maintenance; each type has advantages and disadvantages.

With an intravenous agent:

- No special equipment is needed (but catheters should be used to provide good venous access and oxygen supplied)
- There is no pollution hazard
- Once given, it cannot be taken back (risk of overdose).

With an inhalation agent:

- An anaesthetic machine is required
- There is a potential pollution hazard
- The anaesthetic vapour can be taken back by ventilating the patient with 100% oxygen (overdose potentially reversible).

Anaesthetic gases

Oxygen

- Oxygen is essential for supporting life. It is administered at concentrations of between 33 and 100%
- Oxygen strongly supports combustion. It forms an explosive mixture with some flammable anaesthetic agents, especially ether.

Carbon dioxide

- As an anaesthetic, this gas is mainly of historical interest
- Over-enthusiastic IPPV can cause hypocapnia. The addition of 5% carbon dioxide to the carrier gas will prevent this from occurring.

8.32 Inhalation anaesthetic maintenance agents

Inhalation agent	Usage and effects	Contraindication and warnings
Ether	Mainly of historical interest Premedication with atropine reduces ether-induced tracheal secretions	Major disadvantage is explosion hazard Causes upper respiratory tract irritation
Methoxyflurane (of historical interest only)	Very soluble, so slow recovery Not very volatile: vapour concentrations sufficient to induce anaesthesia cannot be achieved, hence cannot be used as induction agent Good analgesic: high solubility means analgesic properties last well into recovery period	Do not use with patients with renal impairment: its metabolites have been implicated with renal toxicity Do not use in patients that have been given flunixin – will lead to severe kidney damage Produces less cardiovascular depression than halothane
Halothane	Relatively low solubility produces more rapid recovery from anaesthesia compared with methoxyflurane	Produces dose-dependent fall in cardiac output and blood pressure as well as depressing respiration Sensitizes heart to dysrhythmic effects of adrenaline High levels of adrenaline often occur following stressful induction of anaesthesia, in which circumstances fatal cardiac dysrhythmias may be seen. This situation is made even worse if thiopentone has been used as the anaesthetic induction agent
Isoflurane	Less soluble than halothane and therefore produces even more rapid induction of and recovery from anaesthesia Can be used as both induction and maintenance agent Very useful for anaesthetic induction in exotic animals	Produces less severe myocardial depression than halothane (but overall fall in blood pressure similar, due to more profound peripheral vasodilation) Does not sensitize heart to adrenaline as much as halothane, therefore fewer cardiac arrhythmias
Enflurane	Isomer of isoflurane Very similar properties to isoflurane but less popular	Produces seizure-like electrical activity in brain: should be avoided in patients suffering from epilepsy
Sevoflurane and desflurane	Extremely insoluble agents whose effects on veterinary species are still being evaluated	

Nitrous oxide

- Nitrous oxide is a weak anaesthetic agent but has very good analgesic properties
- Synergy with volatile anaesthetic agents reduces the amount of volatile agent needed to maintain anaesthesia
- Nitrous oxide diffuses into gas-filled spaces within the body more quickly than nitrogen diffuses out of them. This means that these spaces can become very distended with gas. For this reason, nitrous oxide should not be used in cases of:
  - gastric dilation and volvulus syndrome
  - uncorrected pneumothorax
  - any other case where there might be a potential gas-filled space
- Because nitrous oxide is not removed by soda lime, it is not suitable for use in the circle circuit or the Waters' to-and-fro canister (unless respiratory gas monitoring is available)
- The uptake of a volatile anaesthetic agent at the beginning of anaesthesia is more rapid if nitrous oxide is included in the carrier gas. This is known as the second gas effect (see *BSAVA Manual of Advanced Veterinary Nursing*, Chapter 3)
- At the end of anaesthesia, nitrous oxide leaving the circulation can displace enough air from the patient's lungs to produce a condition known as diffusion hypoxia. To avoid it, the patient should be allowed to breath 100% oxygen for 2–5 minutes after the nitrous oxide has been turned off
- Nitrous oxide is a significant contributor to theatre pollution.

End of anaesthesia

Steps to be taken at the end of anaesthesia are outlined in Figure 8.33.

Anaesthetic accidents and emergencies

There are many things that can go wrong during anaesthesia. Most can be prevented by good forethought and preparation. The outcome of emergencies depends very much on their early detection, quick and accurate diagnosis and swift treatment.

Observation of the patient is essential if emergencies are to be detected quickly. It is one thing to notice that an anaesthetized animal has stopped breathing, but good monitoring will detect the early warning signs of slowed respiratory rate and reduced depth of respiration, allowing the problem to be corrected before respiratory arrest occurs.

An anaesthetic emergency is anything that poses an immediate threat to the patient's life. The signs of some of

---

8.33 **What to do at the end of anaesthesia**

- Do not allow the depth of anaesthesia to lighten before the end of surgery. It is not ethical to allow a patient to come round as the last skin suture is being placed
- Switch off the vaporizer and the nitrous oxide once the surgery is *finished*. If nitrous oxide has been used, allow the patient to breath 100% oxygen for a couple of minutes to prevent diffusion hypoxia. (Do not forget to increase the flow of oxygen in order to compensate for the reduction in total fresh gas flow being delivered to the circuit.)
- Before disconnecting the patient from the breathing circuit, flush the circuit with oxygen to wash any trace of anaesthetic vapour or nitrous oxide into the scavenging system
- Monitor the patient carefully during the recovery period. Animals are often neglected at this time as everyone is busy with the next patient. (For more details, see section on monitoring.)
- After the last anaesthetic of the day, switch off the gas supply to the machine, clean and put away the circuits and endotracheal tubes and wipe down the anaesthetic machine surfaces with a suitable disinfectant.

8.34 **Anaesthetic emergencies**

Emergency	Signs	Action
Respiratory obstruction	Patient will make extreme respiratory efforts that do not result in any movement of reservoir bag Cyanosis Eventually cardiac arrest	Find and remove obstruction (make sure patient's mouth is safely gagged before trying to remove foreign bodies) Intubate and ventilate with 100% oxygen If obstruction cannot be removed but involves laryngeal/oropharyngeal region perform emergency tracheotomy
Bradycardia	Very slow heart rate	Commonly due to anaesthetic overdose Ventilate with 100% oxygen Use vagolytic agents such as atropine and glycopyrrolate
Apnoea/respiratory arrest	Reservoir bag stops moving No respiratory effort from patient Cyanosed mucous membranes Dilated pupils	Most commonly due to anaesthetic overdose, so ventilate with 100% oxygen Respiratory stimulants may be useful but can have severe side effects
Cardiac arrest	Lack of femoral pulse Dilated pupils Usually (but not always) accompanied by respiratory arrest Pupillary dilation Agonal breathing	Start aggressive CPR

8.35 Drugs used in anaesthetic emergencies

Drug	Effect	Indication	Dose
Adrenaline (epinephrine)	Stimulates heart and increases systolic blood pressure	Cardiac arrest Unresponsive hypotension	0.05–0.1 mg/kg 1 ml of 1:1000 solution per 10 kg i.v., intratracheal or intracardiac
Atropine	Vagolytic	Bradycardia	0.02–0.05 mg/kg 1 ml of 0.6 mg/ml solution per 15 kg
Dobutamine	Increases cardiac output	Hypotension	1–5 µg/kg/min
Lignocaine	Stabilizes myocardium	Used to treat ventricular premature contractions and ventricular tachycardia	Dogs 1–6 mg/kg intravenous bolus 1 ml of 2% solution per 10 kg Cats 0.25–1.0 mg/kg intravenous bolus 0.1 ml of 2% solution per 4 kg cat
Dexamethasone	Anti-inflammatory	Often used after successful CPR	1–2 mg/kg
Atipamazole	Alpha-2 antagonist	Used to reverse sedative effects of alpha-2 agonists	Dogs 0.05–0.2 mg/kg i.m. Cats 0.5 mg/cat i.m.

8.36 Anaesthetic accidents

Accident	Signs and symptoms	Action
Drug overdose	Apnoea/hypoventilation Cardiac arrest Severe CNS depression	Turn off vaporizer Ventilate patient with 100% oxygen If cardiac arrest has occurred, start CPR If drug has reversal agent, use it Institute fluid therapy at high flow rates (10 ml/kg/hour)
Extravascular injection of thiopentone	Swelling around vein as thiopentone is injected Pain on injection	Dilute thiopentone by injecting 2–10 ml of sterile water or 2% lignocaine around vein and massage well

8.37 Antidotes to some anaesthetic drugs

Drug type/examples	Antidote(s)
Alpha-2 agonists: xylazine, detomidine, medetomidine, romifidine	Atipamezole (Antisedan®) Dogs 0.05–0.2 mg/kg i.m. Cats 0.5 mg/cat i.m.
Pure µ agonist opioids: morphine, pethidine, fentanyl, alfentanyl, etorphine, papaveretum (Omnipon®)	Naloxone 0.04–1 mg/kg i.m., i.v., s.c. Buprenorphine 6–10 µg/kg i.m.
Small animal Immobilon®[a]	Diprenorphine (Revivon®) 0.015–0.03 mg/kg i.v. Naloxone 0.015–0.04 mg/kg i.v., i.m., s.c., i.t.

a In case of possible accidental absorption or injection of Immobilon® in humans, before calling the emergency services administer 0.8–1.2 mg of naloxone (2–3 ml Narcan®) by intravenous or intramuscular injection. Repeat dose every 2–3 minutes until the symptoms are reversed. Maintain respiration and heart beat until emergency services arrive. If naloxone is not available, Revivon® may be used in humans.

these emergencies, along with the action to be taken, are given in Figure 8.34. Drugs used in emergencies are tabled in Figure 8.35.

Anaesthetic accidents (Figure 8.36) often occur due to human error. Drug overdose is quite a common mistake. The most important thing is to realize that a mistake has been made and set about correcting it. When a drug overdose is accidentally given, it may be possible to administer another drug that acts as an antidote (Figure 8.37).

Cardiac arrest

Anaesthetic emergencies and some accidents can ultimately lead to cardiac arrest. The heart stops pumping blood to the essential organs and the patient is brain dead within 4 minutes.

Cardiopulmonary resuscitation (CPR, Figure 8.38) is aimed at maintaining a flow of oxygenated blood to the brain in order to keep the animal alive whilst the cause of the arrest is corrected.

Special techniques in anaesthesia

Local anaesthesia

In large animals, where general anaesthesia is risky, local anaesthetics are used for a variety of surgical procedures. In small animal practice they tend to be used to complement

How to perform cardiopulmonary resuscitation (CPR)

 Switch off any anaesthetic agents that are being administered to the patient. Turn off the vaporizer and the nitrous oxide, and increase the flow of the oxygen. Purge the circuit of anaesthetic by flushing it, using the oxygen flush valve.

Use the mnemonic ABCD to remember the correct approach to CPR.

Airway

- Check to see that the patient's airway is patent
- Do not presume that an endotracheal tube coming from the patient's mouth means that it has a patent airway. Check the tube to make sure it is not blocked and that it is correctly positioned within the trachea
- If the patient is not intubated, intubate it if possible
- In some circumstances an endotracheal tube may not be available. It is possible to ventilate a patient adequately using a snug-fitting face mask or mouth-to-muzzle 'kiss of life'.

Breathing

- The animal must be ventilated with 100% oxygen at a rate of 20–30 breaths per minute.

Circulation

- Check the patient's pulse. Note its quality and rate
- If pulse is absent, thoracic massage must be started at a rate of 60–80 compressions per minute
- When performing thoracic massage, the aim is to compress the whole of the chest. Press down on the chest at its widest point, not over the heart
- If possible, place a compression bandage around the dog's abdomen to increase the return of blood to the heart, resulting in a greater cardiac output
- If thoracic massage is working, it should be possible to feel a reasonable femoral or sublingual pulse.

Drugs

- Drugs are administered once a good cardiac output is being generated by the thoracic massage. A list of drugs used in CPR is given in Figure 8.35
- Provided that the thoracic massage is producing a good cardiac output, intravenous injection is the best route for the administration of emergency drugs
- If venous access is not available, many drugs can be given by the intratracheal or intracardiac routes.

general anaesthesia – either as the analgesic component of balanced anaesthesia or to provide analgesia in the postsurgical period – rather than as the sole agents for surgery. Local anaesthetic techniques and their common uses are described in Figure 8.39.

Neuromuscular blocking agents

Although volatile agents all produce a degree of muscle relaxation at normal concentrations, it may not be enough for certain procedures. If a greater degree of muscle relaxation is required, specific neuromuscular blocking agents are used. These act directly on the neuromuscular junction to stop the transmission of motor nerve impulses to striated muscle. The drugs are classified as either depolarizing or non-depolarizing agents (Figure 8.40).

When are neuromuscular blocking agents useful?

High-risk cases
Using neuromuscular blocking agents reduces the amount of volatile anaesthetic agent required to produce

8.39 Local anaesthetic techniques

Technique	Description	Common use
Topical	Local anaesthetic can be applied directly to moist mucous membranes. Absorbable gel containing local anaesthetic is available for use on skin	Applied to the eye to facilitate ocular examination Local anaesthetic cream can be placed over site of intended venous puncture, much less traumatic for patient
Local infiltration	Site of surgery is infiltrated with local anaesthetic	Typically used to suture small wounds
Regional analgesia	Nerves innervating region where surgery is to be performed are blocked by injecting local anaesthetic into tissues surrounding them as they run close to surface	Cornual nerve block used to desensitize horn buds of calves prior to disbudding
Intravenous regional analgesia	Tourniquet placed around limb and local anaesthetic introduced into one of distended veins beneath; local anaesthetic blocks conduction of nerves running in close proximity to veins; results in extremely good analgesia of distal portion of limb while tourniquet remains in place	Used to allow surgery on feet of cattle and occasional limb surgery in dogs
Epidural analgesia	Local anaesthetic can be introduced into fat surrounding spinal cord: blocks nerves as they leave spinal canal, resulting in loss of sensation and motor activity in region of body supplied by affected nerves	Very useful for providing analgesia to anus, perineum and hindlimbs of animals undergoing surgery

Common neuromuscular blocking agents

Group/drug	Usage and effects	Contraindications and warnings
Depolarizing agents:		
Suxamethonium	Very short acting Only of historical interest now	Associated with muscle pain on recovery
Non-depolarizing agents:		
Pancuronium	Only of historical interest now	Long duration of action and cumulative, so top-up doses cannot be used May produce tachycardia in dogs and cats
Vecuronium	Intermediate duration of action (30 min in dog and cat) Non-cumulative Very popular agent but being replaced in most situations by atracurium	
Atracurium	Intermediate duration of action (30–40 min in dog and cat) Major advantage: breaks down spontaneouslyinside body Can be used in animals with poor kidney and liver function	Inactivated by contact with thiopentone and other alkaline solutions Ensure any intravenous catheters flushed thoroughly before using them to administer

surgical anaesthesia. This reduces the degree of cardiovascular depression produced by the volatile anaesthetic agents.

Oesophageal foreign bodies
The oesophagus in the dog contains some striated muscle. Neuromuscular blocking agents can make the removal of an oesophageal foreign body easier.

Corneal surgery
During surgical anaesthesia the eye is rotated ventrally, making corneal surgery impossible. Neuromuscular blocking agents bring the eye back to a central position.

Orthopaedic surgery
Some dislocations can be easier to reduce following the administration of neuromuscular blocking agents. However, these agents do not make the reduction of fractures any easier.

Thoracic surgery
By reducing the muscle tone of the intercostal muscles, access to the thorax is made easier. The intercostal muscles are less severely damaged by the rib retractors, resulting in less postsurgical pain.

8.41 Types of analgesic

Opioids

- Bind to specific receptors within spinal cord
- Use of some opioids restricted by law.

Non-steroidal anti-inflammatory drugs

- Block production of inflammatory mediators
- Also block kidney's self-protection mechanisms – should not be used prior to anaesthesia as this can lead to kidney damage

Analgesia
Analgesia was mentioned earlier in the section on premedication. Using an analgesic before inflicting pain on a patient will produce better analgesia than using it after the event. Types of analgesic are described in Figure 8.41.

Analgesia is very important in veterinary anaesthesia:

- Animals do not have the ability to explain that they are in pain. It is up to us to make sure that they do not suffer following surgery
- It is more humane to use analgesics than not to use them
- Animals eat sooner and recover more quickly if given analgesics following surgery
- Animals do not always show that they are in pain. It is best to assume that they are, rather than wait for signs of distress (Figure 8.42).

Opioid analgesics
Opioid analgesics are subject to abuse and are physically addictive. Because of this, their purchase, storage and use are strictly controlled and detailed records must be kept.

Opioid analgesics bind to specific receptors in the spinal cord. These receptors have been classified into types according to the effects seen when they are occupied. Some are

- Carprofen is exception – does not affect the kidney's self-protection mechanism and so is safe to use prior to anaesthesia.

Local anaesthetics

- Block the transmission of pain impulses along sensory nerves
- Can be administered prior to anaesthesia, thus reducing concentration of volatile agent needed during surgery
- Do not interfere with wound healing as long as they do not contain adrenaline.

8.42 Signs of pain

Dog

- Spontaneous vocalization – whining, growling
- Biting at wound
- Fear – hiding at back of kennel
- High heart rate
- Rapid shallow respiratory rate.

Cat

- Vocalization rare as result of pain
- Hiding at back of cage
- Cowering when approached
- Hissing and growling when wound is touched.

associated with excitement and euphoria (hence their abuse by humans); others are associated with analgesia.

The pain-relieving receptors are called the μ (mu) receptors. Opioid analgesics bind to these receptors and produce analgesia, and are themselves classified as either pure or partial μ agonists, according to the way in which they interact with these receptors (Figure 8.43):

- Pure μ agonists occupy the μ receptor and produce analgesia
- Partial μ agonists occupy the μ receptor but do not stimulate it fully.

The degree of analgesia varies with dose and can even be less when higher doses are used:

- Partial μ agonists tend to be poorer analgesics than pure μ agonists
- They also tend to have a greater affinity for the μ receptor than the pure μ agonist opioids (they stick more firmly to receptors)
- If they are given after pure μ agonists, they will 'knock' some of the pure μ agonists off the receptors. This can result in less analgesia for the patient.

8.43 Pure and partial μ agonists

Group/drug	Usage and effects	Contraindications and warnings
Pure μ agonists		
Pethidine	Short acting. Only 1–2 h in dog Very good analgesic but needs relatively frequent top-up dosing, sometimes as often as every hour Occasional histamine release	Should not be given by the intravenous route Can cause vomiting, though less so than morphine
Morphine	Longer acting than pethidine: 4–5 h in dog and 6–8 h in cat	Will cause vomiting in some dogs if not in pain when given. Can be reduced by administering along with acepromazine Produces pupil constriction, peripheral vasodilation and respiratory depression (respiratory depression seen is rarely a problem in veterinary species) Associated with violent excitement in the cat but *not* a problem at clinical doses
Methadone	Very similar to morphine but less tendency to cause vomiting	Produces less sedation than morphine
Papaveretum (Omnopon)	A mixture of opiate alkaloids Very good sedative, especially when combined with acepromazine	Similar side effects to morphine
Fentanyl	Very potent short-acting pure μ agonist Used as analgesic component of neuroleptanalgesic combination Hypnorm® Used during surgery to provide analgesic component of balanced anaesthesia	Causes profound respiratory depression. When given by the intravenous route, produces several minutes of apnoea, during which time patient must be ventilated
Etorphine	Very potent derivative of morphine Produces greater respiratory depression than morphine does at equipotent doses Used as analgesic component of potent neuroleptanalgesic combinations used in small and large animals. Immobilon SA® and Immobilon LA®	Very dangerous to humans – even tiny amounts can be fatal Can be absorbed through moist mucous membranes of eyes and mouth *Extreme caution should be taken whenever it is used. All personnel should be aware of emergency treatment to be given in the event of accidental administration to humans. (See Figure 8.37 for more information on the treatment of accidental human administration.)*
Partial μ agonists		
Buprenorphine	Provides 8–12 h analgesia	Has a bell-shaped dose–response curve. This means a peak analgesic effect is achieved, after which giving more drug will produce *less* analgesia Do not give top-up doses as this may reduce the level of analgesia Safe to give repeat dose of buprenorphine 12 h after initial dose
Butorphanol	Used in combination with alpha-2 agonists +/– ketamine for sedation and anaesthesia Used as a cough suppressant	Poor analgesic

Partial μ agonists should not be given after pure μ agonists.

Partial μ agonists should be used in patients where the postsurgical pain is expected to be mild. In cases where moderate to severe postsurgical pain is likely, pure μ agonist opioids should be used.

Non-steroidal anti-inflammatory drugs

Non-steroidal anti-inflammatory drugs (Figure 8.44) inhibit the synthesis of prostaglandin (inflammatory mediators) by blocking the action of cyclo-oxygenase, the enzyme that converts arachidonic acid into prostaglandin. By blocking the production of these inflammatory prostaglandins, they reduce pain and inflammation.

Local anaesthetics

Local anaesthetics can be useful for postsurgical analgesia. If they are used, they should be administered prior to surgery to get the best effects. Although all are useful as postsurgical analgesics, bupivacaine is the most suitable because it is the longest acting.

 If local anaesthetic agents are introduced into a wound, preparations containing adrenaline should be avoided as they may impair wound healing.

Combinations of analgesic drugs

Where possible, analgesic drugs from two or more different classes of drugs can be used. For example, following thoracic surgery, infiltration of the intercostal nerves with local anaesthetic can be combined with the use of a pure μ agonist opioid to produce excellent analgesia.

Stages of anaesthesia

In order to judge the depth of anaesthesia, it is important to understand the stages of anaesthesia and the signs a patient will show while undergoing the journey to unconsciousness. There are four stages.

Stage I: voluntary excitement

Stage I begins with induction of the patient and finishes when unconsciousness is reached.

The signs of Stage I are:

- Fear/stress/apprehension
- Pulse/heart rate and respiratory rate increased
- Disorientation
- Muscle activity may be prominent
- May urinate/defecate.

Stage II: involuntary excitement

Stage II begins at the start of unconsciousness. It finishes when the patient is no longer excited and respiration is stable.
The signs of Stage II are:

- Howling
- Excessive movement/struggling
- All reflexes present
- The eye remains open and central
- Pupils are dilated
- Respiration may be irregular but should stabilize
- Vomiting may occur.

Stages I and II can both be made more pleasant for the animal by administration of a premedicant and by giving the correct amount of induction agent. This enables these two stages to pass very quickly; thus they are not seen that often.

Stage III: surgical anaesthesia

Stage III is divided into three planes (Figure 8.45). Minor surgery can be performed at Plane I, such as small lumpectomies, lancing of abscesses or suturing small wounds. More major surgery, such as orthopaedics and thoracotomies, is performed at Plane II.

Stage IV: overdose

Stage IV ends with paralysis of all the respiratory muscles.
The signs of Stage IV are:

- Respiration rate greatly reduced, leading to apnoea; the pattern is irregular and shallow/jerky
- Heart rate reduced along with CRT and blood pressure
- Pulse weak and slow, will eventually diminish
- Reflexes all absent, including corneal reflex
- Eye position centrally fixed with pupil fully dilated and unresponsive to light
- Muscle tone flaccid.

It is important to remember that stages of anaesthesia merge together. The aim of this information is to enable recognition of when the animal is too deeply anaesthetized.

8.44 Non-steroidal anti-inflammatory drugs

Drug	Usage and effects	Contraindications and warnings
Aspirin Paracetamol Phenylbutazone Flunixin Tolfenamic acid Ketoprofen	Longer acting than many opioid analgesics Ineffective against severe pain	Many toxic, especially to cats Should be avoided in patients with cardiac, renal or hepatic disease Should not be used prior to or during anaesthetic: may cause kidney damage Interval between doses should be increased in neonates and geriatrics to avoid toxicity
Carprofen	Very potent analgesic Does not block kidney's self-protection mechanism so can be used prior to anaesthesia	Should be avoided in patients with hepatic, renal or cardiac disease

Plane	Heart rate	Pulse	Respiration	Reflexes	Eye position	Muscle tone
Plane I (Light)	Reduced slightly Regular	Rate is reduced slightly Strong and regular	Regular, smooth, deep Rate increases with painful stimuli	Movement of head and limbs is absent All others present but not as prominent	Nystagmus often seen Eyeball rotates ventrally Third eyelid moves across the eye	Present and responsive, some resistance may occur (e.g. jaw tone)
Plane II (Medium)	Reduced slightly Regular Blood pressure also slightly reduced	Strong and regular	Tidal volume decreased but will increase with stimuli Rate may increase or decrease	Palpebral reflex slow or absent Pedal reflex increasingly slow then absent Corneal reflex present	Nystagmus no longer present Eye has slight ventral rotation Pupil may be constricted	Relaxed Some resistance may be seen in very muscular dogs
Plane III (Deep)	Rate is further reduced along with blood pressure	Weak due to low blood pressure	Tidal volume decreased Rate usually decreased and shallow	All absent except corneal reflex	Eye is central are fixed Third eyelid returns to correct position	Greatly reduced or absent.

Monitoring the anaesthetized patient

Monitoring anaesthesia is a very important role for the veterinary nurse. It is essential that all aspects of monitoring are understood.

Monitoring can be divided into three categories:

- Pre-anaesthesia
- Intra-anaesthesia
- Post-anaesthesia.

Arrival of the patient

- Check that the patient is booked in on the operating list
- The animal must be weighed, as this will determine the amount of anaesthetic drugs to be used
- Take the owner and the patient to a quiet room to begin an assessment of the animal.

Details of the client

Make sure that the following details of the client and patient are correct and up to date on the record.

- Owner's name and address
- A daytime and evening contact telephone number.

Details of the animal

Ask whether the animal has been to another veterinary surgery before. If the answer is yes, take the previous surgery's name, address and telephone number and contact them for the animal's previous history.

The following must also be recorded.

- The animal's name
- The species or breed
- The sex, and whether the animal is neutered
- Date of birth
- Colour.

Pre-anaesthesia

The veterinary nurse should take certain steps when the patient first arrives (Figure 8.46). Any animal that requires an anaesthetic or sedation needs a full physical examination and an account of its previous history to determine its health status. The findings from this examination will influence the type and quantity of the drugs used for premedication and for anaesthetizing the animal, or whether in fact the procedure should take place at all.

The examination carried out by the veterinary surgeon assesses the cardiovascular and respiratory systems, the CNS and hepatic and renal function, all of which are affected by

Questions to ask the client

- Is the animal well in itself? For example, is there any coughing, exercise intolerance, excessive drinking or urinating, vomiting or diarrhoea?
- Note any new information, or recent changes
- Has the animal been starved overnight?
- Has the animal urinated/defecated this morning?
- If the animal is on any medications, were they administered this morning?
- Has the animal had any reactions to an anaesthetic before?

Make sure that the owner is aged over 18. The consent form will be rendered void if it is signed by a minor.

History of the animal

- Is the animal suffering from any illness (e.g. diabetes mellitus, epilepsy, cardiac disease)?
- If the animal is taking any medication: which drugs and how often?
- Are the vaccinations up to date?

anaesthesia. If there is concern regarding any of these systems, further investigation should be carried out (e.g. electrocardiography, radiography or further blood tests).

Once the health status has been determined, the premedication may be given to the patient to produce sedation or tranquillity. This is achieved by giving a combination of drugs, which will be decided by the veterinary surgeon.

The veterinary surgeon may ask the nurse to give the premedication.

- Double-check the drug, the dose and the route via which it is to be administered (this will depend on how quickly it is required to act)
- Record all drugs given and watch for any reactions.

Intra-anaesthesia

After the premedication has taken effect, anaesthesia can be induced. This will be achieved either by an injectable anaesthetic agent (e.g. short/ultra-short acting) or, less commonly, by using one of the volatile anaesthetic agents and a mask (e.g. halothane, isoflurane).

Throughout anaesthesia, measure and record the following parameters:

- Respiration
- Heart rate
- Pulse
- Mucous membranes (colour and capillary refill time – CRT)
- All reflexes
- Temperature
- Blood loss
- Salivary and lachrymal secretions
- Fluid administration and intravenous catheter placement
- Gas flow rates.

Check each parameter every 5 minutes. Higher-risk cases may need more frequent monitoring. Remember to check *all* the parameters – do not rely or make decisions on just one of them.

(Note: When inducing anaesthesia with a small animal chamber, it is important that the chamber is made of clear plastic. This ensures full visibility of the patient at all times.)

Respiration
Note the rate, rhythm and depth.
Normal respiratory rates are:

- Dog: 10–30 breaths per minute
- Cat: 20–30 breaths per minute.

Abnormal respiratory rates are described in Figure 8.47. Abnormal respiratory depths are:

- Hypoventilation
  - Decrease in depth resulting from the intercostal muscles' inability to expand the chest
  - Presents as slow and shallow breathing
- Hyperventilation
  - Increase in depth
  - Presents as deep and rapid breathing.

Respiration should be smooth and regular. Ketamine causes a distinctive respiration pattern in which there is a prolonged pause between inspiration and expiration; this is known as apneustic respiration.

Watch the thorax and the reservoir bag.

- If the circuit is not connected correctly, or if the endotracheal tube has been placed in the oesophagus, there will be no visible movement in the bag
- Also check that the bag is deflating and inflating correctly and causing no resistance.

Heart rate
Normal heart rates are:

- Dog: 60–140 beats per minute (depending on size)
- Cat: 110–180 beats per minute.

Abnormal heart rates are described in Figure 8.48.

8.47 Abnormal respiration

Term	Definition	Causes
Bradypnoea	Respiratory rate lower than normal	Anaesthesia too deep Effects of drugs
Tachypnoea	Respiratory rate higher than normal	Insufficiently anaesthetized Aware of pain
Dyspnoea	Difficulty in breathing	Obstruction in the circuit Obstruction in thorax (e.g. secondary tumours, fluid, stenosis of bronchial tree)
Apnoea	Cessation of breathing	Effects of drugs such as propofol, methohexitone and thiopentone Respiratory arrest

8.48 Abnormal heart rates

Term	Definition	Causes
Bradycardia	Heart rate lower than normal	Increasing depth of anaesthesia Effects of drugs, e.g. acepromazine, medetomidine Illness
Tachycardia	Heart rate higher than normal	Insufficiently anaesthetized Decreasing depth Drugs, e.g. atropine or ketamine
No heart beat		Cardiac arrest

The heart rate can be measured by:

- Auscultation of the heart sounds (using a normal or oesophageal stethoscope)
- Palpation of the apex heart beat on the left side of the patient's chest
- Counting the number of complexes seen on an ECG trace
- Use of a cardiac monitor with an audible bleep.

Heart rate must be analysed along with the pulse, mucous membrane colour and capillary refill time, as the presence of a heart beat does not mean that the circulatory system is functioning correctly.

Pulse

Peripheral pulses can be felt in the following arteries:

- Lingual pulse (found on the ventral aspect of the tongue)
- Femoral pulse (found on the medial aspect of both femurs)
- Digital pulse (found on the palmar/plantar aspect of the carpus/tarsus)
- Coccygeal pulse (found on the ventral aspect of the base of the tail)
- Facial pulse (found in the cheek).

The pulse rate should be:

- Regular
- Of a consistent quality
- Reasonably strong.

Abnormal pulse rates are described in Figure 8.49.

- There should be no pulse deficit (pulse rate lower than the heart rate, denoting a cardiac dysrhythmia)
- Sinus arrhythmia (the rate increasing on inspiration and decreasing on expiration) is normal in the dog.

8.49 Abnormal pulse rates

Pulse	Causes
Lowered rate	Myocardial depression caused by anaesthetic drug, e.g. medetomidine Systemic illness Anaesthesia too deep
Increased rate	Anaesthesia too light Stress Pain Pyrexia Hypoxia Hypercapnia
Weak	Poor circulation, possibly due to hypovolaemic shock Peripheral venous constriction, possibly due to hypothermia Alpha-2 agonists cause weak pulse
Strong and jerky (known as 'water hammer' pulse)	Heart valves performing incorrectly Congenital heart defects, e.g. patent ductus, arteriosis, pulmonary/ aortic stenosis

Mucous membranes

The mucous membranes can be observed by looking at:

- The gingiva
- The conjunctiva
- The anus
- The vagina or penis.

The colour should be salmon pink, indicating good health. Abnormal colours are described in Figure 8.50.

Capillary refill time

This is the time it takes a mucous membrane to return to its original colour after it has been blanched by the application of light pressure. The time taken should be less than 2 seconds. If it takes any longer, this may indicate hypovolaemic shock or cardiovascular depression.

Reflexes

The following reflexes denote the depth of anaesthesia.

Palpebral reflex

Touching of the medial canthus causes the eyelids to blink. As the patient enters Stage III of anaesthesia, this reflex will become increasingly absent.

Eye position

The eye is ventrally rotated during surgical anaesthesia. As the depth of anaesthesia increases further, the eye starts to move back to a central position.

This means that the eye is centrally positioned when the patient is either too lightly or too deeply anaesthetized. If the patient is too deeply anaesthetized, the palpebral reflex will be absent.

The pupil gradually dilates as anaesthetic depth increases but should be responsive to light at all times. A lack of response indicates an anaesthetic overdose. Remember that the pupil will already be dilated if an anticholinergic drug has been given.

Pedal reflex

The reflex caused by pinching in between the digits will gradually diminish as the depth of anaesthesia increases. It is usually lost by Stage III, Plane II.

Jaw tone

This is assessed by stretching apart the mandible and maxilla. Jaw tone will gradually diminish as the depth of anaesthesia increases and is usually lost by Stage III, Plane II.

8.50 Abnormal colour of the mucous membranes

Colour	Causes
Pale	Haemorrhage Hypotension Anaemia Hypovolaemic shock
Cyanotic (blue)	Cardiac arrest Respiratory obstruction Administration of nitrous oxide only will produce navy blue colour
Icteric (yellow)	Indicates hepatic problems
Brick red	Usually brought on by toxaemia or carbon dioxide poisoning

Corneal reflex

This reflex should only be tested as a last resort, as the cornea is extremely sensitive and easily damaged. The reflex should always be present. Its absence indicates an anaesthetic overdose.

Temperature

Normal rectal temperatures are:

- Dog: 38.3–38.7°C
- Cat: 38.0–38.5°C.

The temperature may be monitored by feeling the patient's extremities (ears, paws), which will give adequate information regarding the peripheral circulation. It is also an early warning of hypothermia.

Hypothermia (35°C or below) is most common during surgery, due to:

- Anaesthesia
- The hair being shaved
- The skin being wet from preparation
- The metabolic rate being lower than that of a conscious animal
- Anaesthetized animals being unable to create heat by shivering or movement.

Small animals, such as hamsters, have a high body surface area in relation to their body mass and therefore lose heat more rapidly than animals with a relatively smaller body surface area, such as cats and dogs.

An increasing gap between the peripheral temperature and the core temperature indicates a poor peripheral circulation – more than likely due to shock. Undetected hypothermia increases the recovery time as the liver is slower to metabolize the anaesthetic drugs. Death can occur if hypothermia is not detected.

Blood loss

Haemorrhage from the surgical site will result in a drop in the blood pressure (hypotension). If not treated, this will develop into hypovolaemic shock, producing:

- Weak and rapid pulse
- Tachycardia
- Slow capillary refill time
- Pale mucous membranes.

These signs will be seen when the following amounts of blood are lost:

- Dog: 8–18 ml/kg
- Cat: 6–12 ml/kg.

Figure 8.51 describes how to measure blood loss. Fluids should be given to compensate for the blood loss. Ideally, whole blood should be given, or colloidal plasma expanders. Crystalloids may be used if plasma expanders are not available.

Salivary and lachrymal secretions

Saliva and tears can help to indicate the depth of anaesthesia: production of these secretions becomes less as anaesthetic depth increases, and they are absent during deep anaesthesia.

Ophthalmic solutions (e.g. hypromellose) can be used to prevent the cornea from drying out. These solutions should be especially used in ketamine anaesthesia.

Fluid administration

Monitor the rate of fluid and make sure that the animal receives the correct amount and type of fluid. The catheter should also be checked periodically to ensure that:

- It is still in the vein
- It is not blocked.

Use heparin flush, not fluid from the bag, to flush the catheter through.

Gas flow rates

Always keep a check on the concentration of anaesthetic gas being delivered to the patient. Oxygen and nitrous oxide flow meters should be checked at the same time. Falling of the bobbin indicates that the anaesthetic gas is running out.

Post-anaesthesia

This is the period during which the patient is allowed to regain consciousness and the stages of anaesthesia are seen in reverse.

The recovery period is one of high risk, as patients are often poorly observed. Monitoring and recording of all parameters must continue throughout recovery.

8.51 How to measure blood loss

The volume of blood lost can be measured accurately using the following technique:

1. Calculate the weight of a dry swab
2. Multiply this by the number of swabs used during the surgery (in order to calculate their dry weight)
3. Subtract this dry weight from the weight of the blood-soaked swabs to calculate the weight of the blood lost during the surgery
4. Divide this weight by 1.3 to convert it into millilitres of blood (1 ml blood weighs 1.3 g).

> **Example:**
> 100 dry swabs weigh 230 g. Hence, one dry swab weighs 2.3 g (230/100).
> During an operation, the 20 blood-soaked swabs used are found to weigh 100 g. When dry, the 20 swabs would weigh 46 g (2.3 x 20). Therefore the blood must weigh 64 g (110 – 46). Hence the swabs contained 49 ml of blood (64/1.3).

Alternatively, a good estimate of the patient's blood loss can be calculated using the following technique:

1. Find out the volume of water needed to saturate 10 swabs
2. Divide this by 10 for the volume of water needed to saturate one swab
3. This is roughly equivalent to the volume of blood that will be contained in one swab
4. Multiply the volume of blood contained in one saturated swab by the number of swabs used in the surgery to estimate the volume of blood lost.

> **Example:**
> If 10 swabs will absorb 50 ml of water, one swab will absorb 5 ml. During an operation, 14 swabs become saturated in blood. An estimate of the volume of blood soaked into these swabs is 70 ml (14 x 5).

When using either technique, remember to subtract the volume of any lavage fluids that have been used and that have also been soaked up by the swabs.

Anaesthetic aids

Equipment	Function
Oesophageal stethoscope	Simple device that allows patient's heart sounds to be monitored constantly without disturbing surgical drapes Closed end of stethoscope positioned in patient's oesophagus next to heart Cheap and disposable
Electrocardiogram (ECG)	Monitors electrical activity of heart Produces continuous trace or simple beep when heart beat is detected Existence of electrical activity in heart does not mean that the heart is producing good cardiac output
Respiratory monitors	Measure only the rate Function on temperature difference between inspired and expired gas If further information needed regarding adequacy of respiration, blood gas analysis should be carried out

Monitor the following:

- Return to consciousness
- Heart rate and pulse
- Respiratory rate
- Mucous membrane colour and capillary refill time
- Reflex responses
- Temperature
- Pain (give appropriate analgesic and TLC).

The patient should be allowed to recover in a quiet warm room, where there is easy access to emergency equipment. The length of time taken to recover depends on:

- The type of anaesthetic given and the route of administration
- How long the patient was anaesthetized
- The patient's health status
- The patient's age
- The patient's body temperature
- Environmental temperature.

Monitoring equipment

A number of anaesthetic aids are available for use in practice (Figure 8.52). Although these machines provide information on the parameters to be assessed during anaesthesia, they do not replace the veterinary nurse.

Further reading

Clutton E (1993) Management of perioperative cardiac arrest in companion animals, Part 1. *In Practice* **15**, 267–270

Clutton E (1994) Management of perioperative cardiac arrest in companion animals, Part 2. *In Practice* **16**, 3–6

Clutton E (1995) The right anaesthetic machine for you? *In Practice* **17**, 83–88

Davey A, Moyle JTB and Ward CS (eds) (1997) *Ward's Anaesthetic Equipment*, 3rd edn. WB Saunders, London

Hall LW and Clarke KW (eds) (1991) *Veterinary Anaesthesia*, 9th edn. Baillière Tindall, London

Hall LW and Taylor PM (eds) (1994) *Anaesthesia of the Cat*. Baillière Tindall, London

Seymour C and Gleed R (eds) (1999) *Manual of Small Animal Anaesthesia and Analgesia*. BSAVA, Cheltenham

Short CE (1987) *Principles and Practice of Veterinary Anaesthesia*. Williams and Wilkins, Baltimore

9 Radiography

Deborah J Smith

This chapter is designed to give information on:

- Basic principles involved in the production of x-rays and radiographs
- The application of those principles to ensure a quality image
  - Selection of appropriate combinations of film, screen and grid
  - Positioning and restraint of the patient
  - Selection of exposure factors
  - The identification of film artifacts and factors which may lead to their production
  - Processing the film
  - Principles and practice of radiation safety and protection

Introduction

In many veterinary practices the nurse will act as radiographer and be responsible for taking and processing radiographs. Understanding the principles involved in the production of a radiograph is essential, to ensure that the quality of the final image is as high as possible for the particular patient under examination, with the available equipment. At any stage, poor technique or error may lead to loss of information from the radiograph or the production of artifacts.

Basic principles of radiography

Electromagnetic radiations

- X-rays are a form of electromagnetic radiation. They transfer energy from one place to another without mass and need no medium for their transmission

- X-rays belong to the electromagnetic spectrum, together with other types of electromagnetic radiations (e.g. radio waves, infra-red, visible light, ultraviolet and gamma rays)
- X-rays exhibit wave/particle duality – some properties are explained by considering them as transverse waves, others by considering them as discrete packets of energy known as photons.

Properties of X-rays

- Velocity (v) is constant in free space and equals the radiation frequency (f) multiplied by its wavelength (λ) (Figure 9.1). Therefore, the shorter the wavelength, the higher is the frequency (Figure 9.1a); the longer the wavelength, the lower is the frequency (Figure 9.1b)
- Frequency is variable and directly related to X-ray energy. The higher the frequency (and shorter the wavelength) of the radiation, the greater is the photon energy; the lower the frequency, the lower is the photon energy
- X-rays travel in straight lines. They may change direction but the new path will be in a straight line

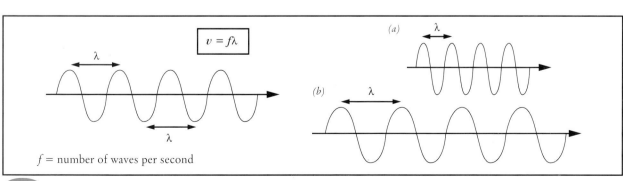

9.1 *Transverse waves.*

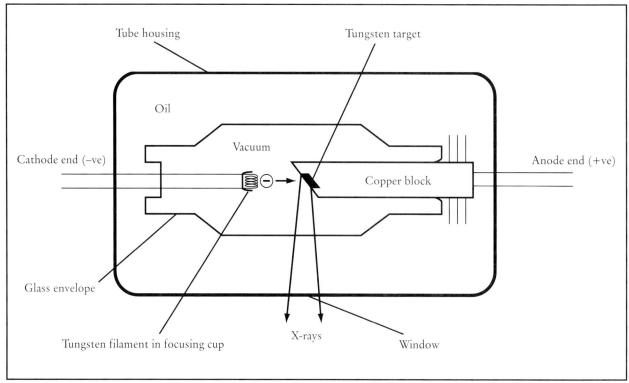

9.2 *Stationary anode X-ray tube.*

- X-rays have no electrical charge and are therefore unaffected by magnetic or electric fields
- X-rays may interact with matter through absorption or scatter. They can produce excitation or ionization of atoms of substances through which they pass. Interaction of matter with X-rays reduces the radiation intensity (attenuation) and can produce:
  - A latent image on photographic film
  - Fluorescence (emission of visible light following X-ray absorption) by phosphors, e.g. rare earth elements, calcium tungstate
  - Biological changes in living tissues
- In free space, X-rays obey the inverse square law. Provided that there is no absorption or scattering, the intensity of a beam of X-rays from a point source is inversely proportional to the square of the distance from the source. Therefore, if the distance from the X-ray source is doubled, the beam intensity will be reduced by a factor of four.

The X-ray machine and X-ray production

The X-ray tube
The X-ray tube consists of a negatively charged cathode and positively charged anode in an evacuated glass envelope (Figure 9.2).

The cathode is a coiled tungsten filament; it produces free electrons by the process of thermionic emission when heated by an electric current passing through it. The size of the current determines the number of electrons produced and, in turn, the number of X-rays produced at the anode. The filament is surrounded by the focusing cup, also negatively charged, which repels the electrons produced by the filament and prevents them from spreading out across the tube.

The electrons are rapidly accelerated to the anode by application of a high voltage (the tube kilovoltage, kV) across the tube. The greater the voltage, the faster the electrons will travel, and this influences the number and energy of X-rays produced.

The electron flow from cathode to anode produces the tube current (milliamperage, mA). The electrons hit a small target area on the anode, where they rapidly decelerate or stop as they interact with the atoms of the target.

X-rays are generated as a result of these interactions. Only about 1% of the electrons' energy is converted into X-radiation; the remainder is converted into heat. The anode must therefore be made from material with a high melting point – tungsten, or a tungsten alloy, is normally used.

Focal spot
The focal spot is the area of the target on which the electrons impinge.

- Focal spot size is important in terms of image quality – the smaller this area, the sharper is the radiograph
- The target is set at an angle so that the area of the target bombarded by electrons (the actual focal spot) is greater than the area projected in the direction of the primary X-ray beam (the effective focal spot) (Figure 9.3)
- The larger the focal spot, the greater is the area over which heat produced during X-ray production is distributed and the greater is the tube current that can be used without causing an unacceptable rise in anode temperature.

Stationary anode tubes
In a stationary anode X-ray machine (Figure 9.2) the target is set into one end of a cylindrical copper block. Heat produced in the target dissipates into the block by conduction and from here passes into the oil surrounding the tube's glass envelope. The inability to withstand large amounts of heat limits the power output of these machines; many have a fixed tube current, often only 20 or 30 mA, necessitating the use of long exposure times. Used in portable and dental X-ray machines and some mobile units, they have no moving parts and should have a long lifetime provided they are treated with care.

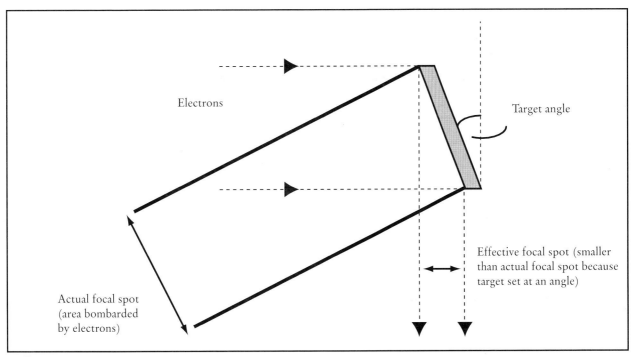

Actual versus *effective focal spot size.*

Rotating anode tubes

In rotating anode machines (Figure 9.4) the target is positioned around the bevelled edge of a disc that rotates at a speed of several thousand revolutions per minute during the exposure. This greatly increases the area over which the electrons hit the target and therefore over which heat is distributed. The heat is radiated to the glass wall of the tube and from there to the surrounding oil. (Conduction of heat would be a disadvantage in these tubes as it could damage the rotor bearings. The stem on which the disc is mounted is therefore made from a poor conductor of heat – molybdenum.)

Output from these machines is much greater than from stationary anode machines but they are much more expensive to produce and are more vulnerable to damage. Rotating anodes are found in fixed X-ray machines and some mobile units. These machines often have two focal spots:

- Fine focus – used to obtain sharper definition but only at relatively low exposures (suitable for extremities)
- Broad focus – used at higher exposures (e.g. chest and abdomen films).

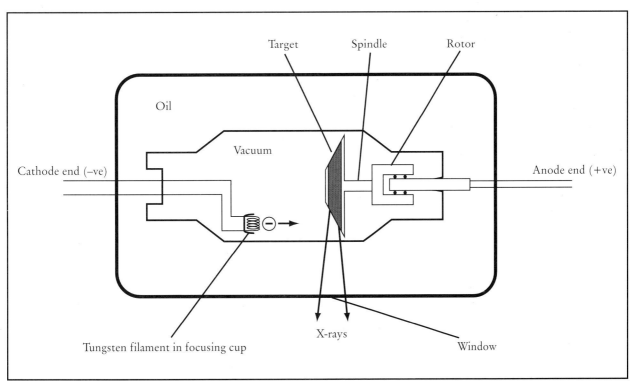

9.4
Rotating anode X-ray machine.

Tube housing

Metal housing provides mechanical support and protection for the tube.

- Lead lining of housing provides protection from X-rays produced in directions other than those that make up the primary beam
- Oil between the lining and the glass tube envelope cools the anode and provides electrical insulation. A bellows system incorporated in the housing allows expansion of the oil as it heats up
- The primary beam exits the glass tube envelope through a window in which the glass is thinner. It then emerges through an opening in the lead lining of the tube housing (Figure 9.5)
- The cables entering the tube housing carry current to the cathode and supply the voltage across the tube. They are heavily insulated to withstand the very high voltages they carry.

Filtration

The primary beam is made up of a range of photon energies. A filter (usually aluminium) placed across the opening in the housing absorbs low energy photons from the beam. These low energy photons do not contribute to image formation, as they are absorbed within the patient and thus only serve to increase the radiation dose to the patient.

Collimation

Close collimation limits the size of the X-ray beam to the area of interest. This limitation:

- Reduces the amount of scattered radiation produced, thus improving image quality
- Minimizes radiation doses to the patient and personnel involved in the radiographic examination, from both the primary beam and scattered radiation.

The *Guidance Notes for the Protection of Persons against Ionising Radiations arising from Veterinary Use* state that all X-ray machines should be fitted with some means of minimizing the size of the primary beam to that necessary for the examination being performed. Modern machines achieve this by using a light beam diaphragm (Figure 9.5), consisting of two sets of lead shutters together with a mirror and a light source, fitted to the window of the X-ray tube housing. The light indicates how far the X-ray beam falls and where the centre of the beam is.

Some older machines may still collimate by using interchangeable cones fixed to the tube head. The beam size is

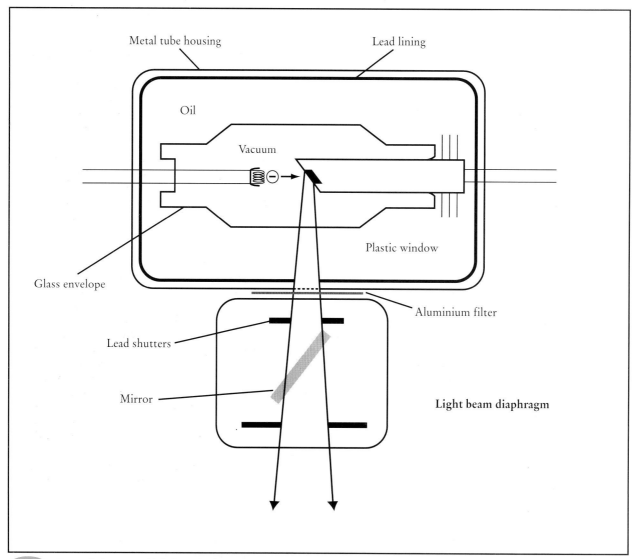

9.5 *X-ray tube housing and light beam diaphragm.*

not infinitely variable (as it would be with a light beam diaphragm) but is restricted by the size of cones available. Restriction to a circular area means that large areas are often exposed beyond the margins of the patient; and because there is no light, it is impossible to know just how far the primary beam actually extends. This has obvious safety implications and the 'Guidance Notes' state that cones should never be used if animals are manually restrained during radiography.

Electrical components

In addition to the tube head, the X-ray machine consists of various circuits:

- A low voltage circuit supplies current to the cathode filament
- A high voltage circuit, consisting of an autotransformer and high voltage transformer, supplies the high potential difference across the X-ray tube
- A timer switch controls how long the high potential is applied across the tube, and hence the length of the exposure.

Control panel

The complexity of the control panel varies considerably, depending on the type of machine and number of variables that can be altered. The smallest portable machines may have only one control allowing choice of exposure, with tube current (often fixed on such machines) and time being automatically selected for a given kilovoltage. On larger machines, some or all of the following controls may be present:

- On/off switch
- Line voltage compensator – to allow for fluctuations in incoming mains voltage
- Kilovoltage (kV) selector – selection may be limited to 5 or 10 kV stops. Increasing kV increases the high voltage across the tube and both the penetrating power (quality) and the intensity of the X-ray beam
- Milliamperage (mA) selector – tube current is determined by the number of electrons crossing the tube from cathode to anode, which in turn determines the number of X-rays produced when these electrons reach the anode's target area. Changing mA affects beam intensity only
- Timer – to allow choice of exposure length. For a given mA, increasing the exposure length increases the number of X-rays produced. Modern machines have electronic timers, which are much more accurate (and safer) than the older mechanical type
- Exposure button – this must be positioned at least 2 m from the tube housing, for the safety of personnel. Rotating anode machines have two-stage buttons: the first stage allows the cathode to warm up and starts the anode rotating up to operating speed (approximately 9000 rpm); the second stage completes the circuit, applying high voltage across the tube.

Image formation

The number and energy of X-rays generated within the X-ray tube are determined by the machine settings selected by the radiographer. X-rays emerge from the tube as the primary beam and go on to interact with the patient's tissues. Individual X-rays may be absorbed or scattered within the patient, or may pass through unchanged. Different parts of the patient absorb different amounts of X-ray energy depending on their composition (mean atomic number), density and thickness and the energy of the X-rays themselves. The X-rays that pass through the patient unchanged go on to affect the X-ray film, usually via an intensifying screen, and produce an image of the patient when the film is processed.

Parts of the patient that are good at stopping X-rays, such as bone, appear white (radiodense) on the final radiograph; those parts that are poor at X-ray absorption and allow most of the X-rays to pass through, such as the air-filled lungs, appear black (radiolucent). Tissues with intermediate ability at stopping X-rays appear as various shades of grey. The reduction in intensity of the X-ray beam as it passes through the patient is known as attenuation. The different black, white and grey tones produced on the film are due to differential attenuation by different parts of the body.

Image receptors

Cassettes

Radiographic film is usually held within cassettes, the purpose of which is to:

- Provide mechanical support for intensifying screens
- Hold film and screens in close contact with each other
- Protect film and screens from physical damage
- Prevent light penetration to the film.

Important features of cassettes (Figure 9.6) are as follows.

- Both sides are rigid, strong and opaque to visible light
- The front cover must be made of a material that allows X-rays to pass through (e.g. aluminium, carbon-fibre, polycarbonate). Carbon-fibre is the best but the most expensive
- The back cover has a lead foil lining to absorb back scatter
- Foam pressure pads within the cassette ensure close contact between the film and screens
- A lead blocker in one corner absorbs X-rays to leave an unexposed section of film, which can be used for film identification.

Intensifying screens

These consist of a layer of fluorescent material (which produces light on interaction with X-rays) applied to a plastic support layer. A single X-ray photon produces many light photons in the screen and these go on to affect the X-ray film. The use of intensifying screens allows a great reduction in the radiographic exposure required to produce an image compared with that required for film alone.

Normally two screens are held within a cassette, with a piece of double-sided emulsion film sandwiched between them. The screen on the front side is slightly thinner than that on the back, so as not to absorb a disproportionate amount of the X-ray beam, to ensure that exposure of the film by light from both screens is equal.

Single-sided emulsion film is available for use with single screen cassettes and is occasionally used for veterinary work.

Screen types

Most new screens use one of the rare earth phosphors as the fluorescent material, though some calcium tungstate screens are still in use. Rare earth screens absorb more X-ray energy than tungstate ones and are more efficient at converting it into

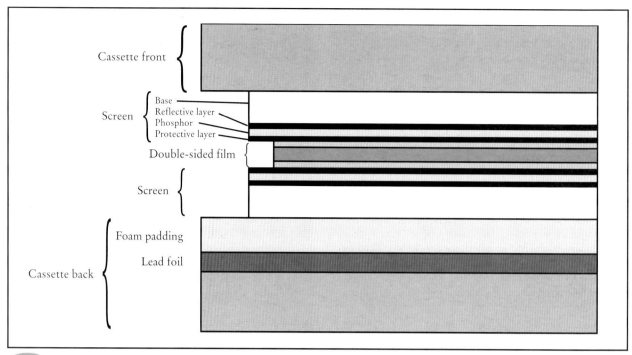

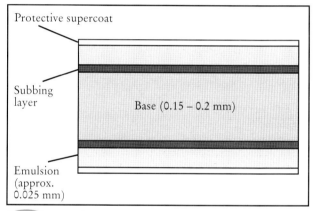

9.6 *Cross-section through film cassette and intensifying screens.*

light. This allows use of lower exposures, therefore exposure times can be minimized and the capabilities of a low power machine may be extended.

Calcium tungstate screens emit blue light whereas rare earth screens may emit green or blue light depending on the type. The radiographic film used, either green or blue light sensitive, must be matched to the type of screen. The wavelength of the darkroom safelight must be matched to the type of film being used, so that the film will not be fogged during cassette loading or processing.

Screen speed

- Fast screens require lower exposures to produce the same degree of film blackening as slow screens
- Faster screens have larger phosphor crystal sizes then slower ones, so resolution is not as good
- Fast screens are used for chest and abdomen radiographs, particularly in larger patients, allowing exposure times to be kept to a minimum to avoid movement blur
- Slow screens can be used to provide superior detail where length of exposure is less important (e.g. skeletal radiography).

Radiographic film

The layers making up a piece of film (Figure 9.7) are:

- Polyester base – increased use of automatic processors nowadays means base strength has become more important
- Subbing layer – thin adhesive that holds emulsion to base
- Emulsion – predominantly silver bromide (AgBr) crystals suspended in gelatin, applied to both sides of base. This is the sensitive part of the film: exposure of silver bromide crystals to X-rays or light produces a latent image within them, which is then made visible by processing the film. Although the crystals are sensitive to light, short exposures to the wavelength of light in the darkroom safelight do not affect them
- Supercoat – a protective layer of clear gelatin.

9.7 *X-ray film construction.*

Types of film

The size of crystals and range of crystal sizes in the emulsion determine film speed (its sensitivity to light and X-rays) and film contrast (range of black, white and grey tones in the image).

- Fast films have larger crystals than slow films and appear grainier
- Fast films require fewer X-rays than slow films to produce the same degree of blackening
- Medium-speed films are most commonly used in veterinary work. They:
  - Allow some room for error in choice of exposure factors and processing
  - Produce a less grainy image than fast films
  - Allow use of much reduced exposures compared with slow, fine-grain emulsions.

Non-screen film

Non-screen film was traditionally used for intraoral work and fine detail (e.g. in imaging digits) but is no longer readily available. Non-screen film:

- Produces images with very fine detail
- Requires much higher exposures than film with screens (approximately 10x)
- Has much thicker emulsion layers than screen film
- Requires increased processing times (many non-screen films are unsuitable for use with automatic processors).

The main disadvantage of using film in a cassette for intraoral use is the bulk of the cassette, which makes positioning it far enough caudally in the mouth virtually impossible. Alternatives include dental cassettes or flexible plastic cassettes.

Scattered radiation

The X-ray photons that either are absorbed by the patient or pass straight through the tissues and go on to affect the film are the ones that contribute usefully to image formation. However, not all of the photons that interact with the patient's atoms are completely stopped by the interaction. Some lose some energy but continue in a different direction from the original. These are known as scattered photons and they:

- May be deflected at any angle from the original
- Contain no useful information about the patient
- Darken the X-ray film more or less uniformly when they reach it
- Cause loss of contrast in the image
- Increase the radiation dose to the patient and any personnel involved in the radiographic examination
- Can also originate from reflection of photons from surfaces beyond the patient after the primary beam has passed through.

The amount of scattered radiation produced increases as the volume of tissue irradiated increases. It is important to limit the amount of scattered radiation produced, for safety reasons and to maximize film contrast. This can be achieved by:

- Collimating the primary beam to the area of interest
- Compressing tissues to reduce thickness (used

occassionally for abdominal radiography)
- Carefully selecting exposure factors (see later)
- Using lead beneath the cassette to reduce production of back scatter from the tabletop.

The amount of scatter reaching the X-ray film can be limited by:

- Use of a grid
- Lead backing in the film cassette to absorb back scatter.

Grids

Grids are used to reduce the amount of scattered radiation reaching the film, thus increasing contrast in the image (Figure 9.8). They are placed between the patient and the cassette which contains the film, and they:

- Are made of very thin strips of lead to absorb scattered radiation, with radiolucent interspacers (e.g. aluminium or plastic) between the strips. Most scattered photons move obliquely and are absorbed by the lead strips
- Absorb a small proportion of the primary beam that has passed through the patient
- Require an increase in exposure factors when used, compared with not using one
- Are normally used if tissue thickness exceeds approximately 10 cm.

Grid characteristics

- Grid ratio – the ratio of the height (h) of the lead strips to the distance (D) between them (i.e. thickness of the interspacer) (Figure 9.9). Typical values for grid ratio are from about 5 to 12 – the higher the value, the more scatter is absorbed
- Grid factor – a measure of the amount by which exposure factors need to be increased to allow for grid use; usually between 2.5 and 3
- Lead strip thickness – usually 0.005–0.008 cm with 20 to 28 strips/cm.

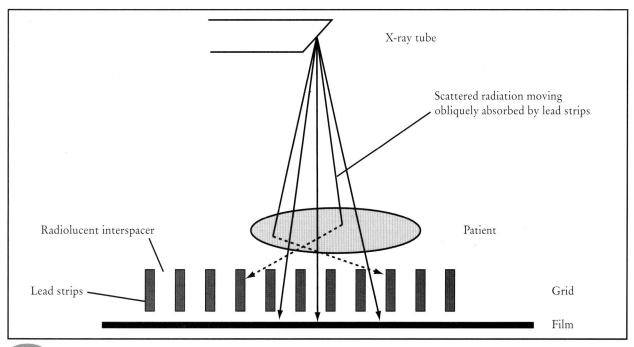

9.8 *Use of a grid to control scattered radiation.*

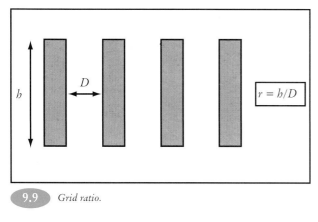

9.9 *Grid ratio.*

Types of grid

Stationary grids

Stationary grids (Figure 9.10) are usually placed on top of the cassette on the tabletop. There are several types:

- Parallel – the lead strips are parallel. Due to beam divergence, more of the primary beam is absorbed towards the edges of the grid, therefore film blackening decreases here
- Focused – the lead strips are angled progressively from centre to edges and point towards the focal spot. This prevents grid cut-off at the edges but it is essential that the correct film-focus distance is used and that the central beam passes through the centre of the grid
- Pseudo-focused – the lead strips are parallel but reduce in height from centre to edges to allow for beam divergence. As with focused grids, correct film-focus distance and accurate centring are essential
- Crossed – two parallel grids with low grid ratio, placed on top of one another at right angles to each other, remove scatter very efficiently. The central axis of the X-ray beam must be exactly at right angles to the grids.

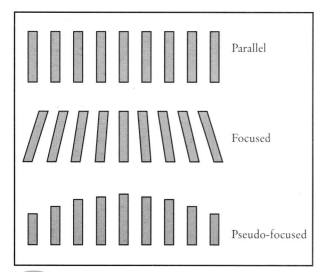

9.10 *Grid types.*

Moving (Potter–Bucky) grid

A moving grid sits between the tabletop and a special tray for the cassette beneath the table. It has the advantage of blurring out grid lines so that they are not visible on the radiograph. The grid moves a distance of three to four interspacers during the exposure. The speed of grid movement therefore depends on grid ratio and exposure length.

Routine radiographic procedures

Patient preparation

- The animal's coat should be clean and dry. Water or dirt can produce misleading white marks on the radiograph
- Collars and leads should be removed for head, neck or thoracic radiography
- For abdominal radiography the animal should preferably be starved for 6–8 hours beforehand and ample opportunity given for defecation. Large quantities of food and faecal material in the gastrointestinal tract can otherwise obscure important details. (Slightly different criteria apply when performing abdominal contrast studies.)
- Dressings, splints and casts should normally be removed before radiography. If this is not to be done for a particular reason, the dressing must be taken into account when selecting exposure factors.

Choice of exposure factors

- Exposure time (s) – the effect of changing this on the number of X-rays produced is simple: doubling the time doubles the exposure to the patient
- Tube current (mA) – as with the time setting, doubling tube current doubles the exposure
- mAs – tube current (mA) multiplied by exposure time (s). These two factors have a direct relationship. Equal mAs settings will produce radiographs of equal density and contrast, provided that all other factors remain constant. For example, a radiograph obtained at 20 mA for 0.1 s (mAs = 2) will have the same exposure as one taken at 200 mA for 0.01 s (mAs = 2)
- Tube voltage (kV) – there is a much more complicated relationship between kV and exposure to the patient and film. As a rough approximation, within the range of tube voltages from 70 to 100 kV, increasing kV by 10 will double the exposure. Outside this range, the relationship does not hold. Below 70 kV an increase of 4–6 kV doubles the exposure, whereas above 100 kV an increase of 14–20 kV is required to have this effect.

Therefore if kV were increased from 70 to 80 kV, the mAs could be reduced by half to produce the same degree of film blackening. The machine settings chosen will depend on the area under examination. Selection of appropriate exposure factors results in a film of optimal density with good contrast between structures and sharp detail of anatomical features.

Density, contrast and penetration

The usual objective is to produce as much visual differentiation between structures as possible.

- The degree of film blackening (density) depends on mAs and kV
- Increasing mAs makes the film darker overall but does not affect contrast between different tissues
- Increasing kV results in a darker film, as tissues are more easily penetrated by higher energy photons. Also, contrast between structures always decreases as kV increases, because:
  - Differential attenuation between different tissues decreases
  - Less scattered radiation is produced but more of it travels forwards and affects the film

- Radiographs taken at low kV values have wide tonal differences, appearing very black and white
- Radiographs taken at high kV values have a longer scale of grey tones, with less difference between each step
- Insufficient penetration of structures if the kV is too low produces an underexposed image with a narrow range of pale tones.

In most situations the kV selected will be as low as possible, to provide maximum contrast between structures, although it must be sufficient to penetrate the tissues properly. This is especially important in the abdomen, as the difference in radiographic density between soft tissue and fat (which is what allows the viscera to be distinguished) is small. However, it also applies to radiography of the limbs and head, where if too high a kV is employed, the soft tissues will be 'burnt out'.

The one exception to this general rule is thoracic radiography. The thorax has high inherent contrast between air-filled lungs, bony margins and soft tissue structures of the cranial abdomen and heart. If the kV is too low, the heart tends to be underexposed or the lungs overexposed. A high kV technique flattens out the white and black tones to give a longer scale of contrast and has the advantage of allowing exposure time to be minimized.

Patient movement

Veterinary radiography normally requires relatively short exposure times because of the problem of patient movement.

- Short exposure times also reduce radiation exposure to any personnel involved in the procedure
- High output machines offer a significant advantage, as the maximum mA is much greater than for small low output machines
- In thoracic radiography, when movements associated with respiration and cardiac function have to be considered, exposure times of 0.03 s or less are required
- Skeletal radiography in anaesthetized patients poses much less of a problem – exposure time may extend to a second or more if required. Good quality radiographs of limbs should therefore be attainable even with low output machines.

Film–focus distance

Film–focus distance influences the radiation intensity reaching the patient and film.

- Use a standard distance – normally between 75 and 100 cm. In small animal radiography, where the tube head is usually positioned over the X-ray table for vertical beam use it is easy enough to check this distance and there is rarely any need to alter it
- Changes in the distance will have a significant effect on film blackening, due to the inverse square law
- Shorter film–focus distances allow reduced exposures but magnification, distortion and image unsharpness will be greater than when a long film–focus distance is used

The increased exposure required for an increase in the film–focus distance can be calculated:

$$\text{new mAs} = \text{old mAs} \times (\text{new distance}^2/\text{old distance}^2)$$

Restraint for radiography

When performing radiographic examinations, one important consideration is patient movement. To provide an image in a standard projection that can be compared with other radiographs of the same area, the patient must stay still in exactly the required position. Any movements, voluntary or involuntary, by the patient during the course of an exposure cause a loss of image sharpness and hence a reduction in quality and loss of information from the radiograph.

Good restraint of the animal and of the part of the body being examined is important and may be achieved by physical or chemical means, or a combination of the two. Manual restraint of animals should always be avoided and is only acceptable in situations where the patient would be clinically compromised by sedation or general anaesthesia. Animals should never be held simply for convenience or to save time.

Where sedation is undesirable, a certain amount of patience is required to try to calm and reassure an animal that is probably in pain or distress and is likely to be frightened by the whole experience. Following these guidelines is likely to result in a cooperative patient:

- Handle the animal slowly and quietly
- Avoid quick or loud movements that may stress and frighten the animal
- Provide analgesia and avoid handling areas known to be painful
- Prepare for the exposure before positioning the patient on the table, to reduce the time for which the animal needs to be restrained. Before lifting the animal on to the table:
  - Select exposure factors
  - Place cassette on table or in Bucky tray
  - Centre X-ray beam to grid and/or film cassette
  - Place markers and labels ready
- If using a rotating anode machine, press and release the first stage of the exposure button while positioning the patient, so that the animal is used to the noise before the exposure is made
- Once positioning is complete, keep reassuring the animal while slowly moving to a position at least 2 m from the primary beam to make the exposure. If possible, stay within the animal's vision to prevent it feeling abandoned.

Some involuntary movements by the patient may be unavoidable – for example, respiratory and cardiac movements in thoracic radiography. Short exposure times help to limit these but it is worth considering that an animal in pain or under stress will tend to have increased respiratory and heart rates. Appropriate use of sedatives and analgesics in such situations will help. If the animal is anaesthetized, the lungs should be inflated for thoracic radiographs. This stops respiratory movement during the course of the exposure and maximizes the volume of air in the lungs.

Chemical restraint

Some form of chemical restraint will be employed for most studies. This may be sedation or general anaesthesia, depending on the circumstances. General anaesthesia is preferred when the study is expected to take some time – for example, when taking multiple views or performing a contrast study – or where positioning is absolutely critical. Similarly, if it is likely that the patient will be going on to surgery after the examination, general anaesthesia is the obvious choice. One important exception to this is contrast studies of the upper alimentary tract, as general anaesthesia has a profound effect on motility.

Suitable sedative protocols for relatively healthy animals for radiography include:

- Dogs: acepromazine (0.05 mg/kg) plus buprenorphine (0.01 mg/kg) – can be mixed in the same syringe and administered i/m or i/v
- Cats: midazolam (0.2 mg/kg) plus ketamine (10–20 mg/kg) – can be mixed in the same syringe and administered i/m.

Patients that are very unwell often do not require any form of sedation, as they will usually lie with minimal restraint from sandbags. If they become very distressed at attempts to radiograph them, it is worth considering using low dose sedation and/or analgesia as this may be less risky than stressing them unduly.

Manual restraint

On the rare occasions when manual restraint is unavoidable, it must be done properly.

- Any personnel remaining in the controlled area (i.e. within 2 m of the primary beam) during the exposure must be protected from scattered radiation by lead gowns and gloves or sleeves
- A single person holding the head and forelimbs may suffice
- If it is necessary to hold both fore and hindlimbs, preferably have one person at each end of the animal, so

that they can stand as far back from the patient as possible, with arms outstretched (one person holding both ends has to stand very close to the primary beam)
- No part of the handler's body must ever be in the primary beam
- To protect eyes, turn head away from the X-ray tube when the exposure is made.

General positioning

Standardizing the position of the animal for a particular view is important, as interpretation of radiographic changes depends to some extent on comparison with normals. Variations from standard positions make interpretation more difficult, as the radiologist may not be sure if changes are due to pathology, or just an unfamiliar orientation of normal structures (Figure 9.11).

Various geometrical effects can produce distorted images of body organs on a radiograph with respect to their size and relative positions in the body. Such effects can be understood by assuming that X-rays originate from a point source and travel in straight lines away from it.

Magnification

Magnification of objects occurs due to divergence of the X-ray beam from the source.

- Objects furthest from the film appear larger than those that are closest
- This can be minimized by increasing film–focus distance and by decreasing object–film distance (Figure 9.12).

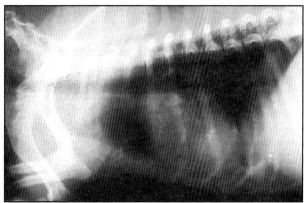
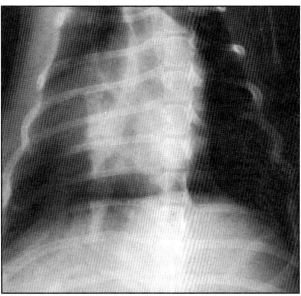

9.11 *Lateral and DV thoracic radiographs, both showing marked rotation which alters the appearance of the heart in particular, with respect to its size, shape and position.*

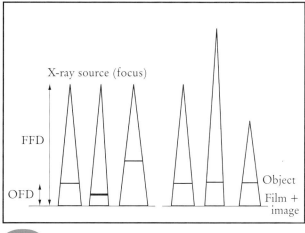

9.12 *Magnification.*

Distortion

Distortion occurs when the object is not parallel to the film and is sometimes inevitable – for example, when trying to obtain craniocaudal images of the femur. The object's position relative to the centre of the X-ray beam then becomes important; the further the object is from the centre (and from the film), the greater is the degree of distortion in the image. For thick objects this is very important (Figure 9.13).

Therefore, when positioning animals for radiography:

- Ensure that the area of interest is as close as possible to the film, to minimize magnification and distortion
- Use as long a film–focus distance as possible (this will be governed by machine output)
- Position the object parallel to the film whenever possible
- Ensure that the area of interest is under the centre of the X-ray beam.

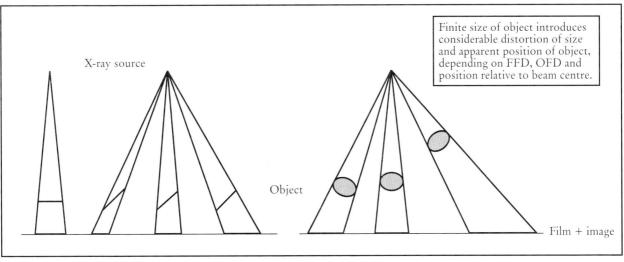

9.13 *Image distortion.*

Centring

Minimal divergence of the X-rays occurs at the centre of the X-ray beam, so the animal should be positioned such that this central beam passes through the required part. It is important that centring is accurate and that the centring points are known for each of the radiographic views. Whilst poor positioning is sometimes unavoidable, there is no excuse for poor centring. There are anatomical landmarks for each projection; in some cases these are superficial and can be seen, in others they are deeper and need to be palpated.

Collimation

Collimation reduces patient dose and scatter (thus improving image contrast).

- Always collimate the primary beam as closely as possible to include all of the structures required, without exposing any unnecessary parts of the patient
- Aim to see four collimated edges on each film (easy to achieve when radiographing a distal limb)
- For a large dog's chest or abdomen, collimate the beam to the cassette before positioning the animal, to ensure that the primary beam falls within its limits, and then collimate further to the animal if possible.

Positioning aids

A good assortment of positioning aids is invaluable to achieve correct positioning of the area under examination. Positioning aids should not be placed over or under the area of interest as none are completely radiolucent and they may produce artifacts on the film.

- Sandbags – essential for positioning and restraint. Long, thin ones are the best shape. They should not be too full, so that the sand can be distributed within them and they can be folded or draped over the animal
- Foam wedges and blocks – a variety of sizes and shapes are useful
- Radiolucent troughs – several sizes to accommodate small and large patients
- Tapes or lambing ropes – with a slipknot in one end for tying limbs. It is best not to use ties in unanaesthetized patients, because of the risk of serious injury if they should attempt to jump off the X-ray table when tied down.

Views

A radiograph is a two-dimensional representation of three-dimensional structures. For the radiologist to be able to build up an impression of the tissues in three dimensions, at least two views of the area are required, at right angles to each other (Figure 9.14). For most examinations, this will mean a lateral view and a second one at right angles to this, although on occasions special views will be taken at a different orientation to highlight a particular area.

When referring to a projection, it is normally named after the path taken by the X-ray beam through the patient to the film (Figure 9.15).

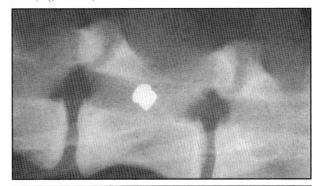

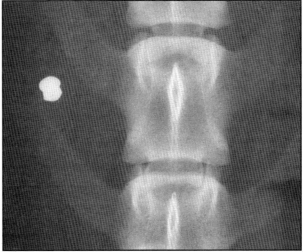

9.14 *The importance of two views. In the lateral, the airgun pellet appears to be within the spinal canal. The ventrodorsal view is required to show that the pellet is in fact lying within the soft tissue lateral to the vertebral column.*

Radiographic projections: terminology.

Lateral	Beam direction may be mediolateral or lateromedial Right or left lateral recumbency refer to thorax and abdomen adjacent to tabletop
Dorsoventral (DV) or Ventrodorsal (VD)	Refers to thorax, abdomen, spine, pelvis, hips
Craniocaudal or Caudocranial	Refers to proximal forelimbs and hindlimbs
Dorsopalmar (DPa)	Refers to forelimb distal to and including carpus
Dorsoplantar (DPl)	Refers to hindlimb distal to and including tarsus
Rostrocaudal	Refers to head

Labelling

A certain amount of information should be included on each radiograph:

- Animal identification (name and/or case number)
- Date
- Left or right side
- Timing of film for contrast studies.

Pre-processing labelling is by far the best option so that information is permanently marked on the radiograph itself, rather than using adhesive labels after processing. Right/left markers, which are placed on the cassette at the appropriate side of the animal when the exposure is made, are readily available. Other information can be placed on the cassette using lead characters or lead-impregnated tape at the time of exposure, or after exposure using a photo-imprinting system in the darkroom.

Use of a grid

A grid is normally used when tissue thickness exceeds 10 cm. The exposure must be increased when using a grid, the amount of increase depending on the grid factor. In some circumstances, particularly where a low output machine is used, the increase in exposure time required to allow grid use may be unacceptable, e.g. thoracic radiography. It may be preferable to sacrifice film contrast for sharpness, particularly for the thorax, which has high inherent contrast. However, for abdominal radiographs of larger patients, a grid is almost always needed to produce films of acceptable contrast.

Care is required when using a grid to ensure that:

- Film–focus distance is correct
- The beam is centred correctly
- The grid is the right way up (Figure 9.16).

Screen/film choice

A slow film–screen combination can be used to provide fine detail for skeletal work, whereas a faster combination will be required for thoracic and abdominal films to allow minimal exposure times and to limit movement.

Care of radiographic equipment

X-ray machine

- Regular servicing is essential for safety and quality control. The *Guidance Notes for the Protection of Persons against Ionising Radiations arising from Veterinary Use* state that servicing should be carried out at least once a year, and more often if frequency of use necessitates this. The service engineer makes a series of checks to ensure the machine is operating safely and that output is as expected
- Check film–focus distance (FFD) regularly. It is convenient to mark the standard distance on the tube stand with a permanent marker so that the position can be easily relocated. If the light beam diaphragm has a tape measure on it, its accuracy should be checked against an external tape measure
- Check that the tube head is level and parallel to the tabletop, using a spirit level (and check this matches the angulation markings on the machine)
- If the plastic covering of the light beam diaphragm becomes dirty it can produce artifacts on radiographs.

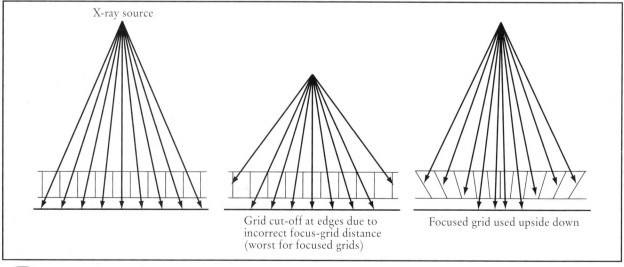

X-ray source

Grid cut-off at edges due to incorrect focus-grid distance (worst for focused grids)

Focused grid used upside down

9.16 *Film faults associated with incorrect grid usage.*

With the machine switched off, any dirt and debris should be cleaned off with mild soap and warm water

- Check light beam diaphragm accuracy regularly (Figure 9.17).

9.17 How to check the light beam diaphragm

1. Ensure that the FFD is set to 100 cm

2. Place a loaded cassette on the tabletop and collimate the beam to an area approximately 3 cm within the edges of the cassette on all sides

3. Place four metal markers (small coins are ideal) at the corner extremities of the field illuminated by the light beam diaphragm. A right ('R') marker placed in the lower right corner of the field will permit orientation if adjustments need to be made

4. Make an exposure at relatively low intensity (e.g. 50 kV/2 mAs)

5. Process the film

6. Compare the position of the exposed area on the film and the position of the objects outlining the illuminated area. It is acceptable if these are within 1 cm of each other at this FFD. If there is a larger discrepancy, the angle of the mirror in the light beam diaphragm requires adjustment and normally a service engineer would be called to do this.

Cassette care

Film cassettes are expensive and must be handled carefully. Care should be taken not to allow leakage of fluid (e.g. blood or urine) or entry of particulate matter (e.g. sand) into the cassette. Dropping a cassette on a hard surface may cause distortion, resulting in loss of film–screen contact and hence image unsharpness; or damage to the edge seal, allowing light to leak into the cassette.

The following measures may be taken:

- Where there is risk of fluid leakage, place the cassette inside a plastic bag
- Use cassette holders to provide some protection from physical damage (they sometimes also incorporate a grid)
- Clean exterior surfaces of cassettes monthly (or more often when needed), using mild soap and water.

If the practice has more than one cassette of a particular type, it is useful to number them. Write an identification number near the corner of one of the screens using a heavy black felt-tip pen and cover with clear nail varnish; write the same number on the back of the cassette. The number will appear on each film taken and a consistently occurring fault can be traced to an individual cassette.

Film faults associated with faulty or ageing cassettes

- A thin blackened edge to the radiograph – caused by light leakage along the cassette edge – may be seen with older cassettes when the felt pad between the cassette edges and hinged back wears with age
- A completely blackened area on the film – at the edge or in a corner – may be caused by damage to the cassette or deterioration of a cassette closure with age, allowing light leakage into the cassette. Also occasionally seen if a cassette is not properly closed (Figure 9.18)

- Unsharpness (blurring) of the image – may be local or involve the whole film. This can be caused by poor film–screen contact due to warping of the cassette (physical damage) or screen (may be due to loss of adhesion between back of screen and cassette) or loss of efficiency of the felt pressure pad in older cassettes. If there is persistent unsharpness when using a particular cassette then the film–screen contact should be checked (Figure 9.19).

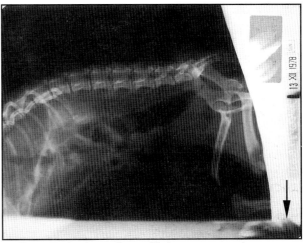

9.18 Fogging (arrowed) caused by improper cassette closure.

9.19 How to check film–screen contact

1. Allow at least 10 minutes after loading the cassette with film before performing the test (to allow any air trapped during loading to disperse)

2. Place the cassette on top of the X-ray table

3. Place a flat sheet of metal gauze or wire mesh over the cassette. If this is unavailable then use paperclips scattered at single thickness over the entire area of the cassette

4. Using a film–focus distance of 100 cm, collimate the beam to just within the edges of the cassette and make an exposure. Use a relatively low exposure: approximately 50 kV and 2 mAs should be suitable, but the exact settings will depend on the machine and cassette being used

5. Process the film

6. Check the film carefully under optimum viewing conditions for any areas of unsharpness.

Poor film–screen contact is of greatest importance when in the centre of the cassette, i.e. where the area of interest is most likely to be. It may be possible to rectify the situation simply by reattaching the screen to the backing felt within the cassette, or the screen and/or cassette may need to be replaced.

Screen care

Intensifying screens, like cassettes, are expensive items of equipment. They are particularly sensitive to damage, e.g. from pressure, abrasion and fluid spillage – such damage is permanent and irreparable. Foreign material such as dust or hair inside the cassette prevents light from the screens reaching the film, resulting in a white mark on the film. Any indentation or abrasion of the screen surface, or prolonged exposure to any type of fluid, can damage the screen, producing an underexposed area in the same location on all subsequent radiographs (Figure 9.20). Screen artifacts can lead to incorrect diagnoses and good screen care is therefore essential.

- Inspect and clean screens regularly (Figure 9.21) – approximately once a month but frequency will depend on workload
- Remove finger-rings when performing darkroom duties, to avoid scratching screens (and film)
- Only open screens to remove and load film and only do this in a clean environment
- Remove film by gently shaking the back plate of the cassette to free the film so that it can be grasped, rather than prising it out with fingers (this also prevents crimping of the film)
- Never touch screens with fingers.

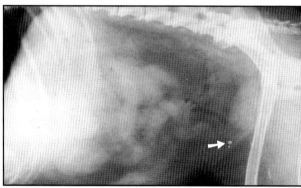

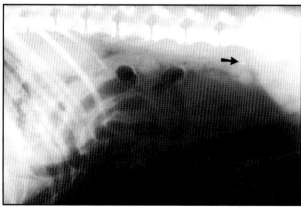

9.20 *Screen marks (arrowed) caused by damage to screens appear on all films taken.*

9.21 How to clean intensifying screens

1. Remove loose fragments of foreign material with a soft dry paintbrush or by pressurized air (camera shops sell small blower brushes for cleaning photographic equipment)
2. Gentle swabbing using cotton wool dampened with a cleaning solution can clean grease and superficial stains on the protective coat of the screens. Mild soap and warm water, dilute ethyl alcohol or proprietary screen cleaners can be used for this purpose
3. After cleaning, the screens must be completely dry before reloading. This should be achieved by propping the cassette open vertically to prevent any dust settling on the screens.

Mounting new screens in a cassette

Most cassettes are designed so that the intensifying screens can be replaced. The new screens will be labelled 'front' and 'back' and it is important that the correct screen is attached to the correct side of the cassette. The screens must be properly secured within the cassette and the screen manufacturer will supply double-sided adhesive tape for this purpose (liquid glue should not be used for this as some chemicals can interact with the screens). The screen surfaces must not be touched during the procedure and the screens should not be pressed into place. The natural pressure applied by the foam pads of the cassette when it is closed will perform this and apply even pressure.

Film storage and handling

As well as being sensitive to light and X-rays, X-ray film emulsion is affected by pressure, temperature, humidity, fumes (e.g. from formalin, ammonia, hydrogen peroxide) and rough handling. The sensitivity of the emulsion increases after radiographic exposure, making the film particularly vulnerable to faults caused by rough handling during unloading and processing. The gelatin of the emulsion becomes soft when it is heated and wet, i.e. during processing, and so it is easily damaged at this time.

When unloading and reloading film cassettes:

- Always check that hands are dry first
- Handle film by the edges only and with care to avoid bending or pressure
- Before closing cassettes, check that film is correctly positioned and will not be trapped at the edges.

Film should be stored:

- In a light-tight container (e.g. film hopper)
- On end rather than flat, to reduce pressure
- In a cool room at low humidity
- Well away from the primary X-ray beam.

Any film that is unlikely to be used before its expiry date can be sealed in a plastic bag and placed in a refrigerator or freezer to extend its shelf-life.

Care of grids

Grids are very expensive and quite delicate items of equipment. If the lead strips get bent or warped, their alignment relative to the primary X-ray beam is altered, resulting in a film artifact (as an underexposed area) every time the grid is used. Potter–Bucky grids are well protected by the tabletop in a dedicated X-ray table. However, stationary grids used on top of the table must be handled carefully and stored where they will not be prone to trauma – dropping a grid, especially on its edge, can cause permanent damage.

Positioning aids

- Dirt or positive contrast agent spilled on positioning aids may cause misleading artifacts on radiographs if the aid is within the area exposed by the primary beam
- Foam wedges can be wrapped in cling film to protect them from fluid spillage and allow them to be wiped clean easily
- Cradles need to be cleaned regularly but especially after positive contrast studies
- Sandbags should be made of waterproof material so that they can be wiped clean
- Any sandbag that develops a leak must be repaired or replaced immediately.

Protective clothing

Lead gowns, sleeves and gloves are expensive items with the very important function of protecting personnel involved in radiographic procedures from scattered radiation. If this clothing is damaged, anybody using it is at potential risk of exposure to radiation in the area of damage. The lead shielding in these items allows a certain amount of flexibility for comfort and movement of the wearer. However, if they are handled or stored inappropriately then cracks can appear in the shielding.

- Aprons should never be folded. When not in use they can be laid flat but it is often more convenient to store them vertically – either with metal hangers on a dedicated rack, or draped over a homemade hanger consisting of a large diameter (at least 4–5 cm) cylindrical bar, attached to the wall or floor
- Sleeves and gloves should not be folded and should preferably be stored on some form of vertical holder to allow air to circulate within them and prevent any build-up of moisture inside
- A regular check should be made of all protective clothing for obvious tears or cracks; this should include feeling both internal and external surfaces for irregularities or defects. A radiograph should be taken of any suspicious areas to check for penetration of the X-ray beam through the lead shielding, which would produce a blackened area on the film.

Processing radiographs

Those X-rays that pass through the patient then go on to affect the X-ray film. Silver bromide crystals in the film emulsion which absorb X-ray or light energy undergo a chemical change. This chemical change is invisible to the eye and the film emulsion appears the same after the exposure as before. The affected crystals are said to contain a latent image, which only becomes apparent to the eye once the film has been chemically processed.

The darkroom

The darkroom should be used solely for processing radiographs. As it is the only place where intensifying screens and X-ray film are exposed to the air, it must be clean. The room should be tidy and well organized so that work can be performed easily in the low light levels required. Obviously it must be lightproof and the door should be lockable from the inside to prevent films being accidentally exposed to light by personnel entering when processing is taking place. The darkroom is organized into two main areas: the dry bench and the wet bench, which must be separate.

The dry bench

The dry bench is where film is loaded and unloaded from cassettes.

- The work surface should be large enough to accommodate the largest cassette when open
- The bench must be cleaned frequently to avoid the possibility of dirt or hairs entering cassettes when open
- Nothing wet should be placed on the dry bench and care should be taken to ensure that no splashes can occur
- Film is usually stored in a film hopper or boxes at the side of, or beneath, the dry bench for convenience. It is helpful to keep film in order of size for ease of selection when reloading cassettes
- For manual processing, a selection of film hangers for each size of cassette available is stored on brackets above the dry bench. Storing different sizes on separate brackets facilitates selection when working in the dark.

Film hangers

Two designs of film hanger are available:

- Channel hangers tend to retain processing solutions and need careful cleaning and drying to prevent fluid spills on the dry bench. Films need to be removed from these hangers for the drying stage
- Clip hangers are more fragile and lose the ability to retain the film taut between the clips with time. The clips puncture the film corners and the edges of the holes created in this way can scratch other films when stored together.

The wet bench

The wet bench is where processing is carried out. If processing is automatic, it consists simply of the processor. If processing is manual, the requirements are:

- Three or four tanks – one containing developer, one containing fixer, and one or two containing water for the rinsing and washing stages
- A close-fitting lid for the developer tank to slow down the rate of deterioration of the developing solution
- A means of heating the chemical solutions – best achieved by standing the individual tanks in a larger tank filled with water warmed by a thermostatically controlled heater
- Thermometer – essential to check developer temperature
- Timer – to time the stages of processing accurately.

Practices with a very low throughput of radiographs may find it more economical to use small volumes of processing solutions in a series of shallow trays. Fresh developer can be made up each time it is required and warmed by a heat pad placed beneath the tray (again, using a thermometer to check when the correct temperature has been achieved). Developer should be discarded after use.

Safelight

To avoid fogging of the film while working in the darkroom, the safelight must meet several criteria:

- The bulb should not exceed 15 watts
- The filter on the light must be correct for the type of film being used:
  - Brown filter for blue light-sensitive film
  - Dark red filter is suitable for both green and blue light-sensitive film
- The light must be at least 1.2 m above the workbench.

Even when these criteria are met, the safelight is only 'safe' for a short length of time. Figure 9.22 shows how to check the light. Film exposed to the safelight for an excessive length of time will become fogged, so personnel performing darkroom duties must be familiar with the procedures.

9.22 How to check the safelight

1. Place a bunch of keys on a piece of unexposed film on the darkroom bench beneath the safelight

2. Leave them for one minute

3. Process the film. If an image of the keys is visible on the processed film then there is a safelight problem.

Stages involved in processing

Development

Developer is a reducing solution that donates electrons to the silver halide crystals containing a latent image. The donated electrons convert silver ions in the crystal into silver atoms, leaving a small black speck of silver on the film, while the bromine from the crystal moves into the gelatin. Crystals not containing a latent image have a barrier of negative bromine ions on their surface that prevents the developer from entering them.

The main components of the developer (dissolved in water) are:

- Alkaline reducing agents (e.g. metol or phenidone plus hydroquinone)
- Accelerators and buffers – to maintain an optimum pH for the action of the reducing agents (e.g. sodium carbonate, sodium hydroxide)
- Preservatives – to slow down oxidation (e.g. sodium sulphite)
- Restrainers – to limit the action of the reducing agents to those crystals that have been exposed (e.g. potassium bromide)
- Hardeners – included in solutions for automatic processors to prevent excessive swelling of the emulsion, which could lead to damage by the rollers
- Fungicides – may be added to deter the growth of moulds.

Developer is normally supplied as a concentrated solution or powder, which is made up with tap water to the recommended strength. Development time, temperature and concentration are critical and should always be according to the manufacturer's instructions. Higher or lower temperatures can be used, with a corresponding decrease or increase, respectively, in the development time if necessary. It is worth remembering that developer oxidizes more quickly at higher temperatures, thus requiring more frequent replenishment and replacement.

Developer deteriorates with time, whether used or not, and should be completely renewed at least every three months, or when the solution has darkened. Oxidation occurs more rapidly on exposure to air, therefore the lid should be kept on the developer tank as much as possible. The developer level can be topped up between replacements, using replenisher. This is not the same solution as normal developer, which is not appropriate for this purpose. Replenishers are formulated to maintain the correct balance of the various components of the solution and are available from the manufacturer.

Rinsing

After development, the film is briefly rinsed to stop the development process and to prevent carry-over of developer into the fixer tank. Ideally the rinse tank will use running water; if this is not available, the water should at least be fresh for each processing session.

Fixation

Fixing the film removes unexposed silver bromide from the emulsion, leaving a clear area on the film. It also stops any continuing development in the emulsion and hardens the emulsion, which becomes soft and swollen during development, to prevent physical damage.

The main components of the fixer are:

- Fixing agent – this dissolves the silver halide (e.g. ammonium or sodium thiosulphate)
- Weak acid and buffers – to neutralize any remaining developer and maintain an optimum pH (e.g. acetic acid, sodium metabisulphite)
- Preservative – to prevent decomposition of the fixing agent (e.g. sodium sulphite)
- Hardener – to prevent further softening and swelling of the emulsion and to increase resistance to physical damage (e.g. potassium alum, aluminium sulphate).

Fixer temperature is much less critical than developer temperature but if there is great variation between the two, it can cause mottling on the final radiograph due to irregular expansion and contraction of the emulsion. Clearing time in the fixer is about 2–3 minutes (the fixer needs to be replaced once clearing time exceeds this) but hardening takes longer and the film should be left in the fixer for approximately 10 minutes. Non-screen film takes considerably longer to clear because of the thicker emulsion.

Washing

After fixing, films are washed to remove all residue of processing chemicals. Washing causes further swelling and softening of the emulsion, so films must be handled carefully at this stage to avoid damage. It is important to immerse the clips and channels of the film hanger completely during washing, otherwise residual chemicals will run down the film while drying, causing streaking on the film.

Drying

Film hangers should hold the film taut, otherwise uneven retention of water causes pale grey water marks on the film. Drying should take place in a clean dust-free environment. Special heated cabinets are available for this purpose but are probably unnecessary unless film throughput is very high.

Manual processing procedure

A step-by-step guidance to this procedure is given in Figure 9.23.

Automatic processing

The sequence of events in an automatic processor (Figure 9.24) is similar to that for manual processing. However, several features of automation mean that the time taken for production of a dry film, ready for viewing, is reduced from well over an hour to somewhere between about 90 seconds and 5 minutes.

- Exposed films are placed on a feed tray
- A roller transport system takes the film through a series of three tanks (developer, fixer and wash) at a controlled speed to ensure that it spends the appropriate length of time in each tank:
  - Developer temperature is between 27 and 35°C, allowing much reduced developing time
  - The rollers squeeze the film as it moves straight to the fixer tank, removing virtually all of the residual developer and removing the need for a rinse tank. The hardening component of the fixer is especially important, as the emulsion is particularly fragile at these higher temperatures
  - Fixer is squeezed from the film by the rollers as it passes through to the wash tank. The wash tank is relatively small but a fast flow rate (at least 6 l/min) carries residual chemicals away rapidly, so washing time is much reduced

9.23 How to process a film manually

1. **Preparation.**
   - Check developer and fixer levels; replenish if necessary
   - Check developer temperature (normally 20°C)
   - Stir processing solutions to distribute chemicals evenly and ensure even development. A separate paddle must be used for each tank
   - Make sure hands are clean and dry
   - Switch on the extractor fan and safelight; lock the door and switch off the main light

2. **Unload the cassette.** Open cassette and gently shake the top so that the film falls free and can be grasped gently between finger and thumb without bending it. Handle film only by the edges. Take care not to touch the intensifying screens. Close the cassette while proceeding with the next step

3. **Load the film on to a hanger.** If a clip hanger is used, hold the hanger upside down and insert the film into the bottom clips first. Then invert the hanger, make sure the film is stretched taut and secure it with the top clips. If using a channel hanger, slide the film into the side channels from the top, check that the bottom of the film is engaged in the bottom channel and then close the hinge at the top

4. **Develop the film and reload the cassette.** Insert the film into the developing tank and agitate a few times to remove any air bubbles from the film surface. Replace the tank lid and start the timer for the required time (usually 5 minutes). Reload the film cassette while waiting. Occasional agitation of the film during development will bring fresh developer into contact with the film surface

5. **Rinse the film.** When the timer rings, remove the film quickly from the developer and move it across to the rinse tank. Try to prevent exhausted developer on the film surface running back into the developer tank. Immerse the film in the rinse tank and agitate for about 20 seconds

6. **Fix the film.** Drain excess water from the film after removing from the rinse tank. Immerse it in the fixer. Agitate a few times to remove surface air bubbles and set the timer for 10 minutes. The light can be switched on after the film has been in the fixer for about 1 minute

7. **Wash the film.** When the timer goes, remove the film from the fix and transfer it to the wash tank quickly so that spent fixer goes into the wash tank. Wash in running water for a minimum of 15 minutes, preferably 30 minutes. After this time a wetting agent can be used for a brief final rinse, if available. Although not commonly used, these agents speed up drying time and reduce the risk of streaky water marks appearing while drying

8. **Dry the film.** If channel hangers are used, the films need to be removed for drying and can be hung by clips on a taut wire. Films must not contact each other when wet, so must be hung carefully to dry. Trim corners off films that have been processed in clip hangers to prevent scratching of emulsion of adjacent film by sharp points.

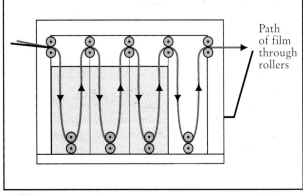

Path of film through rollers

9.24 *Automatic processor.*

- Rollers between washing and drying sections help to remove excess water from the film, which is then dried by blowing hot air on to both sides in a drying chamber.

The chemicals are continuously replenished to keep the solutions at optimum efficiency. As a film feeds into the processor, pumps are activated to infuse replenisher from reservoir tanks of developer and fixer into the appropriate tanks in the unit. Recirculation pumps mix the replenisher with the solutions in the tanks. Excess processing solutions flow from the top of the tanks and must be drained into containers suitable for collection by an approved contractor.

Maintenance of automatic processors

- Always allow the processor to warm up to operating temperature before putting any films through (usually takes 10–20 minutes)
- Once warmed up, put a large exposed unwanted film through the processor to remove traces of dried chemicals from the transport rollers
- Clean the processor regularly – the less the processor is used, the more cleaning is required. Roller racks should be removed on at least a weekly basis, rinsed with warm water and allowed to air dry before being replaced. The tanks also require cleaning on a regular basis (at least once a month)
- Regular servicing by an approved engineer is essential, to avoid costly and untimely breakdowns. In the event of a breakdown, it is helpful if there is some emergency facility (e.g. dish processing) for processing urgently required films.

Safety considerations

The disposal of waste processing solutions is covered by COSHH regulations.

- Discarded developer and fixer must not be disposed of via the drains but collected for appropriate disposal by an authorized contractor. Silver can be recovered from the used fixer solution
- Processing solutions can cause skin irritation in susceptible individuals. It is advisable to wear protective gloves when involved with darkroom duties if there is any cause for concern
- In situations where an automatic processor is enclosed within the darkroom, an extractor fan is required to prevent excessive build-up of heat and fumes from the processor and must always be used while the processor is switched on.

Assessing radiograph quality

A good quality radiograph is one that accurately depicts the structures under investigation. The main factors that contribute to film quality are:

- Film density (blackness of the film)
- Film contrast (differences in density between different structures)
- Resolution (the ability to distinguish small changes in size and shape)
- Sharpness (the clarity with which interfaces between structures can be seen).

These are influenced by many factors, including exposure and processing techniques and choice of film–screen combination.

Any film faults can cause a loss of information and may lead to undesirable repeat exposures being necessary or to incorrect diagnoses being reached. When trying to determine the cause of a particular film fault:

- View the film in both transmitted and reflected light
- Check the film surface for bends, scratches and material on the surface
- Classify the fault as focal or general and as light, dark or cloudy
- Remember that radiographic film is sensitive to X-rays, light, pressure, fumes (e.g. from ammonia, hydrogen peroxide, formalin), temperature, humidity and rough handling. The sensitivity of the emulsion increases after exposure, therefore rough handling at this time causes a large proportion of faults.

Some of the more common causes of poor film quality and faults are listed here.

- Films too dark overall – see Figures 9.25 and 9.26
- Films too light overall – see Figures 9.27 to 9.29
- Causes of poor film contrast
  - Fogging (e.g. by light, chemicals, background radiation)
  - Scattered radiation
  - Incorrect film storage
  - Out-of-date film
  - Overexposure and underdeveloping
  - Developer time too short and temperature too high
- Causes of unsharpness
  - Large focal spot size
  - Movement of patient, table or X-ray tube head during the course of the exposure (Figures 9.30 and 9.31)
  - Poor film–screen contact

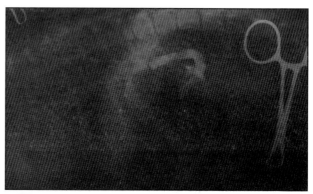

9.26 *Film that is too dark overall and lacks contrast. This may be caused by too high a kV or by overdeveloping.*

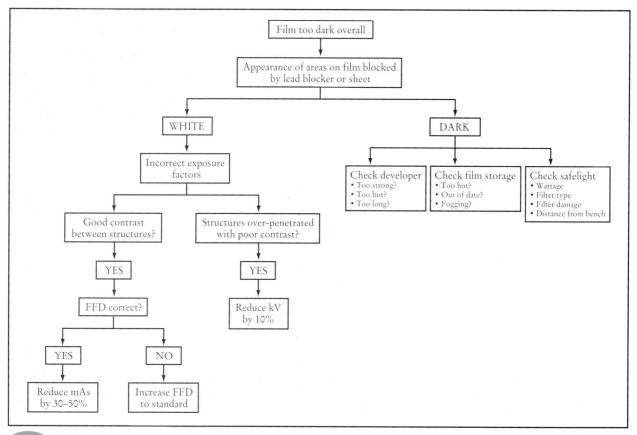

9.25 *Films that are too dark overall.*

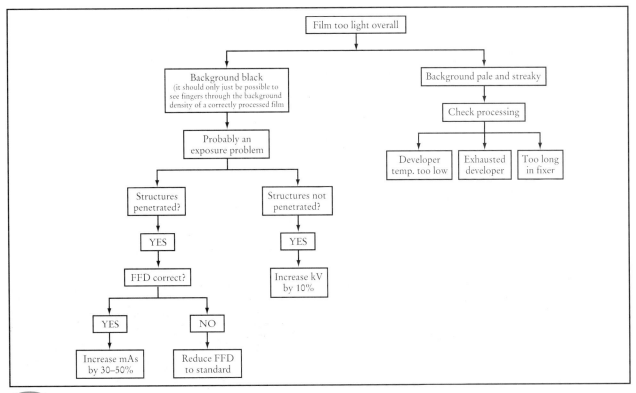

9.27 *Films that are too light overall.*

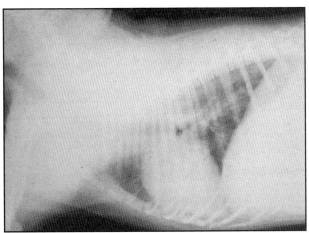

9.28 *Underexposed film; kV too low, producing high contrast film with underpenetration of structures.*

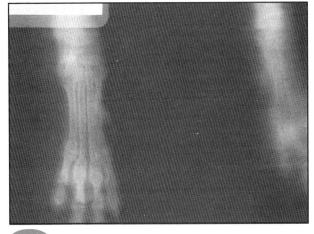

9.30 *Image unsharpness due to patient movement.*

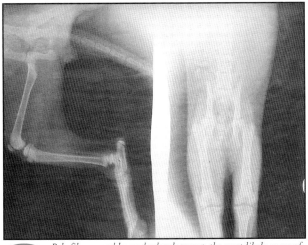

9.29 *Pale film caused by underdevelopment, the most likely cause of which is exhausted developer. The pale streaky background is typical*

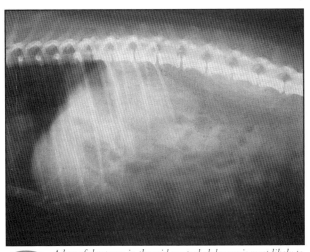

9.31 *A loss of sharpness in the mid-ventral abdomen is most likely to be caused by patient movement but could be due to poor film – screen contact in this area.*

- Film faults – black marks
  - Splashes with water or developer (Figure 9.32)
  - Crescent shaped – caused by poor film handling (Figure 9.33)
  - Fingerprints – caused by film handler having water or developer on hands
  - Static marks – these look like a branching tree and are more likely to occur in very dry weather. They may be caused by drawing film rapidly from the box or sliding it across an intensifying screen, or by discharges from nylon clothing
  - Linear scratches – pressure sensitizes the emulsion
  - Radiation/light fogging at edge or corner of film – may be produced by opening the darkroom door before the film has fully fed into an automatic processor, or by an improperly closed cassette (Figure 9.34, and see Figure 9.18)

- Film faults – white marks
  - Splashes with fixer before development
  - Fingerprints – grease or oil on the film handler's fingers acts as a barrier to the developer
  - Crescent shaped – caused by poor film handling
  - Linear scratches – if deep enough, the emulsion may be completely removed
  - Sharply defined marks – due to hairs and dirt inside the cassette or damaged areas on the intensifying screens (see Figure 9.20)
  - Dirt on the animal's coat
  - Contrast material on the animal's coat, cassette or positioning aids (Figure 9.35)
  - Collars, etc. (Figure 9.36)

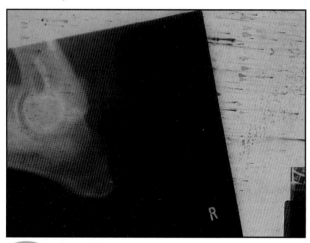

9.32 Film splashed with developer before processing.

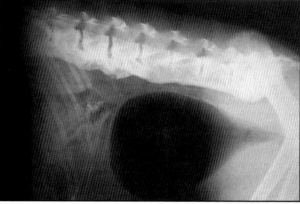

9.34 Light fogging down left-hand edge of film. This could be caused by opening the darkroom door before the film has been fully fed into the automatic processor, or by leaving the film hopper open or leaving the lid off the film box.

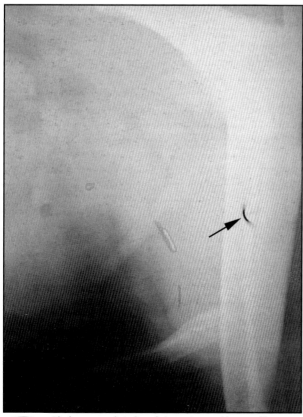

9.33 Black crescent-shaped mark (arrow) caused by poor film handling.

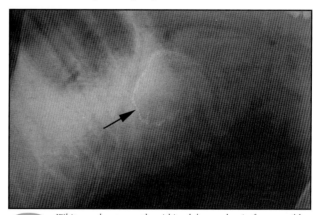

9.35 White marks apparently within abdomen, but in fact caused by contrast spilled on patient's coat.

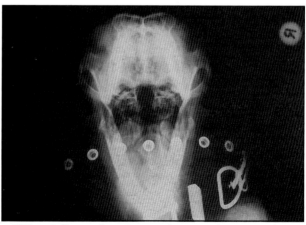

9.36 Collars or other radiopaque objects may obscure areas of interest.

- Film faults – miscellaneous
  - Cassette upside down – film underexposed due to absorption of X-rays by lead in cassette back and metal cassette closures produce white marks (Figure 9.37)
  - Surface marks – caused by algae in the wash tank
  - Dichroic fog – a pinkish stain in reflected light, caused by excess carry-over of developer into the fixer tank
  - Yellow-brown stains – caused by inadequate washing
  - Streaks – caused by inadequate agitation of developer during processing or by processing solutions dripping from dirty hanger clips

- Inadequate processing tank levels
  - Developer – leaves a clear edge at top of film
  - Fixer – leaves an area of uncleared green emulsion at top of film (also seen if two films are fed into an automatic processor too close together and overlap)
- Film faults associated with automatic processors
  - Films stuck together in processor, leaving uncleared emulsion on one side of film (Figure 9.38)
  - Light fogging of film edge (appears black) if darkroom door opened too early (see Figure 9.34)
  - Transport problems – pressure marks from the rollers
  - Sediment on rollers or roughened surface of rollers causing scratches in emulsion.

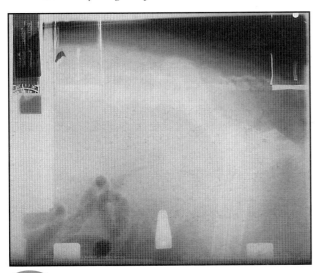

9.37 *Cassette placed upside down.*

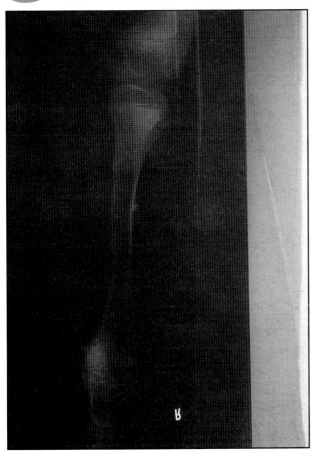

9.38 *Two films stuck together in processor, leaving uncleared emulsion down right-hand side of film.*

Rules governing the taking of radiographs

The Control of Substances Hazardous to Health (COSHH) Regulations (1988) require that employers provide a safe place of work, safe equipment and appliances and a safe work system. They must also exercise due care in the appointment of employees in positions in which the safety of others may depend upon their competence.

The law as it relates to the use of radiation and radioactive materials is defined in the Ionizing Radiations Regulations 1985 and the supplementary *Approved Code of Practice for the Protection of Persons against Ionizing Radiation arising from any Work Activity*. Much of the content of these rather legalistic documents is not relevant to veterinary radiography.

The important points of legislation as applicable to veterinary diagnostic radiography are contained in the *Guidance Notes for the Protection of Persons against Ionizing Radiations arising from Veterinary Use* (1988), which contain practical, readable advice for those involved in this area. Anyone involved in radiography should be familiar with and understand the content of the 'Guidance Notes'.

All veterinary practices using an X-ray machine must notify the Health and Safety Executive, which supplies a specific form for this purpose.

- Most practices are also required to appoint a radiation protection advisor (RPA) – an external expert who will advise on all aspects of radiation safety. The RPA will draw up a set of local rules for the safe use of X-rays within the practice
- There should also be a radiation protection supervisor (RPS) for each practice, who will be a senior member of staff and who is responsible for ensuring that everyone involved in radiography is familiar with the relevant legislation and that the local rules are implemented.

Radiation hazards

The taking of radiographs involves some risk to those involved with the procedure, as ionizing radiations have a harmful effect on living tissues. However, many other work procedures in which veterinary staff are involved carry a much higher risk of injury, such as lifting heavy dogs or handling aggressive animals. The difference between these situations and radiography is that X-rays are invisible and painless and their effects are not apparent at the time of exposure. Also, repeated doses of radiation can have a cumulative effect. The effects of radiation on body tissues depend on the time period in which the radiation is received and the amount of the body exposed to the radiation. Different tissues vary in their sensitivity to radiation injury.

Possible effects of radiation exposure are:

- Somatic (e.g. skin erythema and cataract formation)
- Carcinogenic (e.g. leukaemia)
- Genetic – inherited abnormalities in future generations.

However, provided that care is taken when performing radiographic examinations, the risk to personnel should be insignificant.

Controlled area

An RPA is required where a controlled area has been designated which people enter.

- The controlled area is one in which the radiation dose exceeds a specified minimum. For a typical veterinary practice using a vertical beam, this has been shown to be everywhere within a 2 m radius of the central beam axis
- For permanently installed equipment, the controlled area must be physically demarcated and access to it restricted
- In practical terms, it is usually most convenient if the whole X-ray room is designated as the controlled area, making it easier to restrict access by the use of warning notices and signals
- Personnel should avoid entering the controlled area whenever possible and may only enter under a written system of work, which is prepared in consultation with the RPA and forms part of the local rules
- A copy of the local rules should be displayed in the X-ray room
- The X-ray machine should be isolated from the electrical supply once the radiographic examination is complete and unrestricted access to the room is then permitted.

Principles involved in the safe use of X-rays

The best way to limit exposure to radiation is to keep the use of X-rays to the minimum necessary. For example, it is not satisfactory to radiograph an animal's entire skeleton because it is lame.

- Radiography is not a substitute for proper clinical examination and there must be good clinical justification for its use
- Adequate restraint, together with good radiographic and processing techniques, will avoid the need for repeat exposures
- The use of fast film–screen combinations (rare earth phosphors) to limit exposures and accurate collimation to limit dose and production of scattered radiation, are also important considerations.

It is sensible to maintain as great a distance as possible from the primary beam during exposures, as radiation intensity falls off rapidly with distance from the X-ray source. The safe distance from the primary beam may well be within the X-ray room but the controlled area will usually be to the limits of the room; this means that personnel outside the room are clear and that no special protection precautions need apply.

It will occasionally be necessary for personnel to be present in the controlled area; for example:

- To hold an animal that cannot be safely sedated and will not remain in position with the use of positioning aids
- To inflate the lungs of an anaesthetized patient for thoracic radiography
- To participate in a contrast study.

When this is necessary, adequate protection in the form of lead sleeves, gowns and gloves must be used as appropriate. These items are only intended to protect the body from scattered radiation and no part of the body should ever be in the area exposed by the primary beam. Standing as far as possible from the X-ray machine is advisable. The rules governing entry of personnel into the controlled area will be specified by the RPA in the local rules, under the written system of work.

Protection of the radiographer

- Staff should never be in the primary beam
- Holding of animals should always be avoided if possible
- If it is necessary to hold animals, rotate the personnel involved. No one person should be called upon to do this more than three or four times a year at the most
- Personnel must wear protective clothing in the controlled area
- All staff involved in radiography should always wear a dose meter.

Further reading

Douglas SW, Herrtage ME and Williamson HD (1987) *Principles of Veterinary Radiography*, 4th edn. Baillière Tindall, Philadelphia

Lavin LM (1994) *Radiography in Veterinary Technology*. WB Saunders, Philadelphia

Morgan JP (ed.) (1993) *Techniques of Veterinary Radiography*, 5th edn. Iowa State University Press, Ames, Iowa

NRPB/HSE (1988) *Guidance Notes for the Protection of Persons against Ionising Radiations arising from Veterinary Use*. HMSO, London

10 Reproduction and care of the neonate

Freda Scott-Park

This chapter is designed to give information on:

- The reproductive cycle of the dog and cat
- Mating, pregnancy, parturition
- Lactation and management of the newborn
- Possible problems and complications

Introduction

An understanding of the normal reproductive cycles of cats and dogs is essential for the veterinary nurse in practice. There are many specialized terms that are used to describe the anatomy, physiology and pathology of the reproductive tract. A full knowledge of anatomical structure is required before this chapter is read.

The oestrous cycle in the bitch

Oestrus is the stage of the reproductive cycle when the female accepts the male. An owner often describes this period as a 'heat' or 'season', which includes pro-oestrus as well as oestrus and lasts about 3 weeks (Figure 10.1).

Figures 10.2–10.7 show the changes in vaginal cytology throughout the cycle.

Age at first oestrus is the age at puberty. *Puberty* is defined as the onset of sexual function; it commences at first ovulation. The average age of puberty in the bitch is 8–9 months (range 5–24 months).

The bitch can be described as seasonally monoestrous. Bitches have:

- A heat or season every 4–12 months
- On average, two seasons per year
- Seasons occurring commonly in spring and autumn.

10.1 Oestrous cycle of the bitch

Phase	Duration	Signs
Pro-oestrus[a]	7–10 days (range 4–14 days)	Some vulval swelling Blood stained discharge Attracts dogs but repels mating Sometimes behavioural changes
Oestrus[a]	8–12 days (range 5–15 days)	More swollen and flaccid vulva Discharge more mucoid, less blood Attracts dogs and allows mating Has escapist tendencies
Metoestrus[b] (luteal/post-oestrus phase, also called dioestrus)	Approximately same length of time as pregnancy (55 days)	No external signs Not attractive to dogs Vulva is normal size Possible whitish discharge at start Possible mammary enlargement towards the end
Anoestrus	3–4 months (range 1–9 months)	Period of quiescence following the luteal phase or pregnancy

a *Pro-oestrus + oestrus = heat/season; lasts about 3 weeks*
b *False pregnancy and pyometra occur during metoestrus.*

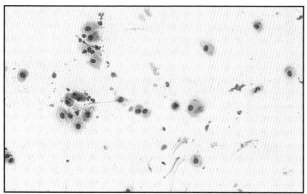

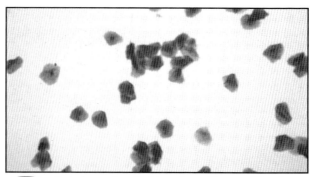

10.2   *Vaginal smear from bitch in anoestrus. Small parabasal cells predominate as they are unstimulated by oestrogens. This bitch was last in season about 5 months previously. Progesterone concentration is basal (< 3 ng/ml).*
Courtesy of Dr M. Harvey.

10.5   *Vaginal smear from bitch in early to mid-oestrus. The cells are almost entirely anucleated. The bitch is very close to ovulating and will be standing to accept the male, with this standing phase lasting about 9 days. Progesterone concentration will be rising (i.e. between 3 and 11 ng/ml) if ovulation is due within 48 hours or will be high (> 11 ng/ml) if ovulation has already taken place.*
Courtesy of Dr M. Harvey.

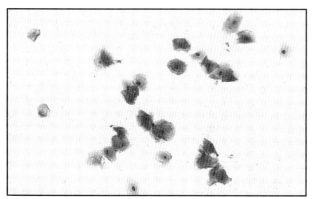

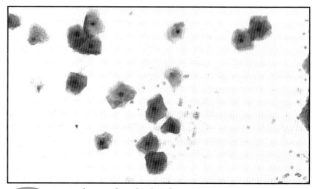

10.3   *Vaginal smear from bitch in early pro-oestrus. Mixture of parabasal and larger oestrogen-stimulated nucleated cornified cells. About 5 days after start of pro-oestrus progesterone concentration is basal (< 3 ng/ml).*
Courtesy of Dr M. Harvey.

10.6   *Vaginal smear from bitch in late oestrus. The appearance is similar to pro-oestrus: the cells are nucleated or becoming nucleated again, due to declining oestrogens. At the very end of oestrus, parabasal cells reappear. The plasma progesterone concentration is high, indicating that ovulation has occurred.*
Courtesy of Dr M. Harvey.

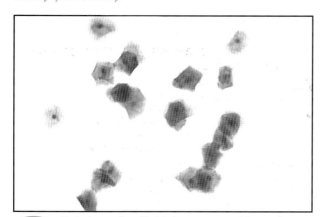

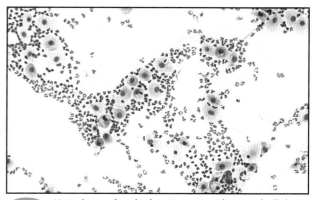

10.4   *Vaginal smear from bitch in late pro-oestrus. Mixture of nucleated and faintly nucleated cornified cells. This bitch started bleeding about 16 days previously. Progesterone still basal (< 3 ng/ml).*
Courtesy of Dr M. Harvey.

10.7   *Vaginal smear from bitch in metoestrus. The vaginal cells have reverted to nucleated parabasal type with a massive inflow of polymorphonuclear leucocytes, indicating that the bitch is past oestrus and no longer receptive or fertile. Progesterone concentration is still very high and will remain elevated for about 2 months whether she is pregnant or not.*
Courtesy of Dr M. Harvey.

Ovulation in the bitch

- The bitch is a *spontaneous ovulator*, which means that she ovulates whether or not mating takes place
- Most bitches start to ovulate 24–36 hours after the onset of oestrus. Many ova are shed and ovulation takes place over hours or days
- After ovulation, the area within the burst follicle luteinizes (forms luteal tissue) and this becomes the corpus luteum. Follicles in the ovary of a bitch luteinize to some degree before ovulation.

Hormonal control of the oestrous cycle

Hormonal control of the oestrous cycle is illustrated in Figure 10.8.

- *Follicle-stimulating hormone* (FSH) from the anterior pituitary stimulates development of follicles in the ovary
- During pro-oestrus, the developing follicles produce increasing amounts of *oestrogen*, reaching a high level at the end of pro-oestrus
- This stimulates a surge of *luteinizing hormone* (LH) from the anterior pituitary, causing:

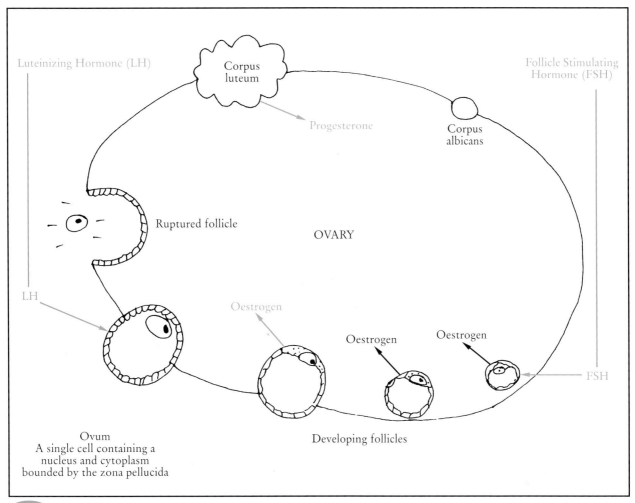

Luteinizing Hormone (LH)

Corpus luteum

Follicle Stimulating Hormone (FSH)

Progesterone

Corpus albicans

Ruptured follicle

OVARY

LH

Oestrogen

Oestrogen

Oestrogen

FSH

Ovum
A single cell containing a
nucleus and cytoplasm
bounded by the zona pellucida

Developing follicles

10.8 *Hormonal control of the oestrous cycle.*

- luteinization of the follicles
- ovulation
- development of the corpora lutea
- The corpora lutea produce *progesterone*, which remains above basal levels until the end of the luteal phase of the cycle
- During anoestrus, oestrogen and progesterone are basal.

Prevention and postponement of oestrus

Suppression (abolition of that particular cycle) or prevention (drugs are given before the oestrous cycle) of oestrus should be effective, reliable, easily administered, reversible and safe.

Reasons for suppression of oestrus:

- To avoid nuisance or inconvenience
- To control abnormalities of the cycle
- To prevent breeding because:
  - There is overproduction of offspring
  - The bitch (or queen) is too old or too young
  - Dystocia is likely to be a problem (pelvic damage, narrow birth canal)
  - The dam is physically or temperamentally unsound.

Pharmacological control

A variety of compounds may be used to inhibit cyclical activity (Figure 10.9). These include progestogens, androgens, testosterone and gonadotrophin-releasing hormone (GnRH) agonists and antagonists. (GnRH products are not licensed for use in dogs.)

10.9 Products commonly used for control of oestrus

Drug	Use
Proligestone	Injection: Temporary and permanent postponement of oestrus Suppression of oestrus
Megoestrol acetate	Oral: Suppression of oestrus Injection: Temporary postponement of oestrus
Medroxyprogesterone acetate	Oral: Suppression of oestrus Temporary postponement of oestrus Injection: Permanent postponement of oestrus
Testosterone	Injection: Suppression of oestrus

The advantages of medical methods are:

- Cheaper than surgery in the short term
- No surgical or anaesthetic risks
- Flexible
- Effective
- Reversible.

The disadvantages are:

- Expensive in large dogs, particularly in the long term
- Owner compliance required for oral preparations
- Not suitable for all animals (e.g. diabetics)
- Unpredictable time of next season
- May cause pain and coat discoloration
- Future problems (e.g. weight gain, pyometra).

There are three ways of controlling the cycle:

- Suppression of the oestrus and prevention of conception: by medication at the onset of pro-oestrus
- Temporary postponement of oestrus to a more convenient time: by medication just before an anticipated heat
- Permanent postponement of oestrus: by repeat medication given in the anoestrus, which has been induced by medication given previously in pro-oestrus (suppression) or anoestrus (temporary postponement).

Surgical methods

Ovariohysterectomy is the removal of the ovaries and the genital tract to the level of the cervix. The term *spaying* is used synonymously but correctly refers to removal of the ovaries only.

The advantages of surgical methods are:

- Permanent
- Owner compliance minimal
- Reduces or abolishes risk of
  - Pyometra
  - Ovarian cysts/tumours
  - Mammary tumours
- Cheaper than long-term use of drugs.

The disadvantages are:

- Irreversible
- Surgical or anaesthetic risk
- Variable risk of long-term effects:
  - Weight gain
  - Urinary incontinence
  - Dermatological problems.

It is preferable that the bitch is in anoestrus when she is presented for surgery.

 If an ovariohysterectomy is carried out during metoestrus and clinical signs of pseudopregnancy are present, then spaying can result in a permanent condition of pseudocyesis (pseudopregnancy).

There is considerable discussion about the optimum age to perform an ovariohysterectomy in a bitch. It is technically easier to operate on a younger animal but there is the possibility of causing early growth plate closure and underdevelopment of the secondary sexual characteristics, leading to infantile vulva syndrome. Some veterinary surgeons operate as early as 4 months; others leave the operation until after the first oestrus.

Abnormalities of the oestrous cycle in bitches

Physiological variation due to the wide variation of normal values in the oestrous cycle can lead to a misdiagnosis of oestrous cycle abnormality. A bitch will achieve the LH peak and therefore ovulation will occur, even if mating has been at an inappropriate time. However, this can cause an owner to suppose that the bitch is abnormal. Vaginal cytology and progesterone assays will help to determine the exact time of ovulation.

Disruption to the normal cycle can cause problems in breeding bitches. Some of the more common problems are as follows:

Silent heat

- No or very weak signs of heat
- Ovarian function is normal
- Ovulation is detected by cytology and plasma progesterone assay
- Condition may be inherited so perhaps bitch should not be bred.

Prolonged pro-oestrus

- Pro-oestrus signs may last as long as 6 weeks
- Bitch remains attractive to dogs
- Considered normal if it occurs during the first oestrous cycle
- Considered abnormal if it is not during the pubertal cycle
- May be associated with LH deficiency
- Most cases resolve spontaneously.
- Vaginal cytology: large numbers of cornified cells and no white cells, which indicate that oestrogen-secreting follicles are present in the ovary.

Split heat (split pro-oestrus)

- Pro-oestral serosanguineous discharge terminates after 4 days
- Discharge then restarts again after a few weeks and progresses to ovulation
- Aetiology is unknown
- Fertility is unaffected
- No evidence of reproductive tract pathology
- Monitor by vaginal cytology and plasma progesterone assay.

Cystic ovaries

- Due to LH deficiency
- Tends to occur in older maiden bitches
- Persistent vaginal bleeding after normal pro-oestrus
- Watery dark discharge
- Attractive to males but bitch is not receptive
- Treatment is by ovariohysterectomy
- Vaginal cytology: epithelial cells are partly cornified with square borders, still containing nuclei reflecting high levels of circulating oestrogens.

Anovulation

- Rare
- Bitches present in pro-oestrus, which lasts an abnormally long time
- Mature bitches come into pro-oestrus but never allow mating

- Bitch progresses to the LH surge but ovulation does not occur
- Chorionic gonadotrophin usually induces ovulation and allows mating
- If not treated the bitch may
  - Either ovulate up to 1 week after the LH surge
  - Or undergo follicular atrophy and return to anoestrus
- Vaginal cytology: 70% cornification.

Retained ovary after ovariohysterectomy

- May be an entire ovary or just a small piece of ovarian tissue
- Signs are those of pro-oestrus with no bleeding but vulva may be more moist
- Plasma progesterone or GnRH stimulation test will later indicate the presence of an ovary
- Treatment is by ovariectomy
- Vaginal cytology: look for cornified cells when bitch is attractive to males.

Ovarian tumour

- Not very common
- Granulosa cell tumours in older bitches
- Often inactive; clinical signs relate to a space-occupying lesion
- Oestrogen-producing tumours will present as pro-oestrus/oestrus
- Some granulosa cell tumours produce progesterone, causing cystic endometrial hyperplasia and pyometra
- Ovariohysterectomy is the treatment of choice.

Abnormalities of the luteal phase

Pseudopregnancy (phantom pregnancy, pseudocyesis, false pregnancy)

This is a common condition in the bitch. Signs occur 6–9 weeks after oestrus, during metoestrus. The animal shows signs of being pregnant although she has not been mated or has not conceived after a mating.

The signs associated with pseudopregnancy are the result of circulating prolactin, which is produced at the end of metoestrus in response to falling progesterone levels. Since this occurs during every oestrous cycle, it has been argued that it is a normal event that occurs in every bitch. It only becomes a problem when the signs exhibited by the bitch become excessive.

Signs

- Mammary development with or without milk secretion
- Behavioural signs of nesting or mothering objects
- Aggression, sometimes associated with the mothering instinct
- Appetite changes
- Sometimes polydipsia/polyuria
- Abdominal straining as though about to give birth (uncommon).

Differential diagnosis

- Most importantly, pregnancy – use ultrasonography or radiography to differentiate
- Other conditions causing polydipsia/polyuria, e.g. pyometra, diabetes mellitus, renal disease.

Treatment

Often the signs regress over 10–14 days without therapy as the prolactin levels return to normal.

- Frusemide (symptomatic treatment that may be used if lactation is excessive)
- Hormones (reduce prolactin levels by negative feedback mechanisms):
  - Progestogens
  - Oestrogen/testosterone
- Prolactin inhibitor drugs (directly reduce prolactin levels):
  - Bromocriptine
  - Cabergoline, the drug of choice
- Ovariohysterectomy (only when the signs have regressed, otherwise it can result in permanent signs of pseudopregnancy)
- Sedation (in extreme cases when aggression is a problem). Note that the use of acepromazine may exacerbate the condition.

Pyometra (cystic endometrial hyperplasia)

This is a serious condition of the uterus that occurs in middle-aged to older bitches. Usually the condition is found in bitches that have not had puppies but it may also occur in bitches after they have had puppies and in quite young animals. Also associated with progesterone therapy.

The uterus develops cystic hyperplastic changes and, during oestrus, the uterus becomes infected. As the corpora lutea develop during metoestrus, the uterus becomes filled with pus. Bitches may become very ill, as toxins are released into the circulation which have a marked effect on the kidneys and other body systems.

Signs

Pyometra should be considered in any bitch that becomes ill 6–8 weeks after her previous season. The bitch is typically dull, inappetent and polydypsic. The body temperature may be elevated initially but as the condition deteriorates it may fall and become subnormal. The animal may become recumbent and collapse.

There is a classification of the condition depending on the presence or absence of a vaginal discharge:

- Open pyometra: open cervix allowing escape of a purulent or bloodstained discharge
- Closed pyometra: closed cervix therefore no vulval discharge.

Closed pyometras can cause severe abdominal distension and be extremely toxaemic. Open pyometras can be equally toxaemic, despite the discharge of uterine contents.

Diagnosis

The history is usually indicative of the condition but other tests include:

- Haematology: leucocytosis, particularly in closed pyometras
- Biochemistry: often blood urea nitrogen is elevated
- Radiography: enlarged uterus is visible cranially displacing the abdominal contents
- Ultrasound: an enlarged uterus is visible and the contents may be floccular.

Treatment

The treatment of choice is immediate ovariohysterectomy. Antibiotic therapy should be given on diagnosis of the condition and the bitch should receive intensive fluid therapy before surgery without excessively delaying the operation.

Very mild cases of open pyometra may respond to antibiotic therapy alone. The use of prostaglandins (to promote luteolysis and uterine contraction) has been tried but should only be used in exceptional circumstances. However, the condition will recur after the subsequent oestrus and ovariohysterectomy is still the treatment of choice.

The oestrous cycle in the queen

The age at puberty in the queen is variable, depending on day length. The first oestrous cycle usually occurs during the first spring after body weight reaches 2.5 kg.

The cat can be described as seasonally polyoestrous. Queens cycle every 2–3 weeks in spring, summer and autumn, but sometimes indoor cats also cycle in winter. Figure 10.10 describes the oestrous cycle of the queen.

Ovulation in the queen

The queen is a *reflex* or *induced ovulator*. The strong spines on the male's penis stimulate the vaginal wall on withdrawal after coitus. This causes a surge of LH; ovulation takes place about 24 hours after mating and continues for several hours.

Occasionally queens ovulate spontaneously and this means that corpora lutea form and the queen progresses through a period of metoestrus (Figure 10.11).

Hormonal control of ovulation

- Follicles develop under the influence of *FSH*
- The follicles produce *oestrogen*, which causes the signs of pro-oestrus and oestrus
- If mating does not take place, there is no coital stimulation and ovulation does not occur. The follicles remain until the end of oestrus and then decline without rupturing (*atresia*)
- If the queen is a spontaneous ovulator, then ovulation occurs without mating with the male. Corpora lutea form and produce *progesterone* until they regress.

Prevention and postponement of oestrus

Medical methods

Inhibition of oestrus in the queen involves the use of similar drugs to those used in bitches (see Figure 10.9). However, queens not required to breed are more commonly surgically neutered.

Surgical methods

Ovariohysterectomy is usually performed at about 6 months of age. In the UK the veterinary surgeon will often use a flank incision.

This approach should not be used in oriental breeds because the hair may grow in a different colour following clipping. In these breeds, a midline incision is advised.

10.10 Oestrous cycle of the queen

Phase	Duration	Signs
Pro-oestrus and oestrus	3–10 days, shortened by mating Difficult to separate the two phases except that the male is accepted when female is in oestrus	Behavioural signs (vocalization, rubbing against objects, rolling on floor) Few physical signs
Interoestrus	About 3–14 days Follows oestrus when no mating has occurred or when mating does not result in a pregnancy	Diminishing behavioural signs No physical signs
Anoestrus	Over the period of winter when there are no hormonal cycles	No physical signs

---

10.11 Ovulation in the queen

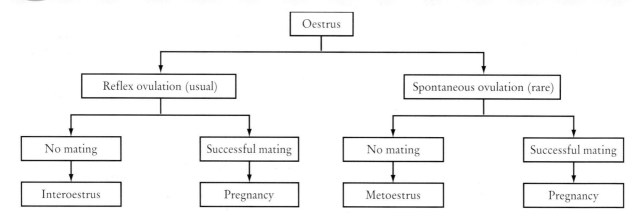

Abnormalities in the oestrous cycle in queens

Pyometra

The nature of the feline oestrous cycle may confer a degree of protection against pyometra. As most queens do not ovulate spontaneously, unmated queens are not exposed to the high levels of progesterone that are prevalent during the luteal phase.

Also, many cats are spayed – if not before breeding, then after they have completed their reproductive phase – and therefore the incidence of pyometra is considerably less in this species than in bitches. However, the condition may occur in spontaneously ovulating queens.

Abnormalities of the male

Most conditions of the male dog are related to prostatic or testicular disease. In tom cats abnormalities of the genitalia, other than trauma, are not commonly reported.

Congenital and hereditary conditions of the male reproductive tract

Intersexuality

A true hermaphrodite animal is characterized by the presence of both male and female gonads in a combined structure (ovotestis) or the animal may have one ovary and one testis.

Pseudohermaphroditism is defined as the animal appearing externally as of one sex but having the internal sexual organs of the other sex. The condition may be difficult to diagnose on external appearance. Males may have some underdevelopment of the penis and testes, or the genitalia may be totally absent. This disorder is more commonly seen in certain breeds, including Beagles, Cocker Spaniels, Miniature Schnauzers, Kerry Blue Terriers, German Shepherd Dogs and German Short-haired Pointers. The condition is very rare in cats. Surgical removal of the reproductive tract is indicated to prevent development of disease.

Hypospadias

This is a congenital abnormality in which the urethral orifice opens ventrally on the prepuce (glandular or penile hypospadias), near the scrotum (scrotal hypospadias) or in the perineal area (perineal hypospadias). The condition is often seen with other congenital abnormalities such as intersex animals. This condition has not been described in cats. The treatment is surgical but reconstruction can be very difficult.

Persistent penile frenulum

The surface of the penis should separate from the preputial mucosa around the time of whelping. In this condition, a thin sheet of fibrous connective tissue remains on the ventral surface, preventing protrusion of the penis or deviating it, if it does protrude when erect. The treatment is surgical.

Cryptorchidism

A cryptorchid animal may have one testis (unilateral cryptorchidism) or both testes (bilateral cryptorchidism) undescended. The testes normally descend around the time of birth and should be present in the scrotum by 10 days in dogs. They are difficult to palpate until around 3 weeks of age. In cats, descent of the testes takes place before birth but the testes may move freely in the inguinal canal and may not be palpable. All male animals should be examined at the time of first presentation to the clinic to ensure that both testes are descended. Owners should be informed if the testes cannot be palpated at this time. A diagnosis of cryptorchidism can be made after the animal is 5-10 months old, around the time of puberty.

The undescended testis/testes may lie anywhere along the tract of testicular descent. It is prudent to advise owners not to breed from these animals since it is thought that there may be a hereditary component to the condition. Cryptorchidism is more common in certain breeds such as Poodles, Boxers, Chihuahuas, Yorkshire Terriers and Miniature Schnauzers.

When the testes are retained, they are at a higher temperature than normally found in the scrotum (2-3°C less than body temperature). This results in reduced spermatogenesis and therefore a diminution of fertility. The increased temperature may also cause increased production of testosterone that may result in the dog exhibiting some inappropriate behaviour such as hypersexuality, excitability or aggression. After some years the retained testes degenerate and may become neoplastic.

All cryptorchid animals should be castrated before puberty, around the age of 6–8 months.

Acquired conditions of the male reproductive tract

Testicular abnormalities

The testes should be roughly oval in shape and firm, but not hard or painful, on gentle palpation. Abnormalities include:

- Cryptorchidism
- Hypoplasia
- Orchitis
- Neoplasia.

One testis or both testes may be affected. A marked disparity in size between the size of the testes should be considered abnormal.

Orchitis

This inflammation of the testicular tissue often occurs in conjunction with an epididymitis. The condition is rare in the cat. The causes can be:

- Trauma – probably the most common cause
- Viral – canine herpesvirus, canine distemper virus
- Bacterial – *Brucella canis* is a problem in Africa and America and other *Brucella* species such as *B. abortus*, *B. suis* or *B. mellitensis* may cause infections. Other ascending or haematogenous infections may affect the testes
- Autoimmune disease – has been shown to be hereditary but is rare.

The signs can include a stiff gait, scrotal enlargement and inflammation, testicular hyperthermia, severe pain, vomiting, anorexia, prostration and pyrexia. The situation may become chronic with the testes appearing irregular and small.

Treatment is based on antibiotics for at least 2 weeks, along with anti-inflammatory drugs to reduce the pain and swelling. As fertility is often lost, castration is often recommended once recovery is complete.

Testicular neoplasia in the dog

Testicular tumours are common in dogs. The incidence of neoplasia is increased in cryptorchid animals. Three types of tumour are found in the testes:

- Interstitial or Leydig cell tumours
  - Not related to retained testes; seen more commonly in older animals; often multiple and bilateral, but cause few problems; may not be diagnosed until postmortem
- Seminomas
  - Cause enlargement of the testicle in middle-aged and older dogs; rarely accompanied by systemic signs; can be locally invasive, particularly when found in the abdominal testis. If unilateral, the other testis will atrophy
- Sertoli cell tumours
  - Testis is normally enlarged, irregular and hard; usually found in dogs aged 7–12 years; not generally malignant but metastasis has been described in cases with retained testes. The other testis is atrophied
  - Produce oestrogen which leads to signs including feminization, penile and preputial atrophy, pendulous sheath, gynaecomastia, bilateral, symmetrical alopecia and hyperpigmentation of the skin, prostatic squamous metaplasia and attractiveness to other males. If the oestrogen causes bone marrow suppression, then leucopenia, pancytopenia and thrombocytopenia may be noted, with resultant petechiae, haematoma or haemorrhage.

Treatment is surgical removal of the affected testis. If a tumour is found in a younger animal, the fertility in the normal but atrophied testis can recover and the dog may continue to be used for breeding.

Testicular neoplasia is rare in cats (a large proportion of the population is castrated). Sertoli cell tumours have been reported but are not associated with significant clinical signs.

Testicular torsion

Torsion of the spermatic cord is rare but may occur at any age. It is seen more commonly in animals with retained testes. There is vascular engorgement and the blood supply to the testis is severely affected. Clinical signs will depend on the degree of torsion. There is often acute pain with reluctance to move, vomiting, anorexia and a rapid decline into shock. This condition may be fatal. Surgical correction may be possible. The early castration of cryptorchid animals is recommended.

Abnormalities of the penis and prepuce

Balanoposthitis

This is a common condition in male dogs but is rare in cats. In young dogs, before or close to puberty, a greenish-yellow discharge may be noted. This is of no clinical significance and is probably related to the hormonal changes around puberty. No treatment is required in these cases.

In adult dogs, the clinical signs include a purulent or haemorrhagic discharge with frequent licking and possible self-mutilation. The prepuce is painful on palpation and the mucosa is usually inflamed or ulcerated. Treatment should be directed at the cause. The possibility of foreign bodies or neoplasia should be excluded. Local or parenteral antibiotics and anti-inflammatory drugs should be used.

Phimosis or paraphimosis

Phimosis is the inability of the male to extrude the penis because of a small preputial orifice. This is usually congenital and resolved by surgery.

Paraphimosis describes the inability of the penis to retract into the prepuce. This is due to a preputial orifice which is sufficient to allow passage of the normal, non-erect penis but once the penis is engorged the orifice acts as a tourniquet preventing detumescence. If left untreated, this condition may lead to severe penile trauma. Tranquillizers are useful in inducing rest and hypotension, which may allow gentle manual replacement. Recurrence is not uncommon and surgery should be considered.

These conditions are rare in cats.

Penile bleeding

This may occur spontaneously or may follow trauma. The source of the haemorrhage should be located and surgery may be required to stop the bleeding.

Fracture of the os penis

This is occasionally broken as a result of trauma, or during a difficult mating. The main signs are pain, bleeding, urethral haemorrhage and sometimes dysuria. Treament is symptomatic unless the patency of the urethra is compromised, when penile amputation or urethrostomy may be necessary.

Abnormalities of the prostate in the dog

Prostate disease is common, particularly in older dogs. The prostate gland may become infected (acute and chronic prostatitis, abscesses) or may be subject to hormonal influences (prostatic hyperplasia) or may become neoplastic (adenocarcinoma). Many clinical signs associated with prostate disease are non-specific, including haematuria, anuria, pain, constipation or stiffness. In all male dogs over the age of 5 years, the prostate should be considered in the differential diagnosis of disease. Infectious prostatic disease should be treated using antibiotics for 4–6 weeks and supportive therapy during the acute phase. Prostatic hyperplasia is only a problem when clinical signs are present. Castration is the most efficient treatment. Prostatic tumours are fortunately rare, since the prognosis is poor and no satisfactory treatment is available.

Breeding

Selection of sire

The definition of puberty in the male is the onset of the ability to copulate and to fertilize. Puberty is attained before full physical maturity and maximum reproductive capacity are reached. Spermatogenesis starts at approximately 5 months of age in both dogs and cats.

Male dog

- In dogs, the age at puberty is 6–8 months (up to 1 year in giant breeds)
- Most dogs are introduced to stud work at 1 year old
- A dog should be used for no more than two or three bitches in the first year. Before increasing use beyond this, the owner should check that the dog is fertile and siring pups with no hereditary defects
- Subsequently, owners should be advised to set individual limits: overuse will adversely affect fertility
- There is no upper age limit but it is known that fertility declines from the age of 7 years onwards

- Before introducing a dog to stud, the owner should ensure that the dog:
  - Is a good example of the breed
  - Works well (if a working breed)
  - Has a sound temperament
  - Has been screened for breed-related hereditary defects.

Male cat

- In the cat, the age at puberty is 9–12 months (purebreds later than cross-breeds)
- Most tomcats are introduced to stud work at approximately 1 year old
- They should be tested for FeLV before being offered for stud
- The upper age limit for stud use is usually 6 years old.

Moral and legal responsibilities

Breeders have a moral and legal obligation to ensure that offspring are clinically healthy and have a sound temperament.

Before mating two animals the following factors should be considered in the selection of a sire:

- Age: should be neither too young nor too old
- Sound temperament
- Good libido and fertility
- Not closely inbred
- Not over-used
- Capable of work (if a working breed)
- Sound general health and free from genetic abnormalities.

Moral responsibilities of owners

All the factors listed above under selection of sire are relevant. Other responsibilities are:

- Honesty with other owners regarding health status
- Stud animal must be the correct one; beware frauds or mistakes
- Animals must be withdrawn from stud if defects become apparent
- An appropriate stud male must be selected for the female.

Legal responsibilities

These are also discussed in *BSAVA Manual of Veterinary Care* (Chapters 5 and 10).

Breeding of Dogs Act (1991)

The main Act was produced in 1973. In 1991 the Act was updated to give additional powers of entry, by local authority personnel, to breeding establishments. The Act defines a breeding establishment as 'any premises (including a private dwelling) where two or more bitches are kept for the purpose of breeding for sale'.

A licence (which is renewable annually) is required to run a breeding establishment and the licensing authority is the local authority. The licence is issued if aspects of welfare, security and fire precautions are satisfactory. Inspections may be carried out by an officer of the local authority or by a veterinarian appointed by the local authority for the purpose. Persons in charge of the establishment must be competent.

If an animal to be used for breeding is not registered with, for example, the Kennel Club or the ISDS, then this must be stated to the owner of the other animal. Progeny will not be eligible for registration.

It is a criminal offence to falsify any document relating to registration, pedigree, vaccination or health status.

Hereditary defects

Hereditary defects are transmitted from one or both parents to the offspring. Transmission is via genetic material and occurs at the time of conception. The defect may not be apparent at birth and only some of a litter may be affected.

Animals that have genetic defects, or who are carriers of genetic defects, should not be used for breeding. Common hereditary defects include:

- Cryptorchidism
- Hip dysplasia
- Progressive retinal atrophy (PRA)
- Entropion
- Cleft palate
- Overshot/undershot jaw
- Spina bifida
- Patellar luxation
- Some congenital cardiac diseases
- Elbow dysplasia.

Congenital abnormalities

These are acquired during uterine development but may not have a genetic basis. They may not have an apparent cause but some may be related to:

- Drugs given during pregnancy
- Live vaccines
- X-rays in early pregnancy
- Infectious agents
- Nutritional deficiencies.

Schemes to control the incidence of hereditary diseases in pedigree dogs

BVA/Kennel Club/International Sheepdog Society (ISDS) Eye Scheme

Dogs are examined every 12 months to ensure that they are free from conditions such as:

- Central and generalized PRA
- Hereditary cataract
- Primary glaucoma
- Primary lens luxation
- Collie eye anomaly
- Retinal dysplasia
- Persistent pupillary membrane
- Persistent hyperplastic primary vitreous.

BVA/Kennel Club Hip Dysplasia Scheme

Dogs are X-rayed on one occasion after they reach the age of 12 months. The radiographs are assessed on nine detailed points and are scored for abnormality:

- Perfect hips score 0
- Scores for affected hips are recorded up to 106

  There is also a scheme for elbow dysplasia.

Other breed societies

Some breed societies have their own control schemes. For example:

- Dobermann Pinscher dogs are monitored for cervical spondylopathy
- Cavalier King Charles Spaniels are monitored for early degeneration of the heart valves
- Boxers are monitored for aortic stenosis.

Mating procedure

It is important to recognize 'normal' mating behaviour and to remember that conditions are often not optimal because the bitch or queen may have had a long journey to meet the stud. Also it is important to know that the mating is planned at the correct time of the female's cycle. If possible, at least one of the animals to be mated should be experienced, i.e. they should have been mated before.

Mating in the dog

Normal mating behaviour is described in Figure 10.12. Tests may have been done to indicate ovulation so that the bitch is at the correct point in her cycle. Mating should be allowed as soon as the bitch accepts the dog. It is common to repeat matings twice or three times on alternate days. A bitch or dog may become aggressive if the bitch is not fully receptive and care should be exercised when introducing strange animals to each other.

Assistance at mating

Interference should be minimal but observation is essential.

- Usually occurs at the home of the stud
- Bitch should be fully in oestrus:
  - Ensure that there is no aggression
  - Introduce on leads
- In long-coated dogs, clip or tie the perivulval hairs
- Allow courtship behaviour
- Try to use at least one experienced animal
- Guide the inexperienced dog to the right end
- May need to guide the penis to the vulva with cupped hand
- Dog sometimes needs gentle support to achieve a tie
- No rough handling or punishment.

Mating in the cat

Mating behaviour is described in Figure 10.13. In controlled breeding, take the queen to the tom to prevent his libido declining in strange surroundings. Multiple mating will occur on one day but the queen will not allow mating immediately after coitus.

10.12 Canine mating behaviour

1. The bitch and dog often exhibit play behaviour, jumping up and chasing each other, as part of the courtship.

2. The bitch will then settle and stand with her tail to one side (flagging).

3. The dog's penis will be partially engorged and extruded from the sheath.

4. The dog mounts the bitch and may ejaculate a small amount of clear fluid.

5. Slow thrusting movements allow the penile tip to enter the vulva.

6. The penis becomes fully erect and enters the vagina (intromission).

7. Thrusting movements become rapid and the second fraction is ejaculated.

8. The dog then dismounts from the bitch and turns through 180° with the penis still in the vagina (the tie).

9. The third fraction is ejaculated into the vagina.

10. The animals remain tied for up to 30 minutes, after which the dog's penis slowly deflates and the pair disengage.

11. Both animals should be allowed to clean and lick themselves.

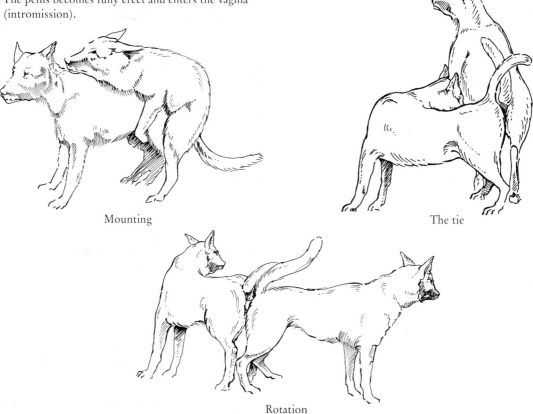

Mounting

The tie

Rotation

Illustrations reproduced from the BSAVA Manual of Small Animal Reproduction and Neonatology. *Artist: Ian Lennox.*

10.13 Mating behaviour in the cat

1. Courtship is variable and often non-existent.
2. Queen adopts the mating position, fore-end crouched and tail up.
3. Male grasps skin on her neck in his teeth and lies over her.
4. Intromission and ejaculation occur quickly.
5. As the penis is withdrawn the queen often howls – coital stimulus.
6. Queen then rolls and licks herself vigorously.
7. She will not allow further mating for about 1 hour.

Assistance at mating

- Allow the tom to be in his own surroundings
- Males in new surroundings require 4 weeks for libido to return
- Check that no fur blocks the preputial orifice
- Virgin queens do not readily accept the tom
- Allow frequent mating over a short time.

Artificial insemination (AI)

AI results in lower fertility (lower conception rates and smaller litter size) than natural mating. However, there are certain situations when AI may be the only way to breed from a specific dog or bitch:

- Situations in which fertilization would not otherwise be achieved
  - Disinterest by male
  - Premature ejaculation
  - Inability to 'tie'
  - Hostility by the bitch
  - Physical deformities
- To increase the distribution of genetic potential from a sire
  - If dog and bitch are separated by long distances
  - If two bitches require insemination by the same dog over a limited period
- To control the spread of infectious disease
  - Unlikely to be necessary because diseased dogs are not used at stud
  - Could be useful if stud contracts mange or ringworm.

Specific permission to use AI must be obtained from the Kennel Club if the progeny are to be registered. The Kennel Club insists that inseminations be made immediately after collection and that both operations are carried out by the same veterinary surgeon. Prior notification of the time and place of the insemination is required and an observer from the Kennel Club may attend.

There appears to be no restriction on AI in racing greyhounds, coursing whippets or lurchers.

For AI to be successful, the use of vaginal cytology or measurement of plasma hormone concentrations should assess the timing of ovulation as accurately as possible.

Collection of semen

- Choose a quiet room with a non-slip floor and minimum people in attendance
- A bitch in oestrus is helpful to increase libido. Failing this, any quiet bitch will do. The bitch should be in the same room. If not in oestrus, she should be restrained to prevent her turning on the dog
- Persuading the dog to ejaculate depends on his experience and temperament but he should be allowed to mount the bitch if one is present. Older stud dogs will ejaculate by digital pressure with no bitch present
- The penis, once erect, should be deflected to the side by grasping the bulbus glandis. Apply digital pressure caudal to the bulbus (Figure 10.14)
- Collection of semen takes place over ejaculation: only the second fraction (see Figure 10.15) should be collected. This sperm-rich fraction is characterized by a milky appearance
- Allow the dog to lick his penis back into the sheath.

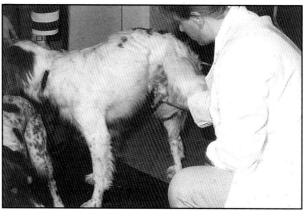

10.14 *Semen collection using a teaser bitch. The prepuce is manually deflected back and the bulbus is held in a firm grip while the collector's fingers are constricting at the point of torsion. Semen may be collected directly into a disposable plastic funnel.*
Reproduced from the BSAVA Manual of Small Animal Reproduction and Neonatology.

10.15 Semen fractions

First fraction

Often ejaculated before intromission
Clear, does not contain any sperm
Originates from prostate gland to flush urine and cellular debris from urethra
Volume: 1–10 ml

Second fraction

Ejaculated into the vagina after intromission
Contains sperm
Volume: 1 ml

Third fraction

Ejaculated during the tie
Flushes sperm through cervix into uterus
Volume: 3–20 ml

Storage of semen

Fresh semen

A small amount (1–2 ml) of prostatic fluid should be collected with the sperm-rich fraction. If the semen is to be used immediately, dilution of the semen is not required.

- The semen should be inseminated on the day of ovulation, with a second insemination 2 days later
- The semen should be deposited directly into the vagina, using 2–3 ml (depending on the size of the bitch)

- Once the semen has been deposited, the bitch's hindquarters should be raised to ensure transport of the sperm through the cervix. The vagina can be stimulated to cause contractions of the reproductive tract to aid sperm transport.

Chilled semen

If the semen cannot be used immediately, it should be diluted with a semen extender and chilled to a temperature of 4°C. It is important that chilled semen contains no prostatic fluid and that the volume of the diluent is greater than the semen fraction.

- Semen is preserved for up to 12 hours by chilling and it should be carefully warmed to 30–35°C before insemination
- The bitch should be inseminated directly into the uterus but it is possible to place the inseminate into the vagina as for fresh semen.

Frozen semen

For prolonged storage and transport, semen should have an extender added and it can then be frozen. The extended semen should be cooled to 4°C and then placed into 0.5 ml plastic straws. The straws are then frozen and stored in liquid nitrogen.

- Sperm that has been frozen is less stable and its longevity in the reproductive tract is reduced. Therefore it is important to inseminate the bitch 24–48 hours after ovulation
- A second insemination is required 24 hours after the first
- The semen should be thawed in a water bath at 70°C and the semen should be examined for sperm quality
- An operator trained in trans-cervical technique directly into the uterus should deposit the semen. A quiet bitch requires no sedation
- Endoscopic visualization of the cervical os may assist the procedure
- If catheterization is not possible, then surgical insemination by laparoscopy may be required.

Misalliance (mismating)

The definition of misalliance is that a female mates with an inappropriate male – usually defined as one not selected by the owner. This can occur in either the bitch or the queen and it may or may not result in conception and pregnancy.

The owner may be unaware it has taken place but sometimes the owner knows immediately that the dam has been inappropriately mated and will come into the surgery for advice. The owner may not know which dog or cat was responsible for the mating. If some time (more than 3 weeks) has elapsed since the suspected mating, it is advisable to scan the dam to confirm pregnancy.

The options for action if pregnancy is confirmed are given in Figure 10.16.

Normal pregnancy

The bitch

Best age for first pregnancy

There is no hard-and-fast rule but usually the third oestrus is considered the best time in biological terms.

Breed characteristics vary and giant breed bitches mature later than smaller breeds. Using the third oestrous cycle to determine the best time for a first mating avoids the danger of mating bitches too early by adhering to an age parameter.

Breeding may be delayed for other reasons; for example, the bitch may be working, or the owners may be on holiday.

Upper age limit for pregnancy

The Kennel Club has imposed a breeding age limit of 8 years, above which a bitch's progeny may not be registered. Special permission may be granted to register pups born to bitches older than this. Some breeds are 'young' at 8 years of age, whereas the giant breeds are geriatric and a pregnancy at this age would be inappropriate.

Duration of pregnancy

If gestation length is calculated from the time of first mating, then there is a considerable variation in the length of pregnancy (56–72 days). However, there is much less variation if the period of pregnancy is determined hormonally by measuring the interval from the pre-ovulatory LH peak.

- Average = 63 days
- Smaller breeds – shorter pregnancy
- Larger breeds – longer pregnancy
- A single fetus results in a prolonged pregnancy.

10.16 Options for action in the case of misalliance

Option	Considerations
Leave animal to whelp	Not advised for females intended for breeding If dam is registered pedigree, this could affect future litter registrations Was sire of suitable size for dam? Is bitch or queen in good health?
Medical treatment (not an option for cats) • Oestradiol benzoate, given 3rd and 5th days post-mating • Prostaglandins, given once the corpora lutea are functional • Glucocorticoids, not consistently effective • Anti-prolactins, limited use so far	Advised for bitches intended for future breeding Treatment of choice is oestradiol benzoate. Side effects (such as iatrogenic pyometra, bone marrow suppression, prolonged oestrus) used to be possible with traditional single high dose of oestradiol. New low-dose regime is given on 2 days; it is possible to give third dose on 7th day if several matings took place
Surgical termination of pregnancy by ovariohysterectomy	Best for females not intended for breeding Operation is carried out 3–4 weeks post-mating

It is difficult to predict the correct date exactly because multiple mating may have taken place and the ova are shed over a period of days. The precise time of fertilization will not be known.

Pregnancy diagnosis

By abdominal palpation

- Can be done at 21–28 days
- Uterus is still high in abdominal cavity
- Conceptual masses are turgid and easily felt
- By 35 days the uterus is lower; difficult to palpate discrete masses
- Accuracy 85%
- Inaccurate for assessing litter size.

By ultrasonography

- Non-invasive
- Positive results from 21 days
- Optimum 28 days
- Can assess litter size reasonably accurately
- Can assess viability of embryo by visualizing movement or heart beat (Figure 10.17).

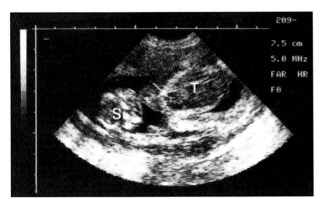

10.17 *Ultrasound image of a fetus demonstrating the fetal skull (S) and trunk (T). The heart (arrowed) can be clearly identified. 5.0 MHz transducer, scale in cm.*
Reproduced from the BSAVA Manual of Small Animal Reproduction and Neonatology. *Photo: Dr GCW England.*

By radiography

- Only done after day 45
- Wait until day 50 in fat bitches
- Can assess number of fetuses
- Causes no apparent harm to fetuses
- Valuable aid in dystocia at parturition.

Auscultation of fetal heart beats

- Fetal heart beat audible during latter part of pregnancy
- Heart rate is much faster than the mother's heart rate.

Blood test (acute phase proteins (APPs))

- Implantation takes place about day 20
- Extremely invasive and damaging process
- Uterus signals this as an 'attack'
- Stimulates liver to produce APPs
- APP rise about day 26; back to basal by day 40
- Detectable in serum samples between weeks 4 and 5
- Accuracy 95%
- APPs can be raised in pyometra.

Care of the pregnant bitch

The anatomy and physiology of pregnancy in the bitch are outlined in Figure 10.18. Changes in her appearance and behaviour are described in Figure 10.19.

10.18 Anatomy and physiology of pregnancy in the bitch

- Fertilization takes place in the oviducts
- Days 5–8: fertilized ova reach the uterus
- Days 16–21: implantation and development of placentae takes place
- Size of conceptual masses:
  - Day 21: pea size
  - Day 25: marble size
  - Day 28: 25–40 mm diameter
- Fetal masses elongate and growth accelerates:
  - Day 35: uterus folds
  - Day 42: fetuses palpated at two levels within the abdomen
  - Day 45: skeletons start ossifying

Note:
Early development is by *cell division* and the conceptus is called an *embryo*
Later, *cell differentiation* begins and organs and limbs become apparent. At this stage the conceptus is called a *fetus*.

10.19 Changes in appearance and behaviour of the pregnant bitch

Feature	Change
Abdominal size	Increases from 5 weeks: can be variable, depending on litter size
Abdominal shape	Changes from round to pear-shaped during the last week
Mammary development	Most pronounced in primigravidae (maiden bitches) in the last 2–3 weeks. In multigravidae (bitches having had at least one litter): last few days
Teat development	Primigravidae: from day 35. Multigravidae: not much change
Temperament	Often quieter and more docile
Appetite	Individual variation but often reduced towards end of pregnancy
Vaginal discharge	May have slight clear mucoid discharge during second half

Feeding

- Diet should be nutritious but amounts should not be excessive
- Bitch should not become fat
- Weight gain during pregnancy should not exceed 30% of non-pregnant weight
- Might need calcium/phosphorus supplementation on veterinary advice
- Protein requirements increase as capacity decreases
- Feed smaller meals and increase frequency of feeds towards the end of pregnancy.

Exercise

- Maintenance of fitness is most important
- Boisterous games should be avoided in latter third of pregnancy.

Whelping quarters

- The area should be quiet and draught-free
- It must be possible to maintain a temperature of 25°C
- There should be sufficient space to avoid pups being squashed
- The area should be enclosed to prevent pups escaping
- The box or area should be lined with newspaper, shredded paper, towels or sheets
- Introduce bitch at least 10 days before whelping.

The queen

Best age for first pregnancy
Cats may be bred from around 12 to 18 months of age but females that mature slowly may start oestrous cycles later than this.

Upper age limit for pregnancy
There is none imposed but most cats show reduced fecundity after about 6 years and most breeders cease to breed from them after this.

Duration of pregnancy

- Average = 65–67 days (range 56–70 days)
- Gestation length can be very variable and difficult to predict accurately due to multiple mating.

Pregnancy diagnosis
Note that failure to return to oestrus during the breeding season is suggestive of pregnancy.

By abdominal palpation

- Can be done from day 21 to day 28
- Abdominal wall is thinner than in the bitch – easy to palpate fetuses
- Cats are less likely to be obese.

By ultrasonography

- Non-invasive
- Positive results from around 21 days
- Can assess litter size and viability.

By radiography

- Use during the last third for fetal safety
- Fetal sacculations evident from 3 weeks.

Auscultation of fetal heart beats

- Often difficult due to the cat purring.

Care of the pregnant queen
The anatomy and physiology of pregnancy in the queen are outlined in Figure 10.20. Changes in her appearance are described in Figure 10.21.

10.20 Anatomy and physiology of pregnancy in the queen

- Fertilization takes place in the oviducts
- Days 3–5: fertilized ova reach the uterus
- Day 14: implantation and development of placentae
- Conceptual masses are smaller than in the bitch but follow the same progression.

10.21 Changes in appearance of the pregnant queen

Feature	Change
Abdominal size	Progressively more evident during second half of pregnancy
Abdominal shape	Appears very round and extended just prior to parturition
Mammary development	Occurs during last 7–10 days of pregnancy
Teat development	Teats become pink during last 2–3 weeks

Feeding

- Feed a nutritious balanced diet with regard to calcium and vitamin A
- Increase the number of feeds to meet demand.

Kittening accommodation

- Introduce cat to the area before parturition is due
- The cat is quite likely to choose her own space.

Abnormalities of pregnancy in the bitch and the queen
Not all conceptions result in healthy offspring being born at term. Anything affecting the health of the pregnant dam can adversely affect the pregnancy. Care should be taken when administering drugs to pregnant females.

If it is necessary to take radiographs of a pregnant female, then her abdomen should be shielded from the beam if possible. Note that a single radiograph, taken in the last third of pregnancy, will not adversely affect the fetuses.

Resorption of embryos
This is the resorption of the entire conceptus during the embryonic phase of development. The true incidence is unclear.

In the bitch, part or all of a litter may be resorbed. This commonly occurs around 28–35 days of pregnancy. There are many potential causes, including:

- Embryonic abnormalities
- Infectious agents
- Competition for uterine space.

If all of a litter is resorbed, it may be difficult to determine whether there has been a failure to conceive (the absence of a pregnancy despite a normal mating) unless the presence of embryos was confirmed before resorption.

Abortion

This is expulsion of the fetus before term, i.e. before the fetus is able to survive out of the uterus. Possible causes include:

- Fetal abnormalities
- Abnormal maternal environment
- Systemic or reproductive tract infection (distemper, feline viral diseases, β-haemolytic streptococci, *Toxoplasma gondii, Brucella canis*)
- Trauma – fights or road traffic accidents.

The dam will usually be presented with a dark red vaginal discharge. If infection is the cause, then the dam may be quite ill and prompt treatment is required. It may be possible to confirm the presence of remaining fetuses by ultrasonography. The expulsion of the fetal material should be encouraged by the use of oxytocin.

Stillbirth

This is expulsion of the fetus close to term, when it is likely to have survived had it been alive. The possible causes are similar to those of abortion.

Fetal mummification

Fetal death without infection *in utero* results in mummification. This only occurs when death takes place well before term. The fetus remains in the uterus, fluids are absorbed and a hard malformed mass remains. If only part of the litter is affected, mummified fetuses will be delivered with live fetuses at birth.

Uterine rupture

Rupture of a gravid uterus can occur following trauma or may occur during parturition. It is a life-threatening condition and should be treated as an emergency. Ovariohysterectomy is indicated in most instances.

Uterine torsion

This is an uncommon complication, more often seen in cats than in dogs. One or both uterine horns will twist, usually close to term. Clinical signs vary from discomfort on abdominal palpation to total collapse. This requires prompt surgical treatment. Although it is possible to reduce torsion, ovariohysterectomy is often the treatment of choice.

Parturition

Parturition is the series of events that terminates pregnancy and bring about the expulsion of the fetuses at a time when they can survive out of the uterus.

Requirements for successful parturition:

- The lower genital tract must permit passage of the fetuses
- The cervix must dilate
- The fetuses must be actively propelled from the uterus to the vulva
- The neonates must be capable of survival.

Hormonal changes at parturition are outlined in Figure 10.22.

Signs of impending parturition

Relaxation of the soft tissue around the pelvis occurs towards the end of pregnancy. The behaviour of the dam changes in response to the hormonal alterations noted in Figure 10.22. Any of the following may be observed:

10.22 Hormonal changes at the time of parturition

- During pregnancy, *progesterone* acts to:
  - Render the uterine environment suitable for fetuses
  - Inhibit strong uterine contractions
  - Promote mammary development
- Increasing levels of *relaxin* are produced by the ovary and placenta, causing the pelvic soft tissues to relax
- At the end of pregnancy, hormonal changes occur in the fetus:
  - Reduction in nutrition from the placenta results in release of adrenocorticotrophic hormone (*ACTH*) and fetal *cortisol* levels rise
  - The rise in fetal and maternal cortisol probably stimulates the release of *prostaglandin F*2a, which is luteolytic (breaks down the corpora lutea)
- As the corpora lutea break down, there is a reduction in progesterone and a swing towards *oestrogen* dominance
- This triggers release of:
  - *oxytocin* (stimulates uterine contractions)
  - *prolactin* (promotes lactogenesis).

- Anorexia
- Seeking solitude
- Nest-making
- Enlargement and flaccidity of the vaginal lips
- Expression of colostrum from the teats
- Fall in rectal temperature 8–24 hours before parturition.

The fall in rectal temperature is the most reliable indicator of impending parturition in the bitch. Body temperature fluctuates during the last week of pregnancy and the sharp drop immediately prior to parturition is mediated by the fall in plasma progesterone. The decrease in temperature varies between 1°C in large breeds and 3°C in small breeds. This drop in temperature is responsible for the shivering recognized during first-stage labour.

Queens show a less marked temperature drop than bitches. Some queens will refuse food but others may continue eating up to parturition. They often seek solitude and may disappear to their choice of nesting site.

Stages of parturition

Parturition can be divided into five component parts:

- Stage of preparation
- First-stage labour
- Second-stage labour
- Third-stage labour
- Puerperium.

Stage of preparation

- Plasma progesterone declines
- Body temperature drops to approximately 37°C
- Relaxation of the vaginal and perineal tissue
- Dam seeks the nesting site
- Colostrum is present within the mammary glands.

First-stage labour

- Onset of myometrial contractions
- Restlessness

- Panting
- Nest-making
- Anorexia, shivering and vomiting may be seen
- Queens may vocalize and groom themselves.

The duration of the first stage of labour is normally between 1 and 12 hours. In primiparous animals (whelping for the first time), this period may be prolonged for up to 36 hours.

At the end of the first stage of labour, cervical dilatation is complete and the *allantochorion* (first water bag) of the first fetus passes through the cervix.

Second-stage labour

- Involuntary myometrial contractions
- Coordinated voluntary contractions of the abdominal muscles
- Dam may crouch, stand or lie in lateral recumbency
- Allantochorion of the first fetus appears at the vulva
- Dam may bite it or it ruptures, releasing allantoic fluid
- Puppy or kitten is contained within the amnion, which is usually intact.

This stage of labour results in the expulsion of the fetuses and is recognized by the first water bag bursting and the start of abdominal straining. The body temperature returns to normal.

The duration is usually 3–12 hours.

The dam will usually open the amniotic sac: if she fails to do so, it needs to be ruptured quickly. Vigorous licking by the dam will stimulate the neonate. The umbilical cord may be chewed to rupture it: it should be ensured that chewing is not excessive.

Veterinary attention should be sought if:

- The puppy or kitten is not born within 30 minutes of the appearance of the allantochorion
- The dam is straining unproductively for longer than 1 hour
- The dam becomes weak and straining is ineffective
- More than 2 hours have elapsed since the birth of the last fetus
- There is a reddish/green discharge and no fetuses are being born
- The dam is in second stage labour for more than 12 hours.

Often the first fetus takes the longest and the subsequent puppies or kittens are born more quickly.

Third-stage labour

- Myometrial and abdominal contractions
- Expulsion of placentas alternating with birth of fetuses
- Production of *uteroverdin* (greenish-brown in bitch, reddish-brown in the cat) from the breakdown of the marginal haematomata (maternal blood trapped between the placenta and the fetal membranes (see Figure 10.23))
- Dam may eat the placentas.

This stage of labour results in the expulsion of the placentas. In the bitch and the queen this stage alternates with second-stage labour. Often fetuses are born without their placenta, which follows after another fetus.

Puerperium

- Uterine involution takes place, rapidly at first, and is completed within 4–6 weeks

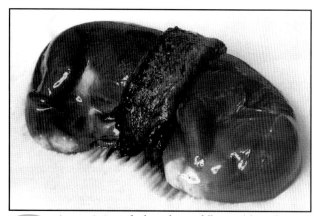

10.23 A puppy in intact fetal membranes, following delivery by Caesarean operation.
Reproduced from the BSAVA Manual of Small Animal Reproduction and Neonatology.

- Uteroverdin production should cease after 1 week
- A mucoid vulvular discharge may be present
- The dam's temperature may be slightly elevated (39.2°C) for a few days.

The reproductive tract returns to its normal non-pregnant state.

Dystocia

Dystocia, or difficult birth, is a frequent problem in both the bitch and the queen. It is defined as the inability to expel the fetus through the birth canal without assistance and is more commonly seen in pedigree cats and in breeds of dogs with large heads.

The causes of dystocia may be maternal or fetal in origin or a combination of both (see Figure 10.24).

10.24 Causes of dystocia in bitches and queens

Cause	Bitch (%)	Queen (%)
Maternal:	75.3	67.1
Primary complete inertia	48.9	36.8
Primary partial inertia	23.1	22.6
Birth canal too narrow	1.1	5.2
Uterine torsion	1.1	–
Uterine prolapse	–	0.6
Uterine strangulation	–	0.6
Hydrallantois	0.5	–
Vaginal septum formation	0.5	–
Fetal:	24.7	29.7
Malpresentations	15.4	15.5
Malformations	1.6	7.7
Fetal oversize	6.6	1.9
Fetal death	1.1	1.1

Uterine inertia

This is the most common cause of dystocia. Both primary and secondary inertia may occur.

Primary inertia

The uterus fails to respond to the requirements of parturition and contractions of the myometrium are absent. Primary *complete* uterine inertia is the failure to initiate labour, whereas primary partial uterine inertia occurs when parturition is initiated but the entire process cannot be completed. Reasons for the failure of contraction may be:

- Insufficient stimulation (from a single fetus or very small litter) to initiate labour
- Over-stretching of the uterine muscle by large litters, excessive fetal fluids or oversized fetuses
- An inherited predisposition
- Older or over-fat animals
- Bitches exhibiting excessive anxiety.

The bitch normally presents as bright and alert with no signs of uterine contractions, even if the cervix is open.

The bitch should be actively encouraged to exercise to induce straining. Manual stimulation of the dorsal vaginal wall may also help to stimulate myometrial contractions. Nervous bitches should be calmed by the owner; occasionally a low dose of tranquillizer is needed to allow parturition to commence.

Secondary inertia

This is always due to exhaustion of the myometrium, generally caused by obstruction of the birth canal. If the condition is diagnosed early enough the bitch may be quite bright; otherwise, she may be depressed and exhausted.

Oxytocin is the drug of choice for treatment of this condition.

 It is essential to check that there is no obstruction of the birth canal before giving oxytocin or uterine rupture may occur.

The recommended dose of oxytocin for the bitch is 1–5 IU given intravenously or 2.5–10 IU i.m. The dose for a cat is 0.5 IU i.v. or i.m. The dose may be repeated at 30-minute intervals but should not exceed a total of 3 IU in the cat. Overdose with oxytocin will cause the uterus to become contracted, preventing expulsion of fetuses and impeding placental blood flow, which will compromise fetal viability.

Oxytocin directly affects the contraction of the myometrium but this requires that the calcium levels in the dam are adequate. If oxytocin does not work alone, then a slow intravenous injection of calcium (calcium borogluconate 10% at 0.5–1.5 ml/kg) should be given prior to the next dose of oxytocin.

If there is no response to a second dose of oxytocin, the dam should be delivered without delay, either by Caesarean section or with the aid of forceps.

Obstruction of the birth canal

The causes may be either maternal or fetal in origin. Maternal causes include:

- Uterine torsion/rupture
- Congenital malformations of the uterus
- Soft tissue abnormalities: neoplasms, polyps, fibrosis of the cervix or vagina
- Narrow pelvic canal.

Fetal obstructions may result from:

- Oversized fetuses: often associated with small litter size
- Malpresentation
- Malformations
- Fetal death.

Malpresentations

The normal presentation of a fetus is either anterior (head first) or posterior (hindlegs first). However, fetuses in posterior presentation may prove difficult to whelp if they are the first of the litter to be born and the cervical dilation is insufficient. Also, if the amniotic membrane ruptures during second stage labour, the fetus is being delivered against the direction of the hair coat. There is also the possibility of the abdominal organs being displaced anteriorly during passage through the pelvic canal, which distends the fetal thorax and can cause the fetus to become lodged in the birth canal.

Breech presentation (posterior presentation with the legs flexed forward) can present a serious problem. Exploration of the vagina will reveal a tail tip or the base of the tail and little else. It is very difficult to manipulate these fetuses manually and surgery is usually indicated.

Lateral or downward deflections of the head are commonly seen in both puppies and kittens. Occasionally, weak or dead fetuses will present with backward flexion of the legs; it may be possible to deliver these normally, depending on the size of the birth canal. Two fetuses can present together, one from each uterine horn; if there is room then they should be manipulated one at a time.

Management

If the fetus is in the birth canal, then manual manipulation may be possible. This should never be attempted single-handed. It is essential to have one person restraining the dam to ensure that the person who is assisting the fetus is safe from being bitten or scratched and to ensure that the manipulation is attempted in optimal conditions. The assistant should ensure that the perineal area is clean from possible fecal contamination or fetal fluids before attempting to aid the fetuses. The usual aseptic precautions (clean hands, gloves and instruments) should be taken to prevent risk of infection of the reproductive tract.

Feline fetuses present problems because of the space restrictions around the obstructing fetus. The fetus should be grasped if possible behind the shoulders or pelvis, gently manoeuvered from side to side and rotated, if space allows.

Puppies should be withdrawn in a ventro-posterior direction in the bitch, to mimic the almost complete somersault that the puppy turns during normal parturition. Kittens should be withdrawn posteriorly because the mother's vagina lies in line with the pelvic floor.

It is important to ensure that adequate lubrication (water-soluble gels, obstetrical lubricants) is present within the pelvic canal, although this makes the fetus difficult to hold. Light cotton gloves may be used to minimize slippage. The assistant should avoid applying traction to the limbs or the tail at any time.

Fetuses that are deeper within the birth canal may require the use of obstetrical forceps, although these can cause severe damage to both the dam and the fetus. Great care should be exercised when using them. The forceps should be guided with a finger and only used if there is one oversize fetus or, possibly, for the last fetus of the litter. The forceps should be used at the neck or cheeks of the fetus or, if the pup or kitten is in posterior presentation, the pelvic girdle should be grasped.

Most bitches and queens with dystocia end up having to undergo a Caesarean section (see below) and therefore manual manipulation should be kept to a minimum.

Caesarean operation

A prophylactic operation may be carried out if a dam has a previous history of unsuccessful parturition. However, most Caesarean operations are related to failure of normal parturition, either because of dystocia, trauma or infection. The indications that a Caesarean might be necessary are:

- Complete/partial uterine inertia that is unresponsive to medical treatment
- Secondary uterine inertia that does not respond to medical treatment
- Fetal oversize causing intractable dystocia
- Fetal malposition intractable to manipulation
- Fetal death with or without putrefaction
- Excess/deficiency of fetal fluids
- Maternal birth canal deficiency (soft tissue/bony pelvis)
- Toxaemia of pregnancy
- Illness/trauma of dam
- Neglected dystocia.

Once a decision has been made to perform a Caesarean operation, then the procedure should be commenced as soon as possible.

Special considerations

The initial consideration is for the state of the dam. If the decision to operate has been taken early in the parturition process, she may be in good health. However, many operations are performed after the dam has been in unproductive labour for many hours and she may be exhausted, dehydrated and toxaemic. Fluids (e.g. Hartmann's solution) should be administered to correct the dehydration and the veterinary surgeon may decide to give preoperative antibiotics.

Anaesthesia

The aim should be to provide adequate surgical anaesthesia for the dam whilst affecting the fetuses as little as possible. It is essential to complete the operation quickly to minimize the depression of the respiratory and circulatory systems of the fetuses. The following points are important:

- The increased volume of the abdomen can result in a reduced thoracic capacity, plus oxygen consumption during pregnancy increases by 20% and the dam is prone to hypoxia
- The acid–base balance of the bitch may vary widely from metabolic acidosis to respiratory alkalosis
- The weight of the enlarged uterus may cause quite marked compression of the aorta and vena cava, if the animal is placed in dorsal recumbency. This may markedly affect cardiac output with resultant compromise of the circulation of the dam and the blood supply to the fetuses
- Pregnancy causes delayed gastric emptying and animals presented for Caesarean section may have full stomachs. There is an increased risk of vomiting and regurgitation during induction or recovery from anaesthesia.

With these considerations in mind, the anaesthetic regimen necessitates the use of low doses of anaesthetic to ensure minimal fetal depression.

Premedication

- Sedative/tranquillizers – avoid using phenothiazines unless absolutely necessary due to their hypotensive effects. Diazepam or midazolam may be used but may not be very effective in distressed animals.

- Anticholinergics – atropine or glycopyrrolate may be useful to counteract the vagal reflex when the gravid uterus is handled. Glycopyrrolate does not cross the placental barrier and therefore is preferable.

General anaesthesia

- Induction
  - Barbiturates such as thiopentone or methohexitone cross the placenta and cause fetal depression and therefore should be used at greatly reduced dose rates
  - Propofol is most useful in the bitch and a single bolus injection should be given before intubation. The animal should then be maintained on oxygen alone until it is necessary to maintain the animal on an inhalational agent. Propofol is less useful in the cat, giving slower recovery and less vigorous offspring
  - Alphaxalone/alphadolone is used in cats, with the minimal dose being calculated to give the appropriate duration of action
  - Induction by face mask is possible but it can cause distress to the animal and may prolong the exposure to anaesthetic agents if the animal refuses to breathe or fights the procedure.
- Maintenance
  - All inhalant anaesthetics cross the placental barrier and the degree of fetal depression is dependent on the agent, the duration and the depth of anaesthesia
  - Isofluorane is the anaesthetic agent of choice due to its high safety margin and the fact that it is almost completely eliminated through respiration (less than 2% is metabolized).

Surgery

All the preparations for a Caesarean operation should be made prior to the dam being anaesthetized. If it is possible to clip the operation site without causing distress to the dam, this will effectively reduce the time under anaesthesia.

The extra requirements for the care of the neonates should be prepared before the start of the anaesthetic procedure. These include:

- Clean, dry towels for drying the neonates
- Respiratory stimulant drops, e.g. doxapram
- Suction device (if available)
- Cotton buds: useful to clean the nostrils and oral cavity of mucus
- Clamps for umbilical cords
- Disinfectant for umbilicus
- Warm area for neonates: use wrapped hot water bottles, heated blankets
- Stethoscope for auscultating respiration and heart beats.

The operation may be via a midline or flank incision depending on the preference of the individual veterinary surgeon. The argument for a midline incision is that the exposure of the abdomen is better and it is more convenient to exteriorize the gravid uterus. However, there will be a suture line between the mammary glands that may be prone to damage by the paws of the litter, as they knead the tissue to induce milk let-down.

A flank incision will avoid this complication. Flank incisions should not be used in pedigree cats because the hair may grow back a different colour.

The surgeon will deliver the fetuses directly from the uterus and will usually open the amniotic sac, to allow respiration to start, and clamp the umbilical cord before handing the fetus to the assistant. The assistant should remember never to touch the surgeon's hands during the transfer of neonates. The surgeon should gently drop the neonate into a warm towel held in both hands of the assistant. The placenta may detach from the uterus at this time and the veterinary nurse may be presented with it attached to the neonate. It is important to ensure that the neonate is breathing and the respiratory passages are clear *before* removing the placental tissue (Figure 10.25).

10.25 Procedure for neonates delivered by Caesarean operation

1. Rub the neonate vigorously, to stimulate respiration and circulation and dry the fetal fluids.
2. Check for vital signs: breathing, heartbeat and colour of the mucous membranes.
3. If respiration is absent or weak, a few drops of doxapram should be administered (2–10 drops in puppies, 2–4 drops in kittens depending on size and respiratory depression).
4. Check the patency of the airway and remove mucus or other inhaled contaminants by suction or cotton bud. If the respiratory tract has a lot of mucus in it, cup the puppy or kitten in the hands and hold it head downwards to allow the fluid to drain out.
5. Blowing into the mouth and nose of the neonate will provide gentle respiratory support.
6. A strong heartbeat should be palpated in the ventral thorax behind the elbow. If not, gentle massage in this area with thumb and forefinger may stimulate the heart.
7. Once satisfied that the neonate is viable, cut the umbilical cord distal to the clamp. Place the neonate into the warm area previously prepared.
8. Check puppies or kittens regularly to ensure they are still without problems. Often you will be dealing with more than one neonate at a time and a good routine will help the procedure progress smoothly.
9. Once the neonates have all been removed from the uterus and revived, check them for congenital abnormalities.
10. It is useful to encourage the neonates to suckle from the dam when she is recovering from the anaesthetic but in practice puppies and kittens are often too drowsy to feed properly at this time. Therefore it is important to maintain constant warmth until suckling can commence, with the provision of a warm drink.

It is essential to ensure that the area in which the neonates are left is neither too hot nor too cold. Hypothermia is the main cause of neonatal mortality. The neonates may be replaced with the dam, under continuous observation, when she has recovered sufficiently to accept them.

Care of the bitch or queen following parturition

The dam will generally clean the perineum after the last neonate has been born. It is advisable to assist the dam if she has a long coat that has become soiled. Allow the young to suckle and then encourage the dam to take exercise and relieve herself. Clean the bedding and offer the dam some food.

Diarrhoea is likely to develop during the first few days if the bitch has eaten an excessive number of placentas. Food intake will increase up to three times during lactation and frequent small meals should be offered.

Although for the first 2–3 weeks the dam will spend most of the time with the young, after this it is advisable to allow her to leave them for longer periods to encourage weaning to take place.

Problems following parturition

Placental/fetal retention
This is not common in dogs and cats.

- Owner should verify that the placentas number the same as neonates born
- Missing placentas may have been eaten by the dam
- Vaginal examination may reveal cord: remove by gentle traction
- Oxytocin may be helpful
- Ultrasonography may help to confirm the diagnosis
- May cause acute septic metritis (see below).

Acute septic metritis
This condition is extremely serious and potentially fatal.

- Often associated with abnormality of parturition:
  - Dystocia
  - Lack of hygiene in environment/examination
  - Fetal/placental retention
  - Uterine prolapse/atony/incomplete involution
- Pyrexia, anorexia, agalactia, purulent vaginal discharge, abdominal pain, diarrhoea
- Intensive nursing required: fluids, analgesics, antibiotics
- Oxytocin may help to evacuate uterine contents
- Remove litter temporarily or permanently.

Haemorrhage
This should not exceed a small drip from the vulva.

- Excess haemorrhage may indicate uterine tract tears or vessel rupture
- Oxytocin may be helpful
- May require exploratory laparotomy
- Treat blood loss if excessive.

Subinvolution of placental sites
Uterine involution should be complete 12 weeks after whelping. Subinvolution is suspected if discharge or haemorrhage persists longer than 6 weeks.

- Aetiology unknown
- Occurs mostly in primiparous animals
- Dam is often unaffected
- Often resolves spontaneously
- Occasionally requires ovariohysterectomy if bleeding is persistent.

Uterine prolapse
This is an uncommon condition, seen in queens more than in bitches.

- Occurs immediately, or within a few hours of the last neonate being born
- May involve both horns or just one plus the uterine body
- Manual repositioning may not be easy and may require laparotomy
- Often dam requires an ovariohysterectomy.

Toxic milk syndrome

- Pathological conditions of the uterus may cause toxins in the milk
- Neonates become vocal and uncomfortable
- May have bloating, diarrhoea, salivation, reddened anus
- Remove litter and give oral fluids
- Return litter to bitch once she has improved.

Eclampsia (puerperal tetany)

This is rare in cats but may be seen in small-breed bitches 10–30 days after whelping.

- Caused by decrease in extracellular calcium levels
- Dam shows restlessness, panting, pacing, salivation, tremors, stiffness
- Progresses to tonic–clonic spasms, fever, tachycardia, seizures and death
- Immediate treatment essential: slow intravenous calcium borogluconate 10%:
  - 2–5 ml for cats
  - 2–20 ml for dogs
- Hand-feed litter or wean older litters
- Prevention: oral supplementation with calcium at 100 mg/kg body weight per day.

 This is a life-threatening condition which requires immediate veterinary attention.

Lactation

Development of the mammary glands

The placenta is the life-support system for the fetus. The mammary glands (Figures 10.26) support the neonates until they are able to find nutrition elsewhere after weaning.

Development occurs in two stages:

- At puberty, FSH and LH stimulate production of oestrogen followed by progesterone from the ovaries
  - *Oestrogen* stimulates growth of the duct system
  - *Progesterone* promotes growth and development of the alveolar (secretory) tissue
- During pregnancy, further mammary development is synchronized with the pregnancy so that lactogenesis coincides with parturition.

10.26 Anatomy of the mammary glands

	Bitch	Queen
Number of glands (pairs)	5 (occasionally 4)	4
Pectoral/thoracic	3	2
Inguinal/abdominal	2	2
Teat orifices	8–20	4–7
Rows (bilaterally symmetrical)	2	2
Arrangement of mammary tissue	Continuous from ventral thorax to inguinal region	Discrete circles around each teat

Mammary changes during pregnancy

In a primigravid female, alterations in the size and shape of the mammary glands are noticed midway through pregnancy. In multigravidae, changes are noticeable only in the last 2–3 weeks before birth.

- Enlargement and pinkening of teats are noticed first. The mammary tissue becomes softer and more prominent under the influence of progesterone (mainly from the placenta) and oestrogen (at around the time of parturition)
- The blood supply to the mammary area increases near parturition and creates a local temperature rise, which creates a vital warm area for neonates. It is possible to express a milky secretion from the teats during the last week of pregnancy.

Other hormones involved in lactogenesis and lactation are:

- *Prolactin* – produced from the posterior pituitary when progesterone levels fall at the end of pregnancy. This ensures continuing lactation
- *ACTH* – high levels produced near parturition enhance the actions of oestrogen, progesterone and prolactin
- *Oxytocin* – brings about contractions of myoepithelial cells within the walls of the mammary alveoli at the time of parturition. Release of oxytocin also occurs in response to the neonates' suckling.

Colostrum

This is the milk produced from the mammary gland over the first 2–3 days after parturition. Colostrum has a special role to play in the early nutrition of the neonate because of the following properties:

- Antibodies to transmit passive immunity to the neonates
- Laxative to aid expulsion of meconium
- Nutrients to protect against hypoglycaemia and start extra-uterine growth
- Warm drink to protect against hypothermia.

Meconium is the term used to describe the contents of the digestive tract that formed during development in the uterus. It is greenish-brown in colour and has a very sticky consistency. If it is not voided soon after birth, the puppy or kitten will become constipated, evidenced by a distended abdomen.

Conditions of the lactating mammary gland

Galactostasis

Milk stasis causes enlarged, oedematous mammary glands.

- Dam is uncomfortable and has warm swollen glands which may be painful
- Pain prevents milk let-down
- Mostly occurs in the two caudal glands
- May occur in glands with malformed teats
- Gentle massage and cold compresses may help
- Fast the dam for 24 hours, then reduce food intake and possibly use a diuretic
- Cabergoline may be used in bitches when the litter has been removed.

Acute mastitis

This may be caused by bacterial infection (*Staphylococcus* spp., *Streptococcus* spp., *Escherichia coli*). It spreads to mammary glands from the blood or through the teat orifice.

- Mammary glands are hot, swollen and painful
- Milk becomes more viscous and the colour is yellow-brown
- Blood or pus may be seen in the milk
- Dam is depressed, pyrexic and anorexic
- Abscesses may develop in the mammary gland
- Intensive nursing (fluids, antibiotics, warm compresses) is essential
- Encourage suckling unless the milk is purulent, in which case use a milk substitute.

Agalactia

The absence of milk after parturition may be failure of either production or let-down.

- Failure of production may occur after a Caesarean section or premature birth
- Failure of let-down is related to oxytocin: often primigravid or nervous bitches
- Treatment: reassurance, sedation, oxytocin or encouraging young to suck
- Other causes may include infection, shock or exhaustion: treat appropriately.

Management of the neonate

The neonatal period covers the first 10 days of life. During this time, the new offspring are totally dependent on the dam. Successful rearing of puppies and kittens depends on a number of factors that include environmental conditions and the state of the dam before whelping.

The design of breeding quarters and catteries is beyond the scope of this chapter but the facilities must be appropriate in terms of privacy, cleanliness, adequate lighting, ventilation and heating.

Care of the dam before and during whelping is essential to ensure that the neonates are not compromised as they are born. An unfit or fat dam will have a prolonged parturition, which may jeopardize the viability of all or part of a litter. Perinatal infection will result in a sick dam that is unable to provide normal maternal care.

Knowledge of the special needs of neonates and their physiology is necessary to ensure their welfare. Many causes of neonatal death are avoidable by application of certain management principles.

Normal neonatal characteristics

Figure 10.27 gives some of the normal characteristics for neonate puppies and kittens.

Care of the newborn

Following a normal delivery the dam should attend to her young by:

- Licking the amniotic membranes away from the nose and mouth
- Biting the umbilical cord
- Nuzzling the neonate to stimulate and warm it

Neonates have little subcutaneous fat and no ability to shiver to protect them from hypothermia. The newborn will find their way to the teats and begin to suck immediately. This will raise the body temperature and help to combat the inevitable heat loss that occurs because of the high ratio of surface area to body weight.

The ambient temperature should be at least 30°C for the first 24 hours. It is important that the dam is allowed to escape from this heat if she becomes uncomfortable. The nest temperature can then be dropped to approximately 26°C over the next few days.

Soiled material from the whelping area should be frequently removed and replaced, but the dam will usually keep the area clean. Initially the dam must lick the perineal area of the offspring to encourage defecation and urination. After 2–3 weeks of age, the young will urinate and defecate voluntarily.

Care of neonates born by Caesarean section

Immediate care from the dam is not available and therefore procedures must be followed to ensure survival of the neonate (see Figure 10.25).

Handrearing of pups and kittens

Wherever possible, offspring should be left with the mother – handrearing is a labour-intensive procedure which requires full-time commitment.

10.27 Normal neonatal characteristics

	Puppy	Kitten
Birth weight	Very variable	Cross-breed: 110–120 g Small breed: 90–110 g Larger breed: 120–150 g
Temperature	Day 1: 36°C Day 7: 37°C	36°C falling to 30°C and rising to 38°C at 7 days
Heart rate	200/minute	200–250/minute
Respiratory rate	15–35/minute after birth	15–35/minute after birth
Eyelids open	10–14 days	5–12 days
Hearing develops	Around 2 weeks	Around 2 weeks
Shivering reflex	Around 1 week	Around 1 week
Suckles	Every 2 hours for first 2 weeks	Every 1–2 hours for first few days
Weight gain	Doubles weight in 8 days	Loses weight to begin with, then gains 15 g/day
Locomotion	Standing: 14 days Walking: 21 days	

It may be possible to foster the litter on to another dam if one is available in lactation. Some females with very strong mothering instincts will willingly accept a new litter but great care is required to ensure that the dam does not become aggressive with her adopted litter.

Reasons for hand-rearing neonates:

- Orphaned or abandoned young
- Dam is unwell or has no milk
- Dam is unsuitable to rear young (e.g. aggressive, nervous, inexperienced)
- Too large a litter
- Eclampsia in the bitch.

Basic requirements for neonates

Warmth
Normally warmth in the early days comes from the dam's mammary area and an additional heat source is rarely required. Orphaned neonates require a reliable alternative source of heat, because hypothermia is one of the main causes of death in the perinatal period. The following may be used, with care to avoid overheating or burns:

- Hot-water bottle
- Heated pad or blanket
- Heat lamp
- Incubator.

Additional bedding will help to insulate the whelping box. The environment should be draught-free. Cold neonates will feed inadequately, thus exacerbating the problem.

Food
Neonates should receive colostrum if at all possible. As well as being a warm drink, it is laxative and will help the neonates to pass the meconium. Colostrum also contains antibodies that are important in the early weeks to help the young combat infections until their own immune systems begin to develop.

Orphaned young may be fed with milk replacer. This should match the composition of the dam's milk (Figure 10.28).

10.28 Comparative composition of milk
(relative percentages of nutrient, as fed)

Component	Bitch	Cat	Cow
Protein	7.5	9.5	3.2
Fat	8.3	4.8	3.9
Lactose	3.7	4.9	4.9

It is possible to make homemade milk substitutes but there are many products on the market that are correctly formulated for the specific needs of the neonate.

- Feed neonates at approximately 2-hourly intervals for up to 2 weeks
- As the quantity taken increases, then the frequency of feeding may be reduced
- The young should sleep well after feeds and should not vocalize
- Weight gains should be checked to ensure that nutrition is adequate
- After feeding, rub the perineum gently with, for instance, a cotton bud to stimulate urination and defecation.

Cleanliness

- Any products of urination and defecation that the bitch does not clean should be removed
- Any bedding contaminated with milk or milk substitute should be removed but, beyond keeping the bedding clean, do not remove it entirely in the early days because the familiar smell gives security to the young
- The neonates must be carefully cleaned if there is spillage of foodstuffs on to their coats
- Utensils should be carefully sterilized using products licensed for use in human babies
- Isolate sick puppies or kittens immediately, being careful to provide an adequate heat source
- Use separate feeding utensils and wash hands after handling affected animals
- Cleanse sticky eyes or noses with warm saline on cotton buds, using separate buds for each eye.

Dewclaw removal
Puppy dewclaws are usually removed at around 48–96 hours after birth. This can be performed by owners but they should be encouraged to use the services of a veterinary surgeon.

- It is important to sterilize the scissors and to ensure that the skin of the puppy is swabbed with an appropriate antiseptic before the dewclaw is removed
- Following removal of the dewclaw, any haemorrhage should be controlled by manual pressure on the site with a piece of cotton wool or a swab
- If haemorrhage is persistent, veterinary advice should be sought
- Any swelling or discharge subsequent to the procedure is a cause for concern and requires veterinary advice.

Complications of the neonatal period

Congenital defects
These arise from disruption to normal development of the blastocyst, embryo or fetus. Some defects may be genetic in origin but, as mentioned in the section on breeding, there is a variety of causes – such as drug therapy, chemical contamination or nutritional abnormalities during pregnancy. Often the causal factor cannot be identified.

Neonates should be examined carefully for defects shortly after their birth. Many defects may not be apparent without careful clinical or pathological examination. Some of the common defects are:

- Cleft palate/lip
- Overshot/undershot jaw
- Spina bifida
- Polydactyly
- Umbilical/inguinal hernia
- Cryptorchidism.

Often these defects are suspected to have a genetic basis and the decision should be taken whether to euthanase the affected neonate.

Fading puppy syndrome
The definition of this syndrome is a failure to thrive despite a normal birth weight. It is followed by death within 3–5 days after birth. The causes for the problem may be multifactorial and wide-ranging. Often it can be very difficult to decide which factors have contributed to the problem.

In order to diagnose the possible causes of the deaths, a post mortem examination should be performed, remembering that pups from the same litter may have died from different causes. The causes of death may be:

- Infections
- Inadequate management and poor facilities
- Poor mothering
- Congenital abnormalities.

Further development of the litter

Following the neonatal period, the young animals continue to grow and enter the transitional period (10–21 days) during which time their eyesight and hearing develop and their thermoregulatory mechanism of shivering becomes functional (see Figure 10.27). Further neurological development increases their independence from the dam.

From 3 weeks to 3 months, puppies and kittens enter a period of socialization (see Chapter 11). This is a period of play and interaction with littermates, adults and other species. It is vitally important that puppies and kittens come into controlled contact with a wide range of species and situations during this period as this will ensure that they are well adapted to cope with their future when they are no longer with the litter.

Basic requirements for young puppies and kittens

Food and weaning

- At 3–4 weeks of age semi-solid food can be introduced (e.g. cereal, baby food, mince, scrambled egg)
- High protein and high carbohydrate foods should be provided
- Puppy food, which is moist, can be introduced in small quantities
- Lapping should be encouraged by dribbling small quantities of semi-fluid food down the nasal surface towards the mouth
- Often bottle-fed young are slow to lap and semi-solids can be fed initially by syringe

- Frequency should be about four to six feeds a day, depending on the age and enthusiasm for the meal.

Worming

Puppies and kittens can be wormed from about 3 weeks of age, depending on the proprietary preparation used.

Protection and safety

Protection from cold, damp and draughts is essential. No additional heating should be required unless the ambient temperature is very low. If the whelping box is in an elevated area, great care must be taken to ensure that the young animals do not fall out.

At this stage, the litter will be very inquisitive: open fires, flexes, cables and toxic chemicals should be well protected from sharp little teeth. Too much exposure to insensitive children or adults should be avoided. Care should be taken when introducing strange animals to the new litter – they will be enthusiastic but the stranger may become aggressive, possibly with fatal consequences.

Facilities for play

A safe confined area much larger than the whelping box is required. If the litter is taken outside, ensure that fences are secure and that fishponds and puddles are out of reach.

Playthings should be plentiful, large and free from easily swallowed removable bits.

Further reading

Arthur GH, Noakes DE, Pearson H and Parkinson TJ (1996) *Veterinary Reproduction and Obstetrics, 7th Edition*. WB Saunders, Philadelphia

Burke TJ (1986) *Small Animal Reproduction and Infertility: A Clinical Approach to Diagnosis and Treatment*. Lea and Febiger, Philadelphia

Jackson PGG (ed.) (1995) *Handbook of Veterinary Obstetrics*. WB Saunders, London

Simpson GM, England GCW and Harvey MJ (1998) *Manual of Small Animal Reproduction and Neonatology*. BSAVA, Cheltenham

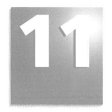

Advice to clients

Kit Sturgess, Janet Parker and Sarah Heath

This chapter is designed to give information on:

- Infectious disease – methods of spread and control
- Immunity – natural and acquired
- Vaccination
- Client information on clinical control measures
- The identification and management of parasitic infections
- Advice to clients on dietary management
- Preparing the client for euthanasia of a pet
- The grief sequence and bereavement counselling
- Counselling on pet behaviour

Introduction to infectious diseases

Methods of the spread of disease

Figure 11.1 shows the main routes of transmission by which disease is spread. The various types of pathogens that can cause disease are listed in Figure 11.2.

Horizontal transmission

Infection can be transmitted not only in the acute phase of infection, when the individual is obviously unwell, but also

11.1 Main routes of disease transmission

Horizontal transmission

- Direct contact
  - direct animal-to-animal contact
  - airborne over short distances
- Indirect contact
  - fomites
  - paratenic, intermediate or transfer hosts i.e. vectors
  - airborne over large distances
  - other body secretions (see later)
  - contaminated food
  - environmental contamination

Vertical transmission

- Transplacental

during the incubation period before the animal has become ill. Following recovery, animals can become carriers, remaining healthy but spreading infection to susceptible individuals. The principal methods of spread of the major infectious diseases in the UK are illustrated in Figure 11.3.

Direct contact

Direct animal-to-animal contact occurs when a part of the body of one animal meets a part of the body of another – for example, when skin surfaces come into contact, when one animal licks or grooms another or during fighting. (Venereal transmission of disease, involving direct contact between the reproductive organs, occurs in dogs and cats but is not a significant route of infection in the UK.)

Infectious agents that are spread by direct contact are frequently fragile and easily killed by heat, light, desiccation and disinfectants. Disinfection is not, however, a major method of control in such infections.

Airborne transmission occurs via droplets produced during coughing or sneezing and is of particular importance in respiratory diseases.

Indirect contact

This is when two or more animals come into contact with the same inanimate object (e.g. bedding material or feeding bowls). Pathogenic organisms can be spread from one animal to another via this inanimate object; contact with the object usually occurs shortly after it has become contaminated with the infectious agent. However, some organisms can remain viable in the environment for long periods, particularly under dark damp conditions or where faecal contamination has occurred. For example, feline and canine parvoviruses can

11.2 Types of pathogen*

Pathogen	Includes	Examples
Bacteria	Specialist intracellular bacteria	*Chlamydia psittaci*
Viruses	'Slow' viruses	Feline immunodeficiency virus (FIV)
Parasites	Endoparasites Ectoparasites	*Toxocara canis* *Ctenocephalides felis*
Protozoa	Intestinal tract Blood borne	*Giardia lamblia* *Haemobartonella felis*
Fungi	Skin Internal	*Microsporum canis* *Aspergillus fumigatus*
Other	Mycoplasmas Rickettsia Unclassified but apparently infectious	Kennel cough *Borrelia burgdorferi* (Lyme disease) Feline spongiform encephalopathy (FSE)

* A pathogen is defined as any disease-producing agent or microorganism.

11.3 Principal methods of spread of the major feline and canine infectious diseases

Direct contact

Feline infectious peritonitis
Feline leukaemia virus
Feline immunodeficiency virus
Chlamydiosis
Feline infectious anaemia
Rabies

Aerosol spread

Distemper virus	Feline calicivirus[b]
Bordetellosis[a]	Canine herpesvirus[a]
Parainfluenza virus[a]	Canine adenovirus 2[a]
Feline herpesvirus[b]	

Indirect contact

Parvovirus	Infectious canine hepatitis
Leptospirosis	Toxoplasmosis

a Infectious agents involved in infectious canine tracheobronchitis (kennel cough syndrome)
b Infectious agents primarily responsible for cat 'flu

survive for up to a year in the environment. Infectious agents that rely on indirect spread are generally hardy and difficult to kill with disinfection.

Some infectious agents do not pass directly from one individual to another but spend part of their life cycle on another host, termed a vector (Figure 11.4).

Vertical transmission

A disease is said to be passed vertically when it spreads from the dam to the offspring whilst they are still *in utero*. Feline parvovirus can be spread vertically if the queen becomes infected whilst she is pregnant. The outcome of such an infection will depend on the stage of the pregnancy. In the case of feline parvovirus it can cause a variety of problems including abortion, giving birth to mummified kittens and underdevelopment of the cerebellum (cerebellar hypoplasia) in which case the kittens are born alive but are poorly coordinated.

Carrier animals

A carrier of an infectious disease is an animal that does not show clinical signs of the disease but whose body harbours the disease-producing organism and may continue to excrete it.

Carrier animals are of great epidemiological importance in the spread of infectious disease in cats and dogs (Figure 11.5).

11.4 Indirect disease transmission

Vector type	Definition	Example
Non-biological (mechanical vector)	An organism in which no development takes place, the vector acting like a moving fomite	Insects carrying infectious agents on their mouth parts
Definitive host	The host in which the organism undergoes the sexual phases of development	The cat is the definitive host for the tapeworm *Taenia taeniaeformis*
Intermediate host	The host in which the infective organism passes its larval or non-sexual phase(s)	The flea acts as the intermediate host for the tapeworm *Dipylidium caninum*
Transfer host	A host that is used by the infection until the appropriate definitive host is reached. A transfer host is not necessary for completion of the life cycle of the infection	Earthworms harbouring *Toxoplasma*
Paratenic host	An animal acting as a substitute intermediate host, usually acquiring the organism by ingestion	Mice can carry *Toxocara* L2 larvae. The life cycle of *Toxocara* is normally direct via the faecal or oral route

A vector is another host which carries the infectious organism and in which the organism can sometimes undergo development. Direct vector-borne transmission is not generally of major importance in the UK but does occur (e.g. Lyme disease (Borrelia burgdorferi) in dogs).

11.5 Major feline and canine infectious diseases for which carrier states are important in the spread of disease

Disease	Continuous excretors	Intermittent excretors
Leptospirosis	> 3 months	
Parvovirus infection	Up to 6 weeks	
Infectious canine hepatitis	Up to 6 months	
Rabies	Up to 1 year or longer*	
Salmonellosis		✓
Feline herpesvirus infection		✓
Feline calicivirus	Up to 18 months	
Chlamydiosis	Up to 8 months	
Feline infectious peritonitis		✓
Feline leukaemia	A true carrier state is unlikely to exist. Persistently FeLV-positive healthy cats are in an asymptomatic disease state which will eventually develop into FeLV-associated disease in virtually all cats. They act like carriers as they can infect susceptible animals	
Feline immunodeficiency	FIV is similar to FeLV; cats can be asymptomatic for long periods up to 5 years	
Feline infectious anaemia	Once infected, cats become lifelong carriers but the organism is not excreted	

* Rarely, animals recover and may then represent a risk to handlers

They may be either 'convalescent' or 'healthy', and each of these two types may be either a continuous or an intermittent excretor of the microorganism.

- *Convalescent carriers* have had the disease, with the usual signs, but do not rid themselves of the organism completely for a long time (sometimes for life)
- *Healthy carriers* have been exposed to the disease and possess an innate immunity sufficient to prevent clinical signs but not to prevent infection. Vaccinated animals can become carriers in this way.
- *Continuous excretors* continuously excrete the infectious agent and can infect other animals at any time; they are easier to identify than intermittent excretors
- *Intermittent excretors* only excrete organisms under certain circumstances, usually periods of stress (e.g. parturition, lactation, rehoming, use of immunosuppressive drugs such as corticosteroids).

Routes by which infectious agents are excreted

Any or all of the following can be infectious, depending on the disease involved:

- Faeces
- Urine
- Nasal and ocular discharges
- Saliva
- Genital discharges
- Fluid from skin lesions
- Blood
- Milk
- Dead animals
- Vomit.

Elementary methods of disease control

Figure 11.6 illustrates the main methods of prevention of the spread of disease.

Treatment

There are four potential aims of treatment:

- To kill the pathogenic organism involved. In the case of viral disease this is rarely possible
- To prevent secondary opportunist infection (usually bacteria) becoming involved and making the situation worse
- To provide nutritional, fluid and other non-specific support (e.g. vitamins) to allow the animal's own immune system to eliminate the organism as rapidly as possible
- To modify the immune response, making it more effective.

Quarantine and isolation

Isolation is the segregation and separation of infected or potentially infected animals from uninfected animals, particularly high risk groups (e.g. neonates, sick animals). Quarantine (the isolation of imported animals) is discussed in *BSAVA Manual of Veterinary Care*.

11.6 Methods of prevention of disease spread

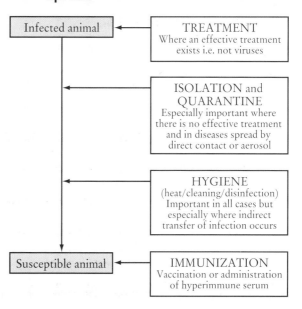

Potentially infectious animals should be isolated in a separate building or room where they can be treated or, alternatively, sent home again to be nursed by their owners. Since few of the infectious diseases of cats (and none of the viral diseases except rabies) are transmissible to dogs, or vice versa, in an emergency an infected cat can be placed temporarily in a room housing only dogs, or conversely an infected dog can be placed in isolation with cats. Ideally animals that are known to have been in contact with infected animals for some time before clinical signs were noted should themselves be isolated in this way and treated accordingly.

Animals in isolation should have their own feeding bowls and bedding (if non-disposable materials are used) and these should be washed separately. Ideally these animals should be attended by different staff to those dealing with other animals, to prevent infectious organisms being transferred on clothing and shoes (see *BSAVA Manual of Veterinary Care*).

It is unwise to house animals in large numbers in a single room or air space, because all are likely to be affected if one of them develops an infectious disease. This is a particular problem in some rescue facilities.

- New animals entering an existing colony (e.g. breeding group) or a multi-animal household should be kept separate for at least 3–4 weeks in case they are incubating an infectious disease. In this time diagnostic testing (e.g. for FeLV/FIV) and vaccination may be carried out. *This will not necessarily identify carriers*
- Young animals usually have no, or poor, immunity to many of the larger parasites, whereas older animals usually have immunity and may carry and transmit the parasites without showing disease signs. Young animals are best isolated from kennels, and particularly runs, used for older animals, in which there can be a gradual accumulation of the infective stages of parasites passed out in the faeces.

Hygiene

The thorough cleansing of all surfaces will remove many of the viruses, bacteria and parasitic eggs/oocysts that may be present. This applies to all feeding and bedding materials as well as all surfaces (including soil) in kennels and catteries. Reducing the weight of infection increases the chances of an animal mounting an effective immune response if it should become infected.

The efficient cleaning of surfaces with soap or detergent plus water (preferably hot), followed by thorough rinsing, is much more effective than using disinfectants to try to kill organisms. Mechanical cleaning in this way actually removes most organisms so that they are no longer present to produce infection. Many disinfectants can kill infective organisms but none will reliably kill bacterial spores or *Toxocara* eggs. Many disinfectants are rendered much less effective by the presence of dirt, blood, pus, faeces or soaps (see *BSAVA Manual of Veterinary Care*). Disinfection alone should not be relied on, nor should it be assumed that all infectious agents will be destroyed.

Methods of decreasing the risk of infection from the environment are summarized in Figure 11.7.

Vaccination/immunization

This is a way of limiting the spread of disease by providing some degree of protection against infection (see later).

11.7 **Methods to decrease the number of infectious organisms in the environment**

- Regular cleaning of the animal's coat (i.e. bathing) will help to reduce the population of infectious organisms that accumulate there
- Heat sterilization of feeding bowls and litter trays is a very efficient way of reducing the burden of organisms
- There should be regular efficient removal of soiled bedding, which should undergo a hot wash cycle or be disposed of as clinical waste
- Either all food should be cooked, or dried and canned foods should be used. This is particularly important in preventing the transmission of tapeworms and *Toxoplasma* to dogs and cats
- Cats and dogs should be discouraged from catching rodents, birds and even slugs and earthworms, as these are intermediate hosts of many internal parasites.
- Rodents and flies should be controlled, since they also act as vectors for infection.

How microorganisms produce disease

In order to establish an infection, an infectious organism must overcome the body's external and internal defence mechanisms. Having done so, it can produce disease in the following ways:

- By direct damage to body cells, leading to loss of normal anatomy and function
- By the action of toxins, which cause cell lysis and death
- By provoking inflammation, which causes many of the signs of disease
- By initiating reaction between antigen–antibody complexes formed by the host, which can lead to severe cell damage and to an allergic reaction
- By damaging the immune system itself (e.g. feline immunodeficiency virus).

Defence against disease

External defence mechanisms

External defence mechanisms are usually non-specific and are designed to prevent any potential pathogen from entering the body.

- The dry horny layer of the *skin* is impermeable; for entry, microorganisms require breaks in this layer (e.g. wounds, burns, bites, injection sites or natural openings such as hair follicles)
- Conjunctivae are constantly washed by *tears*
- Mucous membranes of the body tracts produce *mucus*, to which organisms adhere and are prevented from gaining entry as the mucus is expelled from the body
- The respiratory tract has *cilia* which 'sweep' mucus and bacteria to the exterior
- The high acidity of the *stomach* and enzyme production in the duodenum both act to kill microorganisms.
- *Natural functions* such as coughing, sneezing, sweating, salivating, urinating and defecating help to flush bacteria from the body
- Many *body secretions* contain substances that inhibit or destroy bacteria (e.g. lysozyme, an enzyme that can rupture Gram-negative bacteria).

When the external defences have been breached, it is easier for other microorganisms to invade. These are termed *secondary infections*. In the majority of cases the primary invaders are usually viruses and the secondary infections are bacteria. However, burns, injection sites, surgical wounds and traumatic wounds can act to cause the primary breach, allowing secondary infections.

Internal defence mechanisms

Once inside the body, organisms have to overcome a whole variety of internal defence mechanisms.

Non-specific immune defence mechanisms

Inflammation

Inflammation (Figure 11.8) is the body's response to substances that are produced as microorganisms grow or that are released from damaged cells. It results in:

- Dilation of capillaries and lymphatics (thereby increasing blood flow)
- Increased permeability of vessel walls to fluid, cells and protective substances such as antibodies
- Attraction of phagocytes – at first neutrophils and then macrophages.

The clinical signs of inflammation are heat, pain, swelling, redness and loss of function.

Phagocytosis

See *BSAVA Manual of Veterinary Care*. There are two types of phagocytes, or 'eating cells':

- *Neutrophils* (polymorphs), which circulate in the blood
- *Macrophages*, which are both in the blood and scattered throughout the body in the tissues (when in the blood they are called monocytes).

Neutrophils are the most active at phagocytosis, which occurs in two stages:

- *Attachment* of the neutrophil to the bacterium. If the bacterium has a capsule, it is more difficult for the cell to attach; but it is much easier if it has been coated with antibody
- *Ingestion*. This involves pseudopods ('pretend legs') flowing from the cell around the bacterium and enclosing it.

Once in the cell, the bacterium is killed and broken down by cellular enzymes. Some bacteria evade these mechanisms by being very resistant to ingestion or being resistant to intracellular killing by the phagocyte. When large numbers of dead neutrophils accumulate, this forms pus. At a later stage in the immune response, macrophages appear and phagocytose the dead neutrophils and tissue debris.

Some bacteria are capable of multiplying within the phagocytic cells (e.g. *Mycobacterium tuberculosis*).

Bactericidal substances

These exist within tissue fluids, the most important group being the components of the *complement* system – a complex series of proteins which assists antibodies in destroying bacteria. The attachment of the antibody to the microorganism enables the complement to recognize its target. This sets in motion a progressive increase in the number of attaching molecules of complement in a process called *amplification*. Both inflammation and phagocytosis are increased by the action of complement.

Cytokines

Cytokines, such as interferon, are a complex group of substances synthesized by various types of body cells. Cytokines act to direct the immune response in a cellular or humoral pattern. They are of great importance in the immune response to viruses.

Specific, acquired immunity

These mechanisms are involved in the recognition of specific disease-producing microorganisms and are acquired by an animal during its life, following exposure to the organism or vaccination. There are two different mechanisms:

- *Humoral* response, associated with production of antibodies by B lymphocytes (*B cells*) and defence against extracellular microorganisms
- *Cell-mediated immunity* (CMI), important in response to intracellular microorganisms and mediated by T lymphocytes (*T cells*) derived from the thymus.

Each type of T cell is able to react with a particular type of antigen which it recognizes on the surface of an infected cell. T cells respond by releasing *lymphokines* (a subgroup of

11.8 **Characteristics and consequences of inflammation**

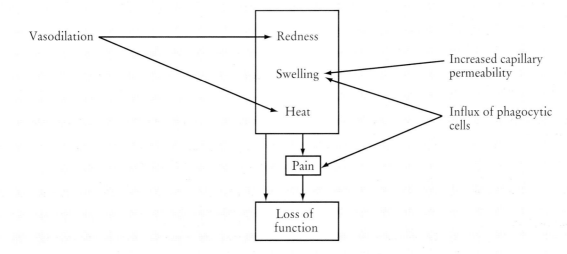

cytokines), which initiate an inflammatory response and attract phagocytes. They have important functions in regulating the type and magnitude of the immune response, as well as activating other T cells that are able directly to kill the infected cell by reacting with cell-surface antigens to produce holes in the cell wall. The cell contents leak through the hole and the cell dies, releasing the microorganism into the extracellular environment where it can be neutralized by antibodies, covered by complement (which facilitates phagocytosis) or ingested directly by phagocytic cells. See *BSAVA Manual of Veterinary Care*.

CMI is most important in combating viral infections, which are unable to multiply outside the host cells as they need to use the cells' metabolic pathways to build new virus particles.

The principles of immunity

Immunity to an infection can occur in a variety of ways (Figure 11.9). A foreign antigen is recognized by the immune system which, depending on whether the antigen is intracellular or extracellular, initiates a cellular or humoral (antibody) response (described below).

Antibodies are protein molecules and can be detected in the blood as part of the globulin fraction. An increase in the globulin fraction of the plasma proteins is often an indication of infection but can also occur as a response to inflammation and sometimes neoplasia.

Once produced, the antibody combines with the antigen. Where the antigen is part of a microorganism or its toxin, this antibody–antigen complex is beneficial to the host, because:

- It makes phagocytosis easier
- It stops viruses entering cells
- It prevents bacteria from attaching to mucosal surfaces
- It neutralizes toxins
- It activates complement, which stimulates inflammation and increases the supply of phagocytes.

When the antigen has been successfully eliminated, the level of antibody gradually falls but some of the B cells become *memory cells* to that particular antigen; if the same antigen reappears in the body the specific antibody response is more rapid and vigorous.

Physiological factors

Physiological factors may make the host more susceptible to an infectious disease. The factors include:

- Poor nutritional status or obesity
- Debilitation due to other diseases or organ failure
- Shock
- Fatigue
- Hypothermia
- Ageing or immaturity (old animals whose immune systems are less active and young animals whose immune systems have not fully matured tend to be more susceptible)
- Immunosuppressive therapy (e.g. corticosteroids)
- Genetic factors also play an important role, some individuals within a group being more or less susceptible.

It is not possible to infect all species of animal with all types of virus and bacteria, as many organisms are adapted to a specific host species. This means that other species are *non-susceptible*, i.e. they have innate protection from that disease due to their genetic constitution. For example, dogs and cats do not contract foot-and-mouth disease and cows do not get distemper.

Immunization

When infection occurs the body responds by producing antibodies specific to the agent responsible. Once recovery is complete the animal is resistant to further infection from that agent and is said to be immune. Immunity can last for variable periods, from a few months to the rest of the animal's life, depending on the immunogenicity of the microorganism involved. This natural process can be copied by the use of vaccines.

Maternally derived immunity

Newborn kittens and puppies have little or no acquired immunity at birth. Further, their immune system is immature and slow to react and their body reserves limited. In order to increase survival in the first few weeks of life, passive immunity is gained from the dam. Immunity can be transferred from dam to offspring in two ways:

- Via the placenta – antibodies pass directly from the mother's blood to that of her fetuses through the placenta. This accounts for less than 5% of immunity transferred to puppies and kittens
- Via the colostrum (first milk) – antibodies are ingested with colostrum and absorbed through the gut wall into the neonate's blood. Colostrum is very rich in antibodies, which are not digested by the offspring in the first 24–48 hours of life but are absorbed into the blood stream. By 48 hours after birth, closure of the gut has occurred; thereafter antibodies are digested as other proteins would be. Colostral antibodies can still provide local protection to the intestinal lining.

11.9 Types of immunity to infection

	Natural immunity	Artificial immunity	Immediacy
Active immunity (antibody or reactive T cells have been made by the animal itself)	Infection	Vaccination or injection of a toxoid	Antibody production after a specific T cell response takes at least 1 week to occur after first contact with a microorganism or toxin, i.e. protection is not immediate. Levels fall gradually after infection as the antigen is eliminated but a memory response remains
Passive immunity (preformed antibodies are received from outside)	Maternally derived (antibodies last 8–20 weeks)	Antitoxin or hyperimmune serum (antibodies last 2–4 weeks)	Protection is immediate, as soon as antibody is transferred. As this is a passive response, no new antibody is produced and no memory cells form

Because of the importance of colostral transfer, it is essential that kittens and puppies suckle in the first few hours of life. Also, as colostral antibodies have been raised against pathogens present in the dam's environment, it is important not to move pregnant bitches or queens to a completely new environment prior to parturition: the offspring may not be protected against the pathogens present in the new environment.

Vaccines

A vaccine is prepared by modifying a bacterial or viral culture grown in a laboratory in such a way that, when the vaccine is introduced into the animal's body, immunity is stimulated but the agent is incapable of producing appreciable disease. This is achieved by killing the organism or by changing it (*attenuation*) so that it loses its *virulence* (ability to cause disease). The protection produced is specific to that particular agent, though some groups of microorganisms are closely related and so immunity to one type protects against another; for example, measles virus and distemper virus; and canine adenovirus 2 being used to protect dogs against infectious canine hepatitis, which is caused by CAV-1.

Vaccines work by eliciting a primary immune response to the pathogen such that when a field infection occurs there is a stronger and more rapid antibody and cell-mediated response (Figure 11.10). Vaccines do not prevent infection but they decrease the severity of the clinical signs.

Vaccination against a number of viral and bacterial infections is available in the UK (Figure 11.11).

Booster vaccination

A memory-immune (anamnestic) response to infectious diseases lasts for variable periods, depending on the immunogenicity of the agent or vaccine. Generally bacteria are poorly immunogenic, as are some viruses (e.g. cat 'flu viruses).

In order to maintain high levels of protective immunity, repeated injections of antigen are given.

- Leptospirosis, parvovirus (dead) and 'flu vaccinations should be boosted annually
- Distemper, parvovirus (live) and canine adenovirus vaccines probably confer life-long immunity, but in the absence of challenge from the naturally occurring pathogen, immunity may wane and booster vaccination is recommended every other year
- Intranasal vaccines should be boosted every 6–10 months but are probably better given 2–3 weeks prior to a high-risk period such as kennelling.

Types of vaccine

The major choice when using vaccines is whether to use a modified live or a killed adjuvanted product. There are potential advantages and disadvantages with both types (Figure 11.12) but, in general, modified live vaccines are preferred for routine vaccination where available.

Live attenuated vaccines

These are made from virulent organisms that have been weakened, usually in cell culture. When injected they undergo limited replication (Figure 11.13a) causing a low grade (usually asymptomatic) infection.

Killed adjuvanted vaccines

These are made from organisms grown in cell culture and then killed (with heat, chemicals or ultraviolet). Dead vaccines do not replicate in the host and therefore require repeated injections to produce a protective immune response (Figure 11.13b).

11.10 Why vaccination works

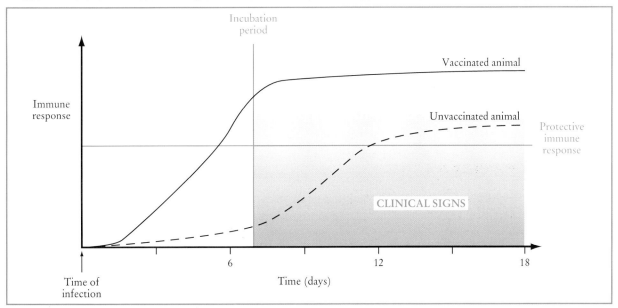

An animal will not show clinical signs if it achieves an immune response greater than that needed for protective immunity within the incubation time. At the time of infection neither a vaccinated nor an unvaccinated animal will have an active immune response. However, the individual that has been vaccinated will mount a stronger and more rapid response to the infection when compared to the unvaccinated individual due to the presence of memory cells that have been produced by its previous vaccination. A vaccinated animal is therefore much more likely to produce a protective immune response within the incubation period and will therefore show fewer or no clinical signs of disease.

11.11 Diseases in the UK for which vaccines are available

Animal	Disease/agent	Vaccine components	Types of vaccine
Dog	Parvovirus	Canine parvovirus	ML; KA
	Distemper	Canine distemper virus Measles virus	ML ML
	Leptospirosis	*L.icterohaemorrhagiae* *L.canicola*	KA KA
	Infectious canine hepatitis Canine adenovirus 1	Canine adenovirus 2	ML
	'Kennel cough'	Canine parainfluenza virus *Bordetella bronchiseptica*	ML i/n
Cat and dog	Rabies	Rabies virus	KA
	Tetanus toxoid	*Clostridium tetani*	KA
Cat	Feline infectious enteritis (feline panleucopenia virus)	Feline parvovirus	ML; KA
	Cat 'flu	Feline calicivirus Feline herpesvirus 1 (feline rhinotracheitis virus)	ML; KA ML; KA
	Feline leukaemia virus	Feline leukaemia virus	KA; GE; SU
	Chlamydiosis	*Chlamydia psittaci*	ML; KA
Rabbits	Myxomatosis	Myxomatosis virus	ML
	Viral haemorrhagic disease	Rabbit haemorrhagic disease virus	KA

ML = modified live vaccine   KA = killed adjuvanted vaccine   i/n = modified live intranasal vaccine
GE = genetically engineered vaccine   SU = subunit vaccine

Genetically engineered vaccines
These are manufactured by a variety of techniques and are aimed at producing the part of the infectious agent which is responsible for inducing a protective immunity. They are essentially similar to killed vaccines and are adjuvanted.

Subunit vaccines
These can be genetically engineered or produced by disrupting the infectious agent into its component parts. They are essentially similar to killed vaccines and are adjuvanted.

Intranasal vaccines
These are temperature-sensitive mutants of virulent organisms; they are only able to replicate at the lower temperatures found in the nares and not at normal body temperature. They produce a rapid (though shorter-lived) local response and protection after a single inoculation and are also not affected by maternally derived antibodies (MDAs). They are of some value in the face of an outbreak of infection as they also act to block receptor sites non-specifically for other infectious organisms. However, there is an increased incidence of vaccine reactions and they can be more difficult to administer.

Autogenous vaccines
These are prepared from bacteria or virus from an individual animal for injection into that same animal. They are most commonly used for dogs with chronic staphylococcal skin infections and horses with viral warts.

Heterotropic vaccines
These are produced from virus affecting a different species and can sometimes be used to produce immunity as they are closely related to a virus affecting the vaccinated animal.

Because there are subtle differences between the viruses, however, they can be used in the face of MDA. Human measles vaccine has been used to produce rapid immunity to distemper in young puppies, and was used to provide some protection for dogs against parvovirus when the infection was first recognized. Feline infectious enteritis vaccines can be given to ferrets to protect them against their own form of the disease.

Vaccination and MDA
The transfer of maternally derived antibodies (MDAs) can be maximized by ensuring that the mother's antibody levels are high around the time of parturition. Vaccination prior to mating is advised. In some situations it is necessary to vaccinate a pregnant bitch or queen and this should be performed a least 4 weeks before parturition.

Live vaccines during pregnancy are contraindicated, due to the risk of residual vaccine virulence causing stillbirths, early fetal death, resorption or birth defects. Concerns have also been raised about the use of live vaccines whilst the puppies or kittens are still suckling.

The presence of MDAs prevents vaccination of newborn puppies and kittens, as the preformed antibodies will bind to the vaccine antigen and prevent it from working. In many cases there is a short period of 2–3 weeks when the residual MDAs are sufficient to prevent vaccination but do not protect against more virulent field challenge (*immunity gap*). This means that offspring at around 5–9 weeks of age are particularly vulnerable to infection. It is at this time that good hygiene practices are particularly important.

Timing of vaccination
As the young animal gets older, MDAs decrease and reach a certain level at which they no longer interfere with

11.12 Advantages and disadvantages of live and killed vaccines

Vaccine type	Potential advantages	Potential disadvantages
Modified live	Fewer inoculating doses required Adjuvants not necessary Less chance of hypersensitivity Induction of interferon and other cytokines Stronger longer-lasting immunity Better cell-mediated immunity stimulation Excretion of vaccine virus may spread the number of animals vaccinated	Risk of developing disease especially if animal immunocompromised Unsafe in pregnancy Tend to be less stable Risks of contamination with other infectious agents greater Unsafe in immunocompromised animals
Killed adjuvanted	Stable on storage Unlikely to cause disease through residual virulence Unlikely to contain contaminating organisms Economic to produce Generally safe in pregnancy or immunocompromised animals More rapid immunity Can be used where no natural infection exists	Tend to be less immunogenic Adjuvants more often associated with local and systemic reactions Do not confer non-specific immunity Adjuvants associated with fibrosarcomas in cats Require repeated dosage to produce immunity

11.13 Live versus killed vaccines

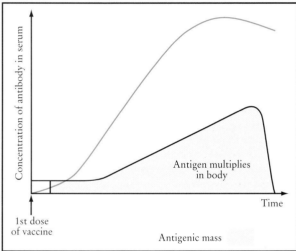

(a) Antibody response to a live vaccine.

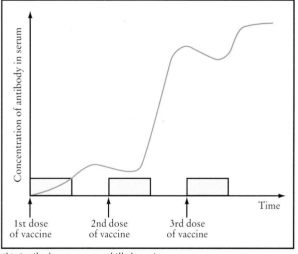

(b) Antibody response to a killed vaccine.

vaccination. It is not practical to find the time at which this decrease will enable an individual to respond (*seroconvert*) to vaccination and so primary vaccination schedules are designed to begin when a significant proportion of animals will seroconvert. The final vaccination is given when virtually all animals will respond.

The majority of vaccination schedules begin at 9–10 weeks for kittens and puppies, with a final injection being given at 12 weeks of age. Parvovirus antibodies can be very persistent in dogs and the final parvovirus vaccination used to be delayed until 16–18 weeks of age, to ensure that the puppy was fully vaccinated. However, owner compliance with this third vaccination was generally poor. Recently introduced vaccines are more immunogenic and can overcome higher levels of MDA, providing full protection earlier; thus parvovirus vaccination can also be completed at 12 weeks of age.

If an animal is vaccinated when its MDA levels are high it will not come to any harm but it will no longer be protected against that disease when its MDA level falls. In animals that are at high risk an extra vaccination may be given at an earlier age (6–7 weeks) to catch the few individuals in which there has been no MDAs or where MDAs have waned early. In some cases where there have been repeated problems with response to vaccination (e.g. Rottweilers and Dobermanns with parvovirus vaccine) a blood sample to measure the antibody response at the end of the vaccine course may be advised.

Suggested puppy vaccination regime
In the majority of situations an initial vaccine given at 6–8 weeks of age followed by a second injection at 12 weeks of age will provide solid immunity to puppies and kittens. The choice of which vaccines to give at 6–8 weeks will depend on the prevalence of the specific diseases in the local area.

All vaccine components should be given at 12 weeks of age. It is important to inform the client that full immunity is not reached until 7–10 days after the second injection; hence puppies and kittens should remain relatively isolated until they are over 13 weeks of age.

Bordetella vaccination is usually given prior to kennelling and not as a routine vaccination.

Suggested kitten vaccination regime

- Aged 9 weeks – feline herpesvirus and calicivirus ('cat 'flu') and feline enteritis +/– FeLV and *Chlamydia* vaccination
- Aged 12 weeks – feline herpesvirus and calicivirus ('cat 'flu') and feline enteritis +/– FeLV and *Chlamydia* if the kitten was vaccinated with these at 9 weeks old.

Intranasal feline herpes virus and calicivirus vaccine can be given from a few days of age (though this is not a data sheet recommendation). Vaccination is recommended at 9 and 12 weeks and may require a booster dose at 6-monthly intervals. Where there is a high risk of infection, intranasal vaccines have been given successfully to newborn kittens.

Storage of vaccines

In order for vaccination to be effective, it is important that vaccines are stored correctly

- Vaccines are damaged by warmth and freezing and should therefore be stored in the refrigerator at temperatures between +2°C and +8°C
- Time out of the fridge should be minimal
- Careful checks should be made to make sure that stored vaccines are not kept beyond their expiry dates, as they may lose their effectiveness.

Administration of vaccines

- A sterile needle should be used
- Chemically sterilized needles are unsuitable as they can reduce vaccine efficacy
- A disposable syringe should be used
- A spirit swab is contraindicated, as it can inactivate a live vaccine.

Vaccines are in the form of either a solution or a freeze-dried pellet. The pellet must be reconstituted with sterile water or with the liquid fraction of the vaccine, so that a multi-component vaccine can be given as a single injection. Once reconstituted, the vaccine should be stored in a fridge and used within a few hours.

- Subcutaneous injection can usually be performed with minimal restraint
- Owners should be warned that their animals may sneeze for a couple of days following administration of an intranasal vaccine.

Vaccination cards

Each vaccinated dog and cat should be issued with a certificate of vaccination. A note of the vaccination should also be kept on the animal's record card, so that a new certificate can be issued if the owner loses the old one.

Record cards are supplied by the vaccine manufacturers and usually have the practice name and address on them. It is very important that *all* details are filled in correctly, especially when groups of puppies or kittens are being vaccinated for a breeder.

Certificates will have to be produced by owners if their animals are going to stud, shows or boarding kennels.

Going to the cattery or kennels

Dogs and cats without a current vaccination certificate will be refused admission to many establishments. Preferably, vaccination should be completed a minimum of 2 weeks prior to kennelling. When time is short, rapid immunity can be produced using intranasal vaccination.

Adverse reactions to vaccination

Adverse reactions to vaccination (such as thrombocytopenia or anaphylaxis) are rare but minor reactions are common and are usually a reflection of the immune response to the vaccine or are caused by the adjuvant.

- Common reactions include small swellings at the site of injection (local reaction) which resolve spontaneously
- Some young animals are reported to be lethargic and depressed with a poor appetite for 24–48 hours following vaccination (generalized reaction)
- Reactions appear relatively more common following leukaemia and rabies vaccination
- Many cat breeders feel that pedigree cats are more prone to vaccine reactions than non-pedigree ones.

More serious vaccine reactions include allergic responses, usually to other components of the vaccine – i.e. small quantities of chemicals and antibiotics which act as preservatives. The reactions include generalized itching or swelling of the face. 'Blue-eye' used to be seen when live canine adenovirus 1 vaccine was used to provide protection against infectious canine hepatitis. This is now very rarely seen as most infectious canine hepatitis vaccines contain canine adenovirus 2 or dead canine adenovirus 1.

There is much current, and often ill informed, debate about the safety of vaccination, particularly with respect to booster vaccinations and long-term health issues. Whilst vaccination is not guaranteed or 100% safe, the benefits of vaccination outweigh the risks and it is easy to forget the severity of diseases like parvovirus or distemper in areas where, because of vaccination, the conditions are now very rare. The following should be considered when giving advice to clients:

- Vaccination should be carried out according to the manufacturer's data sheet instructions
- Vaccination of old animals should be encouraged as their immune system is less effective and, should they become infected, less able to mount an effective immune response
- Whilst dogs or cats living in more isolated areas are less likely to meet infectious disease, their immunity is likely to wane more rapidly than animals in more highly populated areas who are continually being exposed to low levels of infectious diseases which serve to stimulate their immune systems repeatedly. Hence, should an individual from an isolated area happen to meet an infectious disease they may be fully susceptible
- Over vaccination and repeatedly restarting a primary vaccination course should be avoided
- Suspected adverse reactions to vaccination should be reported to the Veterinary Medicines Directorate.

Failure to respond to vaccination

Vaccination can appear to fail for a variety of reasons (listed below) but in most cases it is not the vaccine that is at fault.

- Out-of-date vaccines
- Incorrect storage resulting in the vaccine becoming inactive
- Incorrect administration (e.g. needle passing all the way through the skin, resulting in vaccination of the fur)
- Persistence of MDAs for longer than anticipated (always determine the exact age at first vaccination)
- Animal already incubating the disease. Most animals are presented for first vaccination at the time that MDAs have waned and they are susceptible to disease; in some cases they have already become infected but are asymptomatic. Disease tends to develop very shortly after vaccination (within 2–3 days). Vaccination is unlikely to be harmful but is too late to provide protection
- Sick animals. Administration of vaccine to a sick animal is unlikely to be harmful but the animal may be unable to produce a normal antibody response to the vaccine. A thorough examination should always be performed on animals presented for vaccination
- Corticosteroids. These and other immunosuppressive agents will interfere with the immune response. Animals known to be on such treatment should not be vaccinated
- Stress (e.g. rehoming) can have a similar effect by increasing endogenous corticosteroid production
- Overwhelming infection. The incubation period of a disease is dependent on the virulence and infectious dose. If a vaccinated animal encounters high levels of virulent pathogen, it may not be able to raise a strong enough immune response within the incubation period. In such cases clinical signs will generally be less severe than those in unvaccinated animals
- Strain variation. For example, with feline calicivirus the vaccine protects against around 60% of FCV strains; hence a vaccinated animal will appear unprotected if it should meet a strain where there is no cross-protection from the vaccine strains
- Individual immune deficiency.

It should be noted that the combination of several vaccines given in one injection does not result in a lesser response to any one of them given separately.

Control of parasites

Veterinary nurses are frequently asked to give advice on the control of parasitic infections. They are expected to have a working knowledge of the antiparasitic preparations available, their action and effectiveness.

Parasites are organisms that exist for the whole or part of their life cycle on or in another organism, at its expense.

- An *ectoparasite* lives on the surface of the animal
- An *endoparasite* lives inside the animal.

Ectoparasites

Fleas (*Ctenocephalides felis*)

Fleas are the major ectoparasites of cats and dogs. In order to assist clients in preventing or controlling a flea problem, the nurse should understand the flea's life cycle (Figure 11.14).

This is essential to allow interpretation and explanation of the method of action of the different antiparasitic products that are effective against fleas. Emphasis should be placed on ensuring that the owner has realistic expectations of the effectiveness of the control regime. Encouragement should be given to ensure owner compliance.

Fleas cause problems both to the infected animal and as a zoonosis, i.e. they can be transmitted from animals to humans.

Problems in humans include:

- Bites when there is a household infestation
- Fleas acting as vectors of disease (e.g. cat scratch fever).

Problems in animals include:

- Pruritus, with possible self-trauma
- Development of an allergic dermatitis
- Anaemia in heavy infestations
- Transmission of intermediate stage of tapeworm *Dipylidium caninum*
- Transmission of disease (e.g. feline infectious anaemia, feline enteritis).

Some owners may request regular preventive treatment for fleas. This is relatively straightforward:

- Cats and dogs may pick up a few fleas from outside sources of infestation, mainly by contact with another flea-infested animal
- Prevention consists of ensuring that these few fleas do not breed and produce a household infestation.

A more detailed history should be taken if owners have actually seen fleas on their pet or are being bitten themselves. In assessing the requirement for flea treatment, the nurse must ensure that a veterinary consultation is not required.

An owner who clearly describes the parasite or evidence of flea dirt on their animal should be further questioned to ensure that there is no possibility of the animal having dermatitis or any other complication before considering the supply of any antiparasitic product.

Essential points that should be conveyed to owners requesting antiparasitic products include the following:

- Adult fleas are only 5% of the problem – the rest concerns immature stages (eggs, larvae, pupae), which are in the house
- These immature stages may remain in the house for up to a year before hatching
- Any product used will have very little effect on the pupae, which must hatch out before control is achieved
- Many non-veterinary products may not be fully effective.

If owners' expectations are not correctly met, they may later assume product failure. Only when the owner is aware of the constraints should a product or products be chosen.

Before suggesting a method of flea control (Figure 11.15), certain questions should be addressed:

- Is prevention or control of infestation required?
- Is there environmental contamination?
- Are there other animals in the house that will also require treatment?
- Is there evidence of tapeworm infestation (white segments seen as 'grains of rice' around the anus or on the faeces)?

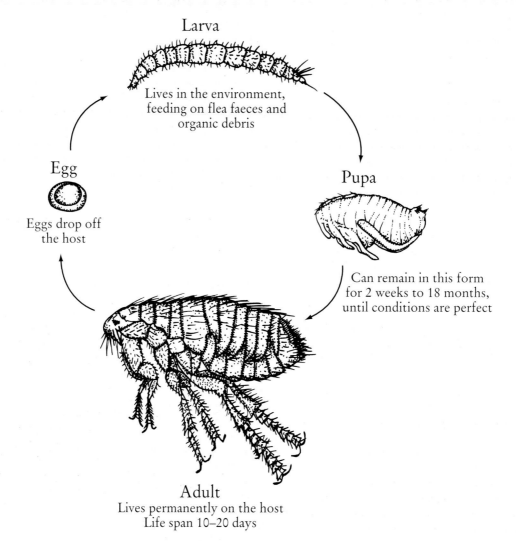

Larva
Lives in the environment,
feeding on flea faeces and
organic debris

Egg
Eggs drop off
the host

Pupa
Can remain in this form
for 2 weeks to 18 months,
until conditions are perfect

Adult
Lives permanently on the host
Life span 10–20 days

11.15 Common flea control products and their properties

Product	Effective against	Method of application
Lufenuron	Eggs, larvae	Oral, injection
Fipronil	Adults	Spot on, spray
Imidacloprid	Adults	Spot on
Insect growth regulators e.g. methoprene, cyromazine, pyriproxifen	Larvae	Environmental spray
Fenitrothion, dichlorvos	Adults	Spray
Pyrethrin compounds	Adults	Shampoos, foams

- Is the suggested product suitable for that particular client? For example, an elderly arthritic owner with a Jack Russell terrier will have difficulties applying some products at home.

  The choice of product should relate to level of infestation and the type of problem.

- Owners requesting flea prevention should be given comprehensive advice. Considerable discussion may be required in selecting the most convenient product to ensure adequate protection
- Owners whose animals have a moderate infestation should be advised:

  – To use a product on the animal to get rid of the adult fleas
  – To treat the environment so that the immature stages are prevented from developing and prolonging the problem

- In the case of severe infestation, owners will need substantial support and will require a mixture of products to ensure total cover. In addition they should:
  – Use a vacuum cleaner daily, applying an environmental spray to the bag of the cleaner to prevent the development of fleas within the bag
  – Wash animal bedding regularly.

Other ectoparasites

Figure 11.16 shows some of the more common ectoparasites (other than fleas) and methods of control. Details of these species are outlined below. Essential points that should be borne in mind when advising owners requesting antiparasitic products include the following:

- The correct product for the parasite present should be selected
- The correct method of application should be described
- The owners needs to be aware that some parasites (e.g. *Sarcoptes scabiei*, *Demodex canis*) may be very difficult to control
- Prevention of reinfestation may be necessary (e.g. ticks).

Ticks

The most common tick acquired by cats and dogs is the sheep tick, *Ixodes ricinus*. Both the nymph and adult forms can be found on animals. They are acquired whilst walking in fields of cattle or sheep, or in areas with high populations of wildlife; as a potential host passes by, ticks jump on to them from grass.

Most owners dislike seeing ticks on their animals. The parasites are quite large and tend to leave blood stains on the owner's carpet if left to fall from the host naturally.

Tick problems in animals include:

- Direct irritation
- Difficulty in removal (if the head is left *in situ*, an abscess may develop)
- Transmission of disease (e.g. tick pyraemia, Lyme disease, ehrlichiosis).

Lice

These parasites spend their whole life cycle on the cat or dog. They are not zoonotic and they are host specific. Transmission is directly from dog to dog (or cat to cat), which means that this problem is often encountered with kennelled dogs and puppies. Environmental hygiene is important in controlling and preventing lice.

Both biting and sucking lice may be found. The preferred site of this parasite is behind the ears and in warm areas of the body. Sucking lice (*Lignognathus* spp.) are often diagnosed by the presence of 'nits' (louse eggs) attached to hairs.

Louse problems in animals include:

- Excessive scratching
- Possible anaemia in severe infestations.

Lice may be visible during a routine check. Confirmation can be made under the microscope and owners are usually impressed when shown their animal's parasites.

Cheyletiella spp.

These mites are known as 'walking dandruff', which immediately describes the way in which they are identified. If in any doubt, a piece of sticky tape will pick up the mites (see Chapter 5). Infestation is commonly seen in longhaired cats and puppies.

Cheyletiella problems include:

- Zoonotic infection of in-contact humans
- Pruritus in some animals.

There are no licensed products for use against *Cheyletiella* mites. Since spread is by direct contact, environmental hygiene is important.

Demodex canis (demodectic mange)

Demodectic mange is diagnosed by a skin scraping in animals with pruritus and alopecia (see Chapter 5). These mites are normal inhabitants of the skin in small numbers. They live in the hair follicles and transfer from the mother to her puppies when suckling. In disease they multiply dramatically. *Demodex cati* is the very rare feline form.

Sarcoptes scabiei (canine scabies)

These burrowing mites cause extreme pruritus. The mite is identified in skin scrapings (see Chapter 5). The mites live on the surface and lay their eggs in the skin; the larvae burrow out. Sarcoptic mange is a zoonosis; there is a need for careful advice to be given on the handling and treatment of infected animals.

Endoparasites

The most common endoparasites in dogs and cats are roundworms and tapeworms, different species of which are discussed below.

Most dogs and cats do not suffer true disease from worm infestation unless they have a very heavy worm burden, when they may suffer from ill thrift. Regular routine prophylactic treatment is recommended to rid the animal of any possible infestation. It is also important to be aware that there may be a risk of zoonosis.

11.16 Other ectoparasites and their control

Ectoparasite	Life cycle features	Possible products
Ticks	Main host sheep, deer etc. Picked up outside	Fipronil, pyrethroids
Lice	Transmitted between dogs, common in puppies and kennels	Pyrethroids
Cheyletiella	'Walking dandruff', spread between dogs	Nothing licensed
Demodectic mange mites	Indigenous in dogs, common in pups, usually don't cause disease	Amitraz
Sarcoptic mange mites	Often spread via foxes	Amitraz

Essential questions to be considered before appropriate control of endoparasites (Figure 11.17) is suggested include the following.

- Is prevention required (routine anthelmintic treatment)?
- Is control of infestation required?
- Is this a young animal that has been infected from its mother?
- Is there evidence of tapeworm infestation (white segments seen as 'grains of rice' around the anus or on the faeces)?
- Is environmental contamination or hunting likely to be a source of tapeworm infection?
- Is there evidence of flea infestation which may lead to tapeworm infestation?

- Are there other animals in the house which will also require treatment?

Toxocara canis and *T. cati* roundworms

The most common endoparasites are the roundworms *Toxocara canis* in the dog (Figures 11.18 and 11.19) and *Toxocara cati* in the cat. These are most important in young puppies and kittens and should be discussed in any first consultation or when advice is given to a new owner. *T. canis* is passed out in a dog's faeces and can cause illness or blindness if a person is infected. Children are most at risk as they are more likely to come into contact with animal faeces or to play in an environment contaminated by faeces.

11.17 Endoparasites and their control

Product	*Toxocara canis*	*Toxocara cati*	*Uncinaria*	*Trichuris*	*Dipylidium caninum*	*Echinococcus granulosus*	*Taenia* spp.
Pyrantel + praziquantel +febantel	✓	✓	✓	✓	✓	✓	✓
Pyrantel, praziquantel	✓	✓	✓	✓	✓	✓	✓
Fenbendazole	✓	✓	✓	✓	✗	✗	✓
Piperazine	✓	✓	✓	✓	✗	✗	✗
Nitroscanate	✓	✓	✓	✓	✓	✗	✓

11.18 *Toxocara canis* in puppies

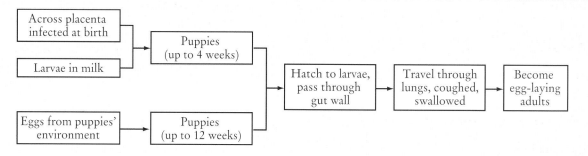

11.19 *Toxocara canis* in adult dogs

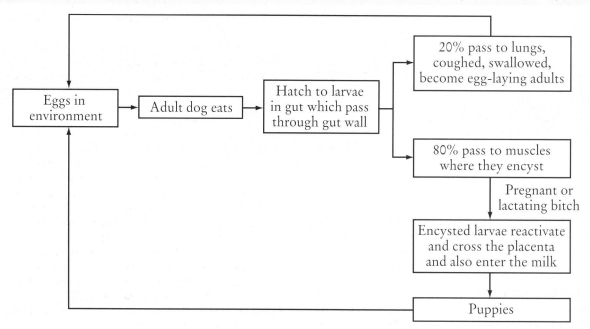

Essential facts that must be conveyed to dog owners requesting anthelmintic products include the following.

- Puppies can be born with *T. canis* passed to them from the mother in the womb
- Further infection can occur in puppies through milk
- The worms move into the lungs, are coughed up and swallowed; they then produce egg-laying adults until the puppy is about 14–16 weeks old
- All puppies, regardless of which anthelmintic product is used, should be wormed at 2, 4, 6, 8, 10, 12 and then 16 weeks of age. This regime is designed both to decrease environmental contamination and to prevent build-up of *Toxocara* numbers in puppies
- After 16 weeks, dogs should be routinely wormed two to four times a year
- More frequent treatment is required in pregnant bitches to reduce the level of infestation in their offspring
- *T. canis* infection is zoonotic.

The *Toxocara cati* life cycle is essentially the same, but there is no transplacental transmission. Essential facts that must be conveyed to cat owners requesting anthelmintic products include the following.

- Kittens become infected through their mother's milk
- All kittens, regardless of which anthelmintic product is used, should be wormed at 5, 7, 9, 11 and 13 weeks of age (as there is no placental transmission, a later start can be made in kittens)
- After 13 weeks cats should be routinely wormed two to four times a year
- There is less risk of zoonosis, as cats bury their faeces.

The nurse must emphasize that all anthelmintics kill only the worms present in the animal at the time of administration. Therefore their effect is transient and depends on the potential for reinfestation and the immune status of the animal.

Other roundworms

Other roundworms of some importance in the dog, especially in kennelled animals such as greyhounds, include *Uncinaria stenocephala* (hookworm) and *Trichuris vulpis* (whipworm).

- Hookworm infection occurs after ingestion of infective larvae or by larvae penetrating the skin; it can cause skin reactions and mild anaemia
- Whipworm infection is by ingestion of the infective larvae; it can cause diarrhoea.

Some anthelmintics are not effective against these parasites. When either species is suspected, faecal sampling should be undertaken to provide a definitive diagnosis so that the correct treatment can be prescribed.

Tapeworms

Tapeworms are segmented parasites, flat in cross-section, and require an intermediate host in which to undergo a stage of their development before being ingested by the dog or cat. Infection is therefore by ingesting all or part of the intermediate host.

Dipylidium caninum

Dipylidium caninum is the most common tapeworm of cats and dogs. Its intermediate host is the flea and this fact should

be explained to the owner of an animal infected with either *D. caninum* or fleas: even if the infected animal is wormed, tapeworms may return unless the flea infestation has been controlled. Flea larvae eat tapeworm eggs. Adult fleas ingested by the dog or cat then release the immature stage which then develops to the adult in the gut. The tapeworm's life cycle can be completed in as little as 3 weeks, so infection can recur very quickly if fleas are not controlled.

Taenia spp.

The intermediate hosts of several *Taenia* spp. are either large ruminants (e.g. sheep, cattle) or small rodents (e.g. mice, voles). *Taenia* infestation is therefore more common in farm dogs and hunting cats, where infection occurs due to ingestion of carcasses or prey.

Echinococcus granulosus

Echinococcus granulosus occurs in only certain parts of the UK, such as Wales and some parts of Scotland. It is fairly uncommon but extremely important as it is a serious zoonosis. An infected egg ingested by a human will develop into a hydatid cyst. This can cause severe disease, depending on where in the body it is situated, and it requires surgical removal.

- The normal intermediate host for *E. granulosus* is the sheep; therefore, the proper disposal of sheep carcasses is an important control measure
- Regular worming with an appropriate product should be undertaken in at-risk areas
- The local office of the Ministry of Agriculture can identify areas where *E. granulosus* is a problem
- If a dog has no access to sheep carcasses or hillside areas, it is very unlikely to become infected.

The role of diet in the treatment of disease

Nutrition is vital to life. It is becoming increasingly clear how important good nutrition is and the far-reaching effects it can have on the long-term health and well-being of pets.

Figure 11.20 summarizes the types of diet available for a healthy animal.

The body is able to store a surplus of many nutrients so that it can function normally during short periods of starvation or nutrient deficiency. In the long term, adequate nutrition is essential for formation of the body structure, the provision of energy, the transportation of substances around the body, metabolism, homeostasis and the normal functioning of the immune system.

As an animal grows, develops and then ages, its nutritional requirements will change. Similarly the demands for the various major dietary components will vary with activity and, in females, reproductive status: non-pregnant, pregnant or lactating (Figure 11.21). Maintenance energy requirements will also vary with life stage and activity (Figure 11.22).

At each stage of life therefore, energy requirements must be calculated. The following formulae are assumed when calculating the energy requirements in the examples below. It must be remembered that each case should be assessed as an individual and that figures calculated using standard formulae are a guide rather than absolute.

11.20 Types of diet

Diet type	Features
Complete	Formulated to meet all the dietary needs for that group of animals. Some diets are complete for all life stages whilst others will only be complete for one life stage, e.g. maintenance
Complementary	Unsuitable as a single source of food as they lack one or more essential dietary component and are not necessarily balanced in terms of vitamins and minerals. May be intended to be fed with another diet component to produce a complete diet or as a minor dietary component as a treat or to add textural variety
Moist foods	Contain a high water content, usually 70–80%. Tend to be meat based. Preserved by heat sterilization, vacuum packing or freezing. Tend to be highly digestible and palatable. Energy content is generally low so a large volume needs to be fed, with a tendency towards protein excess
Semi-moist foods	Contain a moderate water content (15–30%) with a shelf life of several months. Preservation is achieved by the use of humectants (sugar, salt or glycerol which bind water), mould inhibitors and low pH. Can be made from a variety of products and have a fairly high nutrient density, digestibility and palatability Propylene glycol used as a preservative in some semi-moist foods can be toxic to cats.
Dry foods	Contain a low water content (around 10%). Preservation is achieved by drying, storage life is short. Many are complementary foods, such as mixer biscuits containing high levels of cereal. Nutrient density is high with lower digestibility than moist or semi-moist diets. Palatability is very variable. Animals, particularly cats fed dry food, may be at greater risk of developing urolithiasis, depending on the formulation used

11.21 Life stage nutrition

Life stage/activity	Advice to clients
Growth	*Pre-weaning* Ideally the bitch's or queen's milk, if this is not possible then fostering is the next best approach. If kittens or puppies are to be hand reared then a proprietary milk substitute is required in the long term as both cow's and goat's milk give inadequate levels of nutrients. *Post-weaning* Most puppies attain 50% of their adult weight by 5-6 months, but maximal growth does not mean optimal growth. The energy demands of a growing puppy are high and need to be met by frequent meals to enable the necessary volume to be consumed (e.g. a 20 kg, 12-week-old puppy needs about 2.5 kg of wet food per day). Puppy feeds need to be energy dense, and highly digestible, with a suitable amount and balance of vitamins and minerals, particularly calcium and phosphorus. Kittens, unlike puppies, are better fed *ad libitum*. Energy requirements/kg peak at about 10 weeks of age but tend to be lower than those of puppies, as the percentage increases over birth weights are smaller, though they achieve a higher percentage of adult weight (75%) by 6 months of age.
Maintenance	There are few requirements for maintenance except a balanced diet. Cats and small dogs have achieved adult requirements by 12 months of age, medium-sized dogs mature at around 15–18 months and giant breeds 18–24 months. In the majority of dogs, overfeeding (causing obesity) is the major concern. Owners should be encouraged to weigh their pets regularly and restrict their food as necessary or use a less energy-dense product.
Gestation (pregnancy)	Most fetal weight gain occurs in the last 3 weeks of canine pregnancy. To this point little extra feeding is required. A palatable balanced maintenance diet is suitable, fed at normal rates. From the fifth week onwards, the ration should be increased by 15% per week. In late pregnancy, feeding small meals of higher density diets may be required due to the reduced space available in the abdomen for the stomach to expand. Cats tend to require a steady increase in food intake from conception. As they rarely overeat, *ad lib* feeding can occur. Alternatively a 4–5% increase in ration can be given weekly.
Lactation	This is the biggest nutritional test of a bitch or queen. Energy requirements depend on litter size, with the maximum demand occurring 4 weeks after the litter is born. Small meals of highly palatable, highly digestible food are required for bitches; *ad lib* feeding of queens is recommended. Supplementation of vitamins and minerals is not necessary if a balanced diet is used. In general it is necessary to feed a diet that is more tightly formulated than for maintenance, preferably one specifically designed for lactation (increased energy density).

Figure 11.21 continues ▶

Life stage/activity	Advice to clients
Activity	Few dogs, despite many owners' beliefs, are truly active. A 5 km run will increase a dog's daily requirements by around 10%. Maximum demand occurs in dogs travelling long distances in cold conditions, where they may have an energy requirement of 4–5 times maintenance. Diets should meet the needs for muscular work and stress. For short-burst athletic dogs such as greyhounds, increased carbohydrates are required; for sustained effort, particularly at low temperatures, energy needs are best met through high-fat, low-carbohydrate diets. There is no evidence that an increase in dietary protein is required. It has been suggested that working dogs may have a higher requirement for iron, vitamin E and selenium. Generally working dogs need a highly palatable, energy-dense, highly digestible and nutritionally balanced diet.
Old age	The requirements for ageing cats and dogs are poorly defined. Intestinal function starts to decline from around 8 years of age. It is general felt that lower nutritional density is desirable. Energy demands also decrease, due to reduced levels of activity and a lower lean body mass. The requirement for vitamins, particularly water soluble (B and C) vitamins, may be increased, due to increased water turnover. A decrease in energy requirement and nutrient density needs to be balanced against the tendency to poorer appetite. A compromise of a highly palatable diet with mildly reduced nutrient density and increased vitamin levels is currently recommended. Increasing the number of feeds per day is also desirable.

11.22 Estimated energy requirements in healthy cats and dogs in various physiological states

Physiological state	Dog (x MER)	Cat (kcal/kg body weight)
< 3 months (growth)	2	250
3–6 months (growth)	1.5	130
6–12 months	1.2	80–100
Inactive adult	0.75	70
Active	1	80
Working 1 hour/day	1.1	N/A
Working full day (mild–moderate work)	1.5–2	N/A
Gestation (<42 days)	1–1.1	88
Gestation (> 42 days)	1.1–1.3	88–104
Peak lactation (3–6 weeks)	1 + (0.25 x number of puppies)	80 x [1 + (0.25 x number of kittens)]
Cold weather (pet outside)	1.25–1.75	na

N/A, not applicable; na, figures not available

As a metabolic by-product of cellular processes, 10–16 g of water are produced for every 100 kcal of energy metabolized. The examples below have used a mid-range figure of 13 g/100 kcal.

Resting energy requirement (RER) – this is the basic energy expended by an animal at rest in a thermoneutral environment

RER (kcal) = 70 x (body weight in kg)$^{0.75}$

For animals weighing between 2 and 48 kg then this approximates to

RER (kcal) = 30 x (body weight in kg) + 70

Maintenance energy requirement (MER) – this is the amount of energy that is used by an active animal in a thermoneutral environment. This does not include the energy required for growth, pregnancy, lactation or heavy work. A variety of ways of calculating MER have been suggested:

Dogs
MER (kcal/day) = 1.8 x RER
= 132 (body weight in kg)$^{0.75}$
= 1500 x body surface area (m^2)

Cats
MER (kcal/day) = 70 x body weight in kg

Dietary deficiency and toxicity

Dietary deficiencies and toxicities sufficient to cause clinically significant disease are generally rare and usually associated with neglect or an owner feeding a home-prepared diet. Disease states, usually of the intestinal system, can lead to deficiencies in some or all dietary components. Diseases that cause malnutrition and weight loss can be grouped into one of four headings:

- Lack of nutrient intake (inappetence or dysphagia)
- Lack of nutrient absorption (vomiting, diarrhoea, small intestinal disease, exocrine pancreatic insufficiency)
- Cachectic states (increased nutrient demand in animals with a variety of diseases such as neoplasia, congestive heart failure or hyperthyroidism)
- Excessive nutrient loss, e.g. protein-losing nephropathy, diabetes mellitus (glucose lost in urine), protein-losing enteropathy.

A few breed-associated vitamin and mineral deficiencies have been reported and are thought to be associated with specific carrier molecule deficits (e.g. zinc deficiency in Alaskan Malamutes) or renal tubular dysfunction (e.g. Fanconi syndrome).

The fact that a nutrient is essential does not mean that it cannot be toxic in excess. If a little is good, a whole lot can be very dangerous; for example, an excess of vitamin A or D can become toxic. Dietary deficiency can occur due to a lack of a particular nutrient in certain diets. For example:

- Skeletal muscle (meat) is deficient in calcium, riboflavin, vitamin A, iodine and copper
- Cereals are deficient in calcium, taurine, riboflavin, niacin and fat.

Dietary imbalance can occur when an excess of one nutrient prevents the absorption of another:

- Nutrients are bound so that they are no longer available for digestion; for example:
  - fat-soluble vitamins (A, D and E) bound to mineral oil used as a laxative
  - egg white (avidin) binds biotin (B vitamin)
  - phytates in plants bind iron, copper and zinc
- Nutrients may compete for carriers, particularly divalent ions
- Free nutrients may bind with other components when combined in the gastrointestinal tract; for example, aluminium hydroxide can be used to lower the available phosphate content of a diet as it binds the phosphate to form an insoluble salt
- Animals can be more or less sensitive to dietary imbalances, depending on their breed and the state of development; for example, large-breed dogs are particularly sensitive to imbalances of calcium, phosphorus, magnesium and fluorine during skeletal development as puppies.

The manifestations of common dietary deficiencies or excesses are shown in Figure 11.23.

11.23 Manifestations of common dietary deficiencies or excesses

Nutrient	Causes and consequences of deficiency	Causes and consequences of excess
Protein	Rare, as low protein diets are unpalatable. Most serious in growing animals which are undergrown with poor joint cartilage and bone mineralization. In adult animals, protein malnutrition is reflected in a dull coat, skin lesions, lethargy and hypoproteinaemia	None in healthy animals. There is no evidence to link the feeding of high protein diets to dogs or cats with normal kidney function to the onset of renal disease
Carbohydrate	None as long as energy requirements are met by fats and proteins	Digestive disorders (e.g. lactose intolerance). If the capacity for carbohydrate digestion is exceeded then the excess is fermented by bacteria in the large bowel, producing fatty acids and lactate resulting in an acidic osmotic diarrhoea. Carbohydrates are poorly tolerated in animals needing high energy diets (e.g. lactation, work) and by puppies/kittens who have low amylase activity
Fat	Sufficient energy levels can rarely be provided by a fat-deficient diet, hence the animal will lose weight Essential fatty acid deficiencies include hair loss, fatty liver degeneration, anaemia, infertility	Obesity
Taurine	CATS ONLY: deficiencies can lead to blindness, dilated cardiomyopathy, reproductive failure and developmental abnormalities in kittens. Deficiency is seen in cats fed dog food or vegetarian food	None known
Calcium and phosphorus	Highest requirements in young fast-growing dogs. Ratio is as important as absolute amounts and should be between 0.9:1 (cats), 1:1 (dogs) and 2:1 *Nutritional secondary hyperparathyroidism* – usually seen in animals fed all-meat diets (calcium deficient) and results in the reabsorption of bone. Affected animals have problems walking and in severe cases standing; there is pain on palpation. Ghost-like bones and pathological fractures can be seen on radiography *Eclampsia* – occurs at whelping (large breeds) and mid lactation (small breeds) and is seen as muscle twitching and tremor. Can occur in animals fed too little or too much calcium	Excess is usually only a problem in young rapidly growing dogs and is seen as skeletal abnormalities In adults, particularly cats, there may be an increased risk of calcium oxalate crystalluria or uroliths Eclampsia
Potassium	Seen mainly in cats fed on low-potassium vegetarian diets. Affected cats are intially stiff and have poor hair coat; this progresses to weakness and an inability to raise the head. Renal failure has been reported in cats fed high-protein acidifying diets, which require higher levels of potassium supplementation	None known

Figure 11.23 continues ▶

Nutrient	Causes and consequences of deficiency	Causes and consequences of excess
Magnesium	Usually occurs in animals fed a poorly formulated 'struvite prevention' diet. Causes depression and muscle weakness	Increased risk of struvite urolithiasis, especially if water turnover is low
Iron	Seen in puppies and kittens fed inappropriate milk substitutes. Causes a non-regenerative anaemia	May impair the availability of other elements. Excessive supplementation tends to cause vomiting
Copper	Puppies and kittens fed home-cooked diets based on milk, milk products and eggs Excessive zinc supplementation Causes anaemia, depigmentation of hair and skeletal disorders	Chronic toxicity not reported
Zinc	Poor bioavailability due to high calcium levels or diets based on soybean or cereals Causes parakeratosis (scaly skin) and depigmentation of hair	Rare, secondary to ingestion of zinc-containing coins Causes vomiting, weight loss, anaemia and anorexia
Iodine	Animals fed meat or cereals produced in iodine-deficient areas. Cooking also reduces iodine Causes enlargement of thyroid gland (goitre), lethargy, alopecia, disorders of growth and fertility, weight loss and oedema	None reported. Cyclical high and low iodine-containing diets have been suggested as a cause of hyperthyroidism in cats
Thiamin	As there are poor body reserves, deficiency can occur quickly. Most commonly seen in cats fed high levels of uncooked fish (which contain thiaminase), cats and dogs fed uncooked meat preserved with sulphur dioxide, or poorly formulated cooked diets where the thiamine is destroyed by heating and not replaced In young animals, causes poor growth progressing to weight loss, neurological signs and death. Neurological signs seen in cats include abnormal posture, neck weakness, ataxia and seizures	Not reported
Niacin/tryptophan	Dogs fed corn-based diets Causes severe tongue (black tongue) and buccal ulceration, drooling saliva and halitosis	Not reported
Biotin	Excessive feeding of raw eggs where the avidin binds biotin produced by intestinal microorganisms, particularly in combination with oral antibiotics Causes dry scurfy skin, alopecia and dried secretions around the nose, mouth and feet	Not reported
Vitamin A	Dogs fed cereal or offal-based diets or cats fed vegetarian diets Causes skin and eye lesions, increased susceptibility and poor response to infection, problems with bone development and reproduction	Cats or dogs oversupplemented with cod liver oil or cats fed predominantly liver-based diets Causes weakness, anorexia, pain, lameness and stiffness associated with bony hyperplasia, particularly affecting the neck (in cats) Changes are not reversible if the diet is discontinued, although some improvement in clinical signs occurs with time
Vitamin D	Rarely seen Causes ricketts and osteomalacia	Usually associated with oversupplementation (vitamin D is also used as a rodenticide) Causes calcification of the soft tissues, including the skin, and can lead to organ failure (e.g. of the kidneys)
Vitamin E	Deficiency is usually relative where high fat (dry) diets have become rancid or in cats fed diets based predominantly on fish, particularly tuna Causes steatitis (inflammation of the fat) associated with lethargy, fever, pain and palpable subcutaneous masses	Not reported

The role of diet in the treatment of disease

A major focus for nutrition in veterinary practice has become the value of dietary modification in the treatment of disease in cats and dogs. In some cases dietary change can lead to a resolution of clinical signs (e.g. dietary allergy, struvite urolithiasis) whilst in others it can reduce the requirements for potentially toxic drugs (e.g. inflammatory bowel disease) or improve the quality of an animal's life (e.g. chronic renal failure).

The major roles for diet in the treatment of disease in cats and dogs are outlined in Figure 11.24. It is important to remember that any changes in diet should be made slowly over a number of days to allow the animal to become used to the new flavours, textures and nutrient content.

11.24 Dietary therapy in small animal disease

Condition	Suspected cause	Dietary requirements
Gastrointestinal disease	Non-specific vomiting and diarrhoea	Dietary rest followed by frequent small meals of a highly digestible low-residue diet
	Dietary allergy	Feed a single, novel source of protein (hypoallergenic[a]) and avoid gluten and lactose. The diet should be highly digestible
	Dietary intolerance	Avoid that component of the diet (e.g. lactose or gluten)
	Exocrine pancreatic insufficiency	Highly digestible and palatable diet with restricted fat and moderate levels of high quality protein
	Pancreatitis	Highly digestible diet with restricted fat and moderate levels of high quality protein
	Small intestinal bacterial overgrowth	Highly digestible diet with restricted fat and moderate levels of high quality protein
	Motility disorders	Low fat and low fibre diets promote gastric emptying
	Gastric dilation–volvulus (dogs)	None of the surveys into the influence of diet on the occurrence and recurrence of GDV has established a clear link with diet type. However, it is generally recommended that high-risk dogs (deep chested) are fed three times daily with a highly digestible wet diet
	Inflammatory bowel disease	Diets similar to those used for dietary allergy are recommended, as an allergic component to the disease has been postulated. A 'sacrifice' diet can be used. A new diet is introduced whilst the intestinal inflammation is being controlled, during which time it is possible that the animal will become intolerant to the new diet. Once the inflammation is controlled, a second novel protein diet is introduced for long-term management
	Colitis	Two approaches to dietary management are taken: 1. Initially low-residue, single-source protein diets used in cases of dietary allergy are preferred 2. Long-term management can use the same diet but some animals are better managed on a diet containing increased levels of soluble and insoluble fibre, vitamins and minerals, and restricted fat
	Constipation	Increased faecal water content can be achieved by using high fibre diets with increased levels of vitamins and minerals
Obesity	Overfeeding and lack of exercise	Restriction of calories to 40–60% of calculated maintenance requirements is aimed at producing weight loss of around 1% per week in dogs. Calorie intake of less than 60% MER should be avoided in cats, due to risk of hepatic lipidosis. Levels of protein, essential fatty acids, minerals and vitamins should be balanced to a low energy density diet of high palatability
Liver disease	Chronic liver failure or portosystemic shunt (dogs)	Diets should be designed to meet protein requirements of an inappetent animal whilst slowing the post-prandial rise in nitrogenous waste. This can be achieved using moderate levels of high quality protein. High energy density from non-protein, mainly highly digestible carbohydrate. Increased zinc, B-complex and vitamin E levels, restricted copper. Moderate fat restriction and increased fibre
	Chronic liver failure or portosystemic shunt (cats)	High palatability with moderate protein restriction which ensures adequate levels of arginine, taurine and B vitamins
	Hepatic lipidosis (cats)	Feeding is essential and may require a naso-oesophageal or gastrostomy tube. Suitable diets which can be fed via a tube need to contain adequate energy levels to prevent further mobilization of body fat and adequate high quality protein
Kidney disease	Chronic renal failure	Uraemic cats and dogs are often inappetent, hence high palatability is important – eating something is better than catabolizing further body protein. Restricted phosphorus with medium levels of high quality protein is sufficient in the majority of cases. High energy density from non-protein sources. Moderate sodium restriction and increased B-complex vitamins. Potassium levels increased for cats

Figure 11.24 continues ▶

Condition	Suspected cause	Dietary requirements
Lower urinary tract disease	Idiopathic cystitis (cats)	Diets that encourage a high water turnover (i.e. tinned food) and a urine pH between 6.0 and 6.5
	Struvite urolithiasis	Reduce magnesium (< 20 mg/100 kcal diet), ammonium and phosphate (ash < 3%). Preferably an energy-dense diet with protein levels moderately restricted designed to produce acidic urine (high cation:anion ratio, increased sulphur amino acids) in high volume
	Ammonium urate, sodium acid urate, uric acid urolithiasis	Diet designed to produce an alkaline urine (pH > 7) which is moderately protein restricted can lead to calculolysis
	Cystine urolithiasis	Low-protein urine-alkalizing diet; long-term dietary management usually necessary
	Calcium oxalate urolithiasis	Surgical removal then avoid diets high in salt, protein and calcium and with low or high levels of phosphorus
Cardiovascular disease	Cardiomyopathy	Feline taurine-deficient dilated cardiomyopathy cases should be treated with taurine supplementation and feeding a balanced diet. L-Carnitine (synthesized from lysin and methionine) may be of value in treating canine dilated cardiomyopathy
	Congestive heart failure	Many dogs and cats with congestive heart failure have poor appetites and weight loss (cardiac cachexia). Diets that are highly palatable, highly digestible, moderately restricted, high quality protein and of moderate nutrient density are desirable. The value of salt restriction is less clear but is generally felt to be beneficial. Current recommendations suggest 0.1–0.3% on a dry matter basis for dogs and 0.4% for cats. Magnesium supplementation and potassium supplementation or restriction may also be helpful, depending on serum levels
	Hypertension	There may be some value in feeding diets with a high omega-3 PUFA content
Endocrine disease	Diabetes mellitus in dogs	Ideally feed a diet high in complex carbohydrates, no simple sugars, restricted fat and moderate protein. Dietary fibre has been shown to reduce the rate of digestion and absorption of carbohydrates following feeding and therefore decrease post-prandial hyperglycaemia. Diets formulated to the above criteria tend to have lower palatability; in some cases better diabetic control is achieved by feeding a diet that the dog will eat consistently. Feeding should occur at specified times and the same amount and type of food be given each day. Obesity increases insulin resistance so weight loss in obese animals is important
	Diabetes mellitus in cats	Cats tolerate high-fibre high-carbohydrate diets poorly as well as being able to supplement their intake by catching prey or getting fed next door. There is no clear evidence for a particular dietary type in cats, though semi-moist foods should be avoided. The aim should be for dietary consistency in terms of amounts and times. Weight reduction in obese animals is also important
Skeletal disease	Protein–calorie malnutrition or excess	Feed a palatable, balanced, highly digestible high-density diet
	Vitamin/mineral deficiency or excess	Feed a palatable, balanced, highly digestible high-density diet
	Renal osteodystrophy	Treat as for chronic renal failure
	Hip dysplasia and osteoarthritis	If animal is overweight then treat as for obesity
Skin disease	Protein–calorie malnutrition	Feed a palatable, balanced, highly digestible high-density diet
	Vitamin/mineral deficiency or excess	Feed a palatable, balanced, highly digestible high-density diet
	Manifestation of systemic organ failure	See relevant treatment above
	Dietary allergy	Feed an exclusion single-source protein diet for a minimum of 8 weeks

a *The term 'hypoallergenic' when used to describe a single-source novel protein is misleading. The proteins used are suitable because of their novelty but are not innately less allergenic than the animal's current diet.*

There is a tendency for 'prescription' diets to be less palatable, due to restriction of protein and salt content. Whilst a particular diet type may be desirable, it is of no value if the patient refuses to eat it. In some disease states (e.g. chronic renal failure) it is more important that the animal eats something rather than what it eats. Acceptance can be improved by slow introduction and warming of the new diet.

The majority of prescription diets are formulated such that they will provide adequate nutrition for a normal adult dog or cat. However, a significant number are inappropriate for feeding at certain life stages; for example, low protein diets are unsuitable for rapidly growing puppies. It is important, therefore, to consider not only the disease process that is being treated but the life stage and activity of the animal concerned when making a suitable dietary choice.

Dietary choices for cats are fewer and the modifications that have been made are less profound, this has occurred for a number of reasons:

- In general, less is known about the dietary needs of cats in different disease states
- Cats have an higher absolute requirement for protein
- Cats have significantly lower pancreatic amylase activity and therefore can not tolerate high carbohydrate diets, thus limiting the extent to which fats can be restricted in a diet
- Cats are generally less 'food driven' than dogs, hence low palatability diets are poorly accepted e.g. high fibre products.

Management of obesity

Many practices have instituted obesity clinics as a central component in the management of the overweight pet population.

Obesity

Obesity is the most common nutritional disease of dogs and cats. Estimates vary but it is generally accepted that between 25 and 44% of dogs and 10–40% of cats are overweight. In man obesity is defined as a person who is greater than 10–20% above their ideal weight. Less data exist about ideal weight for dogs and cats, even for pedigree animals. For the purposes of this discussion, obesity is defined as an animal's being overweight to the point that there is a significant risk of developing weight-related health problems. Practically, this will be animals who have a significant fat layer covering their ribs and dorsal spinous processes and whose waist and abdominal tuck is being lost.

Traditionally cats are thought to be less likely to suffer from obesity as they 'regulate' their energy intake better than dogs. The validity of this argument is questionable and obesity in cats is a growing problem, probably related to the increase in indoor living (and therefore lack of exercise) and *ad libitum* access to highly palatable energy-dense dry diets. Increased exercise as part of a diet programme should be strongly encouraged as it has two major advantages:

- Increased caloric demand
- Increased metabolic rate.

As with most disease problems, prevention is better than cure and good dietary advice given to new kitten and puppy owners is the point at which the management of obesity should begin. This is particularly important in those breeds of dog that are susceptible to obesity (Figure 11.25).

11.25 Breed susceptibility to obesity

Breeds most likely to become obese	Breeds least likely to become obese
Labrador Retriever	German Shepherd Dog
Cain Terrier	Greyhound
Shetland Sheepdog	Yorkshire Terrier
Basset Hound	Dobermann
Cavalier King Charles Spaniel	Staffordshire Bull Terrier
	Lurcher
Beagle	Whippet

A variety of disease risks have been suggested to be associated with obesity; however, only circulatory disease and articular/locomotor problems have been clearly linked to obesity and then only to dogs that are grossly obese. Other disease considerations should include: fatty change in the liver (and an increase risk of developing hepatic lipidosis in cats); respiratory embarrassment; increased surgical problems (anaesthetic risk, surgical access, slow wound healing, increased risk of wound infection); problems with parturition; poorer immune response; heat intolerance; urinary incontinence; and increased risk of diabetes mellitus.

Management

It is not sufficient to tell an owner that their animal is obese, as nearly all owners are fully aware of the problem. Practical advice and, most importantly, long-term support needs to be given. Owners easily become despondent and give up trying to control their pet's weight which is frequently associated with unrealistic expectations and a lack of support. It must be emphasized at the beginning of a weight loss programme that health benefits usually lag behind weight loss. Once the owner is able to see clear health benefits, usually in terms of a brighter, more active pet, then there is usually less need for support.

Setting a target

Regardless of how overweight the pet is, an initial target of around 15% loss should be set. This is usually achievable over an 18–20 week period.

How much weight loss to expect

Around 1% per week is a good, and safe, rate of weight loss. This means that a 6 kg cat will lose around 60 g (0.06 kg) per week so, unless you have very accurate practice scales, it is pointless weighing such a cat weekly as it will only serve to dishearten an owner.

How much to feed

Caloric intake should be restricted to 45–55% of the maintenance requirements for the target weight (see Example below).

What to feed

Essentially it does not matter what diet is fed. However, potential problems can arise if an energy dense diet is used, as the quantity given becomes small and this may lead to micronutrient deficiencies. It also is more likely to lead to diet failure as:

- The pet is more likely to beg (and worry the owner) as it does not feel full
- The owner is more likely to feed extra or give titbits as the suggested amount 'seems such a small amount'.

Commercial calorie-controlled diets tend to have low nutrient densities which are achieved by increasing fibre or water content and using non-fats as an energy source. For these reasons palatability tends to be less high.

What about treats?

Treats are allowable, and often desirable, as owners feel less 'mean' to their pet and are more likely to stick to other dietary restrictions. *But* the caloric content of the treat should be taken into account when calculating the size of the main meal(s). Where possible, low-calorie treats should be used, e.g. raw carrot for dogs.

Example of calorific calculations

A 30 kg Labrador is obese and needs to be dieted. Calculate her caloric requirement to achieve a 15% weight loss over 20 weeks.

Target weight	=	30 – (30 x 0.15)
	=	30 – 4.5
	=	25.5 kg
MER (25.5 kg)	=	1.8 [(30 x 25.5) + 70]
	=	1.8 [765 + 70]
	=	1.8 x 835
	=	1503 kcal/day
45 to 55% of MER	=	1503 x 0.45 to 1503 x 0.55
	=	676 to 827 kcal/day

A low calorie diet contains 52 kcal per 100 g of tinned food or 315 kcal per 100 g of dried food. Assuming a caloric requirement of around 750 kcal/day for the dog above, calculate the amount of food that the owner should feed to give half the calories as dry food and half as tins. Each tin contains 400 g of food, calculate the number of tins/day required.

Kcal of each type of diet	=	750 ÷ 2
	=	375 kcal
Amount of dry food (g)	=	(375 ÷ 315) x 100
	=	1.2 x 100
	=	120 g dry food
Amount of wet food (g)	=	(375 ÷ 52) x 100
	=	7.2 x 100
	=	720 g wet food
Cans of wet food	=	720 ÷ 400
	=	$1^3/_4$ – 2 tins

Approach to a pet that fails to lose weight

Failure to lose weight is the most common reason for owners to give up dieting their pets. Owners should be invited to attend regular weigh-ins for their pets and, if available within the practice, obesity clinics organized to encourage and support them. When an animal starts a diet it is important that the owner should be aware that:

- When an animal is calorie restricted, it will reduce its basal metabolic rate and therefore its caloric requirement will be reduced, making weight loss harder
- There are two phases to weight gain, a dynamic phase when the pet is gaining weight and a static phase when weight is constant. Frequently, caloric requirement at the

new weight is *less* than when the pet was thinner, so cutting the food back to the original amount fed is unlikely to lead to weight loss and could result in further weight gain.

If a pet is failing to lose weight, check:

- Owner compliance with diet, particularly the feeding of scraps/treats and the type of fluids being given
- For alternative feed sources, particularly when dieting cats (hunting, being fed next door)
- If sufficient time has been given to show a change within the accuracy of the practice scales
- Calculated requirement and recommendations to client
- The possibility of a medical reason, e.g. an endocrinopathy, as a cause of the obesity.

If the client appears to be following the diet adequately then the caloric intake should be reduced by 15%.

Vegetarian diets

The construction of a well balanced, nutritionally complete vegetarian diet for dogs is an established concept. However, serious nutritional consequences can occur if owners try and feed vegetarian diets to cats. Cats are obligate carnivores and have 'lost' the ability to manufacture a number of essential dietary components which are present, preformed in meats. Of particular concern is the availability of arachidonic acid, vitamin A and taurine, which are deficient in vegetarian diets. Other concerns with a vegetarian diet is the low biological value of the proteins and the amino acid profile, in particular the level of arginine. The inclusion of these components as synthetic additives has been tried but experience of groups who have fed cats semi-purified, well balanced diets to meet all their currently know nutritional needs has been that the cats are not as healthy and active as those fed on conventional cat foods. This suggests that there may be other micronutrients that are important for long-term health of which we are, as yet, unaware or that the complex interactions between food components are an important feature of a diet that is difficult to mimic with synthetic additives. As a final, and personal note, if one elects to look after an obligate carnivore such as a cat, it seems inappropriate to then try and feed it a non-carnivorous diet.

Nutrition of the hospitalized animal

Feeding of hospitalized patients is often overlooked in the management of complex medical and surgical cases. It is vitally important to begin nutritional support as soon as is practicable.

When to feed

No animal should go for more than 3 days without serious considerations of their nutritional needs.

What to feed

In general, hospitalized patients should be offered highly palatable, highly digestible nutrient dense foods in *small* quantities. Frequent feeding (four to six times per day) is essential for critically ill or anorexic patients.

There is probably nothing more unappetizing for a hospitalized animal than a large bowl of food that is left to go stale in the kennel and from which they cannot get away. It is far better to offer a small quantity of food which, if it is not eaten in 15–20 minutes, is removed and fresh food offered 2–4 hours later. If the patient eats all of its ration, then slightly more can be offered at the next feed.

11.26 Approximate illness energy factors

	Minor disease	Surgery	Trauma	Systemic disease and neoplasia	Sepsis	Major burns
Dog	1.0–1.2	1.25–1.35	1.2–1.5	1.4–1.6	1.5–1.7	1.6–1.8
Cat	1.0–1.1	1.1–1.2	1.1–1.3	1.2–1.3	1.3–1.4	1.3–1.4

How much to feed
Calculations should be based on the resting energy requirement multiplied by an illness energy factor (Figure 11.26). On the first day, between one-third and one-half of that calculated amount should be given; it should be built up to the full calculated amount over 2–3 days.

How to feed
Many animals will eat voluntarily, especially if given highly palatable warmed and odorous food. Time should be taken to encourage a hospitalized animal to eat by sitting with the patient and offering food by hand. Sometimes inviting the owner to feed the animal can have positive benefits. Chemical appetite stimulants can be of value in the short term but only when the underlying problem causing the inappetence is being resolved.

If an animal refuses to eat, then consideration should be given to alternative feeding methods. In general, force feeding is counterproductive – it only increases an animal's aversion to food and is stressful for the patient and staff. Recent advances in tube-feeding methods have made force feeding unnecessary. In extreme cases parenteral nutrition may be required.

Tube feeding and management
For information on assisted feeding see Chapter 4.

Euthanasia and bereavement counselling

Loss of a pet is a significant life event but in many circumstances euthanasia can be vital to relieve the suffering of a dying animal. Many owners who have lost a close relative to chronic illness appreciate the humanity and privilege of euthanasia.

Around 2% of patient contacts at the veterinary surgery will result in euthanasia. In a busy multivet practice this means that several euthanasias occur each day and it is easy to forget that, for the owner, this is a rare and often highly emotional event.

No two euthanasias will be exactly the same. The need to euthanase can profoundly affect the client, veterinary surgeon and nurse, particularly if that pet has spent a lot of time at the practice being treated before the decision for euthanasia is made.

Much of the advice that follows is time consuming and difficult to organize in a busy practice, but it is an important part of veterinary care. It has a profound influence on the way a client will view the practice in the future and on the way that the public views the veterinary profession in general.

Taking the decision
Because euthanasia is allowed in veterinary practice, it is the cause of death of around 75% of animals and is therefore the most likely way in which a pet is going to die. It must never be taken lightly. 'Convenience euthanasia' should be strongly discouraged.

No matter what nurses may think or feel about whether or not a pet should be euthanased, they *must* not appear judgmental. Often there are many complex issues involved that may not be obvious at that time.

This can be particularly difficult when euthanasing a young healthy animal for what appears to be a fairly trivial matter. Under these circumstances, nurses should ask to speak to the veterinary surgeon concerned to find out whether it is appropriate to offer to rehome the pet – a gesture for which some clients will be immensely relieved.

Many owners have difficulty with the decision to euthanase their pet and will ask the nurse: 'What would you do if it was your pet?'

- The nurse should not make some off-the-cuff answer. Many clients are extremely vulnerable at this stage and will take the advice very literally. It can also sound as though the nurse is disinterested.
- A nurse who is not familiar with the case should say so and should advise the client to talk further with the veterinary surgeon concerned
- Under no circumstances should a client be told what they ought to do
- In virtually all cases the client has actually made a decision and is looking for support. The nurse should try to find out what that decision is and support it
- In general, the nurse should try to make the client understand that this is an individual and personal decision and that there are no right and wrong choices. They know their pet best and so are in the best position to make the decision.

Arranging the environment
The professionalism with which a pet is euthanased has a profound influence on the way that the client feels about their pet's treatment and their use of the practice in the future.

The practice should be organized so that, where clients are having pets euthanased, the following occurs:

- The client should have to wait as short a time as possible. In most instances an appointment shortly before the beginning of a surgery is preferred, as appointments at the end of surgery can mean a long wait if the veterinary surgeon is running late
- If waiting is unavoidable, somewhere outside the main waiting area should be provided
- It may be helpful to arrange for a nurse or receptionist to wait with the client, allowing them to recount stories of their pet's life. Nurses should always appear sincere and interested in what the client is telling them, no matter how many times they have heard the story before. Talking about the good times in a pet's life will often help the grieving process, as the client feels that their pet has had a happy life

- When the pet has been euthanased the client should be able to leave the surgery without walking through a waiting-room full of people
- Removal of the body should not involve carrying the bag through the waiting-room or being unable to use the consulting room for the rest of the session.

Arrangements for disposal of the body

The method of disposal of the body can be a big decision for the client. It is important to be honest with the client so that they can make an informed decision as to what they would like done. If it is mass cremation, then this should be made clear; if it is a mass grave, then owners may want to visit the grave site (a potential problem if this is a landfill site).

It is essential that:

- The client's instructions regarding post mortem, disposal of the body or return of ashes are clearly understood, preferably in writing
- Great care is made in identifying bodies for individual cremation
- The disposal service is supervised when the body is collected, particularly if bodies are going to more than one place.

Note that euthanased animals are treated as clinical waste and disposed of only to licenced organizations. However, where an animal is euthanased at home, it may be buried on the owner's premises.

Paperwork

Signing the euthanasia form

Many owners find signing a euthanasia form upsetting but it is an important legal document (owners have been known to deny having given permission, particularly during the grieving process). A signed consent form is particularly important when the client is not well known to the practice or if there may be differing family opinions as to whether the pet should be euthanased. A consent form cannot be signed by a minor (person less than 16 years old) and should usually be signed by a person of over 18 years of age.

Settling the account

Settling the account can add great stress to the situation, particularly if the bill is large for what eventually has been unsuccessful treatment. Nurses should not be afraid to ask for money at the time of euthanasia – many clients prefer to sort everything out quickly. Where possible, all the paper work and, if it is a standard charge for euthanasia, the account should be settled before the animal is euthanased.

There should be a clear practice policy as to whether accounts can be sent out following euthanasia or must be settled at that time, and nurses should know what their practice policy is. If there are problems, they should ask the veterinary surgeon who has performed the euthanasia to talk to the client immediately.

Practice records

When a pet has been euthanased it is vitally important that practice records are updated. On no account should an owner receive a reminder about a booster vaccination a few weeks after the pet has been euthanased. If for any reason such a reminder has already gone out, the owner should be informed that it will be arriving and apologies should be made accordingly.

Condolence cards

Owner contact after a pet has been euthanased can be important in retaining and increasing their trust in the practice. Personalized condolence cards can be much appreciated; they also give the client an excuse to telephone the practice, ostensibly in thanks for the card but in reality to discuss other issues regarding their pet's death that may have been bothering them.

The euthanasia process

Different owners react very differently to having a pet euthanased and their wishes should be accommodated if possible. For example, some clients arrive, hand over their animal and leave immediately. They are not openly emotional but usually the reason for not staying is that they are afraid of breaking down in public. If it seems appropriate, the nurse should reassure them that crying is understandable and natural.

Preparing the owner

It is helpful to the owner if they are warned what to expect during euthanasia; it will then be easier to keep them calm when some of the following happen:

- The majority of animals lose urinary continence; some also defecate
- There may be reflex gasping movements, even after the animal is dead
- Dead animals do not close their eyes.

Problems during euthanasia

Euthanasing difficult pets can be particularly stressful, especially if the veterinary surgeon is inexperienced or the euthanasia is being conducted at home. The key is to remain calm.

- Sedation of the patient may help but many sedatives reduce blood pressure, making finding a vein more difficult
- Before starting the procedure, all equipment should be to hand – for example, scissors/clippers, swabs, euthanasia solution, needles, syringes
- If a dog needs to be muzzled, tape should be avoided
- If the nurse feels that the needle is not in the vein or that the injection appears to be going perivascularly, the veterinary surgeon should be alerted immediately, because:
  - The animal will not die
  - Perivascular injection is painful
  - The animal may become hyperexcitable if only a small amount of barbiturates has been given intravenously before the injection becomes perivascular.

After euthanasia

Some owners like to stay a few minutes with their pet after it has died. To give them that time, the consultation room should not be booked immediately following a euthanasia appointment.

If the nurse does not know what to say to the client at this stage, it is often better to say nothing but simply remain quietly with the client. No matter how busy the practice is, it is important not to appear to rush the client.

If it is necesary to place the animal in a plastic sack in front of the client, this should be done carefully. Even though the animal is dead, the client will be very sensitive about it being knocked. The animal should be left lying flat; there should be no attempt to curl it up.

The grief sequence

The grieving process normally lasts at least 4–8 weeks and frequently as long as a year. Among pet owners, 15% say they will never own another pet as they cannot bear to go through the loss again. It is sometimes helpful to suggest that the owner focuses on the good times they have had with their pet rather than the end of its life.

There are five well recognized stages of grieving, though they do not necessarily occur as distinct phases and there is considerable variation between how different people cope with their grief:

1. Shock
2. Anger and guilt
3. Bargaining
4. Depression
5. Acceptance.

It is important to reassure the client that grieving for a beloved pet is a normal and healthy process. The most serious problems arise when people fail to progress through to acceptance of their loss and remain 'trapped' in one of the earlier phases.

Shock

Shock is usually exhibited by a refusal to accept that euthanasia is the only option. Shock and disbelief most frequently occur following a traumatic accident in a young animal, or where the owner believes that the problem is trivial and is told that their animal has serious, advanced and terminal disease. Often owners will request a second opinion and this should be provided, wherever possible, from within the practice.

Shocked people tend to become pale, weak and confused and may have difficulty grasping simple information. It is important that initial explanations are given slowly and as simply as possible. Any decisions that are made should be recorded in writing.

Shock tends to be a brief phase, lasting a few hours and rarely more than a day. Figure 11.27 describes how the nurse should approach owners in shock.

11.27 Dealing with shocked owners

- If clients are expressing disbelief they should not be contradicted directly. Sympathize with their situation
- If a second opinion is requested try to provide one from within the practice (shocked owners with dying pets travelling distances by car are a danger to themselves and other road users). If it is unavoidable, persuade the client to rest for a short while, make them a drink and stay with them if possible
- If an animal is brought in following a road traffic accident:
  - It may have died *en route*, it may be necessary to call in a veterinary surgeon to confirm death
  - If the owner is convinced that the animal has been recently breathing, then resuscitation should be attempted until help arrives – even if it appears hopeless
- Ambiguous phrases such as 'put to sleep' (which some owners interpret as needing an anaesthetic) or 'I think you should leave …… with us' should be avoided.

Anger

This is a common emotion and is frequently directed at the practice, or at a neighbouring practice that has previously treated the pet. In many cases owners are feeling guilty (see below) and are seeking to blame someone else for their pet's misfortune. The type and quality of treatment are often questioned and such complaints, however unjustified, can sometimes lead to more serious actions such as litigation. Figure 11.28 describes how to deal with angry owners.

11.28 Dealing with angry owners

- Verbal attacks may be directed against the practice or nurse. They are still hurtful, particularly where the practice has put considerable time and effort into a case
- It is important to stay calm and courteous and not become too defensive. Any failings on the part of the owner (such as time taken to seek veterinary advice) should not be raised
- Where possible, try to explain that what has happened is normal procedure (such as asking for the account to be settled). If the client refuses to be placated:
  - Try to find a quiet place for them to sit
  - Locate someone more senior to talk to them, preferably the veterinary surgeon who has dealt with the case and already knows the details – even if this is the person with whom the client appears unhappy
  - If it is impossible to find that particular veterinary surgeon, make sure that the person who does talk to the client has full case notes and as much other detail as possible (including the nurse's impression as to why the client is upset). Computerized records are characterized by brevity and it can be difficult to gain a real impression of the case and in particular discussions that have occurred with the owner
  - If no one else is available, then either book an appointment for the client to come back or arrange for the veterinary surgeon involved to telephone them to discuss the case. *In the latter situation, it is essential that the veterinary surgeon should make the call. If they cannot, the nurse must phone the client to rearrange the contact.*
- Avoid making statements that could be interpreted as an admission of carelessness, neglect or error.
- In many cases sincere expressions of sympathy and understanding at their loss may be all that the client requires. For many clients it is not so much whether the practice was right or wrong but more that they cared and tried
- If an error has been made then it is the responsibility of the veterinary surgeon, not the nurse, to explain the circumstances to the client.

Guilt

Most pet deaths are surrounded by a degree of guilt on behalf of the owners, who may feel that if the pet becomes ill prematurely then this is due to a failing on their part. Common guilt areas are:

- Not spotting how unwell their pet had become
- Seeking veterinary advice too late
- Being unable or unwilling to afford more extensive investigations and treatments

- Failing to bring the pet back when requested or when its condition deteriorated
- Not requesting euthanasia at an earlier time
- Being responsible for a traumatic injury.

Figure 11.29 gives guidelines for nurses dealing with owners dealing who express guilt.

11.29 Dealing with owners who feel guilty

- It is important not to intensify feelings of guilt, as this can lead to the guilt being transferred to aggression, blame or depression
- Reassure the owner that it is not their fault – for example, if the pet developed cancer. It is also helpful to sympathize with the owner and reassure them that it is always easier to see what would have been best after the outcome is known, or that accidents do happen and they are by no means alone in leaving the gate open which led to a pet being run over.

Bargaining

This phase is often not obvious in the grieving process. It may be seen as the client bringing gifts for the nurses in an effort to influence the advice that they have been given by the veterinary surgeon. Some clients will ask for special access to their pet or some other favour which has already been expressly refused by the veterinary surgeon dealing with the case.

- Gifts, within reason, should be gratefully accepted. It is good policy to say that they will be shared with all the people looking after the client's pet, as this helps to emphasize the team and caring aspects of the practice
- If asked to do something that is not normal practice policy, such as allowing the client into busy areas of the practice, check with the veterinary surgeon first
- The nurse's primary responsibility is to the welfare of the animal. It is important to support decisions made by the veterinary surgeon and not to suggest treatments that may be expensive, involve considerable discomfort to the pet and have little chance of success.

Depression

Sadness following the loss of a pet is natural. In some cases, particularly where there is a single pet belonging to a person living on their own, then clinical depression can occur. Such cases are rarely simply about the pet but involve other personal experiences, particularly the loss of relatives. Guilt can also play a part in the onset of depression.

Depressed people can become physically ill, not eating or sleeping properly and losing interest in their daily responsibilities and appearance. Many become confused about the circumstances surrounding their pet's death and still feel their presence at home. Such owners are prone to break down in tears for no apparent reason.

Depression usually occurs within a few days of the loss, reaches a peak in about 2 weeks and then subsides. Action that can be taken by the nurse dealing with depressed owners is suggested in Figure 11.30.

Acceptance

This is essentially the recovery phase, when the client can rationalize their loss and view the circumstances of their pet's death objectively. The client is able then to talk about their pet more rationally without excessive emotion.

11.30 Dealing with depressed owners

- Sometimes the client will telephone the surgery with an apparently trivial enquiry, or becomes a frequent visitor with other pets with minor problems. A third party will occasionally contact the surgery for help
- Care must be taken to make sure that the client does not become emotionally dependent on the nurse or the practice, as neither has the time or training to be of long-term help
- In many cases the client wants to talk to someone who understands their loss. They may have questions or want to have situations explained again as they were unable to take in the details at the time. The nurse should find time to answer these enquiries in a quiet place where there is no obvious interruption. Sometimes the veterinary surgeon should speak to the client, particularly if it has been a complex case
- Clients should be assured that their feelings are normal and to be expected. Where appropriate, they should be reassured that they have done everything for their pet
- The grieving process will be helped by encouraging a client to make a memorial gesture (for example, a charity donation, or sponsoring a rescue animal)
- On rare occasions, professional help may be necessary. The practice should be aware of any local support group so that it can be recommended
- In extreme cases of profound depression, continuing for more than 3 weeks, and where there is a risk of self-harm, professional medical help should be sought. It is the responsibility of the veterinary surgeon dealing with the case to make the initial contact with the client's GP or with social services.

During the acceptance phase:

- No action may be required
- This is the time when suggesting a new pet is sensible, unless the previous pet died of an infectious disease which may still be present in the owner's home
- The practice should advise the client where to find a new pet, what will be most suitable and what to look for. The client should be encouraged to present the new pet to the practice for a check-up, preferably 4–5 days after it has been brought home
- Many owners are keen to adopt rescue pets at this stage. Having gone through the emotional turmoil of a sick pet, taking on a new animal with problems may not be the best solution. A young healthy pet may be more appropriate.

Assessing the client's needs

Assessing a client's needs is often a matter of experience, which is helped by previous contact with that client. For newly qualified nurses or those who have recently joined the practice, help from senior nursing colleagues can be invaluable.

Situations that tend to suggest an owner will have problems coping with the death of their pet can be identified:

- Lack of time to prepare for, or come to terms with the loss (e.g. severe traumatic episodes, rapidly advancing disease, or disease that has gone unnoticed until a crisis occurs)
- The owner has suffered problems following the death of a pet in the past
- The owner lives alone and it was their only pet

- The pet has been nursed through a period of intense care and dependency (this may not necessarily relate to the current illness but have occurred in the past)
- The pet has helped an owner through a personal crisis such as divorce or loss of a close relative
- The pet belonged to someone close to the owner who has now died – the last living link
- The owner is forced to opt for euthanasia for financial reasons or because they are unable to provide the necessary support at home.

Such clients should be contacted, where appropriate, a few days after their pet's death or encouraged to phone the practice if they have any questions or 'just want a chat'. When contact is made the conversation need not be prolonged but should appear sincere, concerned and unhurried. Asking how the client is feeling can then allow them to express their grief or give clues to their state of depression. Reassurance is the key, particularly if it is necessary to suggest that they contact a support agency. The nurse should always end the conversation by saying that they can contact the surgery again for a chat.

Grief within the practice

Grief at the loss of an animal may not be confined to the owner but may profoundly affect other members of staff within the practice, particularly where an animal has been hospitalized for a long period and has undergone intensive treatment. Support should be provided where possible, particularly to trainees and less experienced staff. Older staff may appear less affected but this is usually due to the necessity of developing coping strategies; it does not mean that they do not care about an animal's death.

Behaviour counselling

The level of interest in companion animal behaviour within a veterinary context has increased substantially in recent years. With this interest has come the realization that animal behaviour is a field in which the veterinary nurse can play a vital role within the general practice. When considering the areas in which veterinary nurses are requested to give advice to clients, behaviour is near the top of the list.

The relevance of behaviour counselling to general practice

There are a number of potential causes of so-called behavioural problems (Figure 11.31) and in order to differentiate between them the veterinary nurse needs to be familiar with the natural behaviour patterns of the common companion animal species, as well as with the possible link between human behaviour and inappropriate animal responses.

11.31 Possible causes of behavioural problems

- Normal species-specific behaviour in an inappropriate context
- Inappropriate learned responses
- Behavioural changes resulting from physical or mental illness
- A combination of the above

An understanding of the link between disease and behaviour is also essential. When dealing with specific cases it is important to ensure that the animal undergoes a full veterinary examination before behavioural advice is given. Veterinary involvement in the work-up of individual behavioural cases should be sought and knowledge of the medical differential diagnoses for the commonly presented behavioural symptoms is essential for anyone working in this field. It is not possible to explore the links between disease and behaviour here but those wishing to work with behavioural cases can gain this information from other sources (see later and Further reading). The theory of veterinary behavioural medicine is also not within the remit of this book, but there is adequate material available for those who wish to broaden their knowledge base and this is essential before beginning to offer specific advice in behavioural cases.

It is important to realize that the skill of knowing when to refer is as important as the ability to offer advice. In cases of behaviour problems which are potentially dangerous, it is important to recognize when it is time to hand the case over to someone else!

Dealing with specific behavioural cases is only one aspect of providing a behavioural service, however, and veterinary nurses can significantly increase the rapport between clients and the practice by offering behavioural advice in a variety of other ways.

Preventive behavioural advice

This is an area where the veterinary nurse can be invaluable. Owners of puppies and kittens are often at a very receptive stage in their relationship with their pets, making this an ideal time to get the message across. Advice on dealing with common behavioural problems can also form an important part of the information offered by the veterinary practice, either as a first aid approach or as a prelude to referral. It is important to remember that owners are crucial to the success of behavioural modification and that if the owner does not understand or agree with the suggested approach to the pet's behaviour they will not cooperate with the advice that is given.

When considering establishing a preventive behavioural service within general practice there are three main target groups to be considered:

- Breeders
- Prospective owners
- New owners.

Working with breeders

As breeders are involved from the beginning, they have a tremendous responsibility to ensure that prevention of behavioural problems occurs from the earliest opportunity. Puppies and kittens may eventually lead many different kinds of lives, for example as show animals, working animals on a farm or family pets. The common aim of the breeder and veterinary practice should be the development of emotionally stable puppies and kittens that can adapt to whatever lifestyle they are offered and can successfully coexist with their own and other species. Veterinary practices are well placed to offer the necessary advice to achieve this aim and working with breeders in this area can be very rewarding.

Providing preventive behavioural advice for the breeder will involve studying both the breeding programme and the rearing methods and considering these from a behavioural viewpoint.

It is generally recognized that the temperament of the dam and sire must be considered when deciding on breeding programmes but it is not uncommon, for a number of reasons, for other factors to take precedence. The veterinary practice can offer useful advice in this area, especially to the novice breeder, and it is the responsibility of every veterinary practice to help to dispel the myth that breeding from nervous bitches will help to calm them down. It also falls to the veterinary practice to give clear advice on the suitability of individuals for use in breeding programmes. Such advice must be clearly justified and a knowledge of genetic influences on behaviour is required.

In order to advise breeders on appropriate rearing methods, veterinary nurses need to have a good level of knowledge of kitten and puppy development and the ability to convey the information in a tactful, relevant and practical manner. Information on the importance of adequate and appropriate socialization and habituation has been available for decades but there are still many puppies and kittens being raised in conditions which make it impossible for this to be achieved. It is important to be aware of the sensitive period of socialization and the importance of experiences that animals have during that time. For puppies the period runs from around 4 to 14 weeks of age, while for kittens this important phase of development occurs much earlier, between 2 and 7 weeks.

The prime concern of the veterinary profession is the welfare of the animals committed to its care. Consequently it has a responsibility to ensure that the vital information about exposing kittens and puppies to appropriate experiences within the sensitive socialization period is made available to every breeder in a way that makes sense and appears relevant to them. Socialization and habituation take time and effort and it is important to emphasize the rewards in terms of emotionally stable puppies and kittens who will be easier to home and unlikely to be returned. Far from being an added burden, the institution of an imaginative and effective socialization and habituation programme (Figures 11.32 and 11.33) should be seen by the breeder as being a way of increasing their professional image whilst improving the welfare of the animals. This will only be achieved if veterinary practices take the time to give the appropriate advice.

11.32 Important experiences for puppies and kittens at the breeder's premises

- Adequate interaction with dam and possibly sire
- Adequate interaction with litter mates
- Exposure to appropriate and adequate handling by a variety of people including men, women and children
- Exposure to a wide range of auditory, visual and tactile stimuli through the provision of toys and the encountering of normal everyday human activities
- Exposure to solitude on a temporary basis

11.33 Special considerations for kittens

- Handling by at least four different people in order to ensure generalization of socialization
- Handling by a variety of people including men, women and children in short frequent sessions with a minimum total of one hour every day
- Appropriate handling, which should include lifting the kitten, touching it all over and gently restraining it

Providing advice on pet selection

When working with prospective owners the main objective is to assist people in choosing a pet which is best suited to their requirements and which offers them the best potential for a long and mutually rewarding relationship (*see BSAVA Manual of Veterinary Care*). In order to achieve this it is worth taking time to determine the prospective owner's expectations and help them to assess the commitment of pet ownership in realistic terms. There will be a number of factors that need to be considered and it is important to steer people away from misguided choices and give clearly justifiable reasons for the selection that is advised. Prospective owners may not have taken the time to evaluate their reasons for wanting a pet and it can be very helpful to talk them through this process. Pointing out the possible considerations in terms of the species, breed, age and sex of the potential pet can help to put the decision in perspective and can prevent distressing mismatches.

Providing help for new owners

Once owners have acquired their new pet the veterinary nurse has an essential role in providing preventive behavioural advice. Advising clients on how to socialize and habituate their puppy or kitten successfully (Figures 11.34 and 11.35) needs to be given as soon as the new owner contacts the practice. It is important to emphasize that these vital processes can begin while the vaccination programme is in progress. A high percentage of behavioural problems can be prevented if puppies, kittens and young of other companion animal species are given the correct experiences early in life.

Ways in which new owners can be assisted in learning how to deal with their new pet include the provision of 'puppy parties' and kitten information evenings. Owners are invited to the practice to attend a class with other new owners, where they are given advice on preventive health care, including prevention of the most common behavioural problems.

11.34 Behavioural issues for new puppy owners

Providing suitable socialization and habituation
House training
Teaching appropriate greeting behaviours
Teaching recall
Providing suitable toys
Preventing specific behaviour problems
Preparing the puppy for life in a complex environment
Accustoming the puppy to being home

11.35 Behavioural issues for new kitten owners

Providing suitable socialization and habituation
Litter training
Explaining the importance of feline play
Teaching the kitten to use a cat flap
Teaching the kitten to come when called
Accustoming the kitten to wearing an appropriate collar
Accustoming the kitten to appropriate handling
Preventing specific behaviour problems
Preparing the kitten for life in a complex environment

Nurses need to be able to devote an adequate amount of time to each client and running behaviour prevention clinics where owners can be given one-to-one appointments can be a very useful way of providing information. Puppy parties offer an opportunity to convey the important messages of early training and adequate socialization and habituation, but for many owners the presence of other owners makes it difficult to ask questions or to raise specific concerns.

In order to assist new owners in avoiding common pitfalls when dealing with their pet's behaviour, it is necessary to teach them about the species-specific behavioural responses of the animal they have chosen to live with. Understanding the social behaviour and communication systems that their pet's wild relatives display can go a long way toward making sense of the behaviours that they encounter on a daily basis.

Teaching new owners the very basic principles of learning theory is essential in order to assist them in understanding how their pet learns, but this is complicated information and it takes time and patience to get the message across. Explaining the meanings of reward and punishment and showing how rewards need to be delivered in order to change an animal's behaviour will help to avoid the common problem of unintentional reinforcement leading to the development of undesirable behaviours.

Basic principles of learning theory

The two methods of learning that are important to understand are:

- Classical conditioning
- Instrumental (operant) conditioning.

Classical conditioning

The two main features of classical conditioning are:

- It involves involuntary or reflex responses
- There is no involvement of reward.

The best known example of this is the famous experiment by Pavlov where the *unconditioned stimulus* of food gave an *unconditioned response* of salivation in dogs. By pairing the food with the previously neutral stimulus of a sound, Pavlov was able to make that sound a *conditioned stimulus* which would eventually lead to a *conditioned response* of salivation, even if there was no food present.

House training

The unconditioned stimuli are the internal sensations, mediated via the nervous system, which communicate to the brain the need for the animal to urinate or defecate. The unconditioned response is elimination. In the process of house training we aim to associate the internal triggers with certain conditioned environmental stimuli, namely outdoor stimuli. Eventually these conditioned stimuli should lead to the conditioned response of elimination so that the animal will only eliminate when it is outside.

This sounds simple but in order for the training to be successful the desired conditioned stimuli (outdoor signals) need to occur at the same time as the unconditioned stimuli (internal sensations). As internal nervous signals are not readily apparent to the owner, it is necessary to arrange for the conditioned stimuli to be present at those times when the unconditioned stimuli are most likely to occur, such as after meals, after sleep and when sniffing around in search of scent marks. The most important rule is to give the animal the maximum opportunity to get it right and the minimum opportunity to get it wrong. In addition, owners should resist the temptation to punish a young animal when it 'makes a mistake' but, rather, should take the blame for not getting the timing right.

Instrumental (operant) conditioning

This involves the integration of:

- Stimulus
- Response
- Reward.

Instrumental conditioning forms the basis of animal training and much of behaviour modification. One of the main implications of this type of learning is that animals will go on learning even when no one intends to teach them anything. Provided a stimulus and a response occur in conjunction with some form of reinforcement, then learning will take place and in this way a lot of so-called problem behaviour is learned inadvertently.

Jumping up

This is an example of learned behaviour. A dog jump ups when people greet it: the stimulus is the approach of a person; the response is jumping up; and the reward is social interaction (however negative that may appear).

In order to rectify this behaviour, the owner first needs to decide what sort of behaviour they want their dog to display when people approach. The owner then needs to ensure that this appropriate response is rewarded, while the inappropriate response is ignored. It needs to be emphasized that a dog will learn more readily if the required response occurs spontaneously, and the required stimulus and reinforcement can be arranged to occur in conjunction with it, than if the response is forced. This can make training a slow process and increases the requirement for patience on the part of the owner.

Sitting to greet

A food reward can be used initially to lure the dog into the sit position. As the dog sits (to all intents and purposes voluntarily) the owner can say 'Sit!' and then immediately give a reward of greeting and food. Eventually the food is no longer used. As the lure involved the owner slowly raising their hand above the dog's head, this gesture can be continued as a visual command to sit and the appropriate response can be rewarded by owner praise and affection.

Reinforcement and punishment

- Reinforcement: The increase in response probability that results from the presentation of a reinforcer
- Positive reinforcement: An increase in the frequency of a behaviour when a positive reinforcer (an appetitive stimulus) is presented at the same time as the behaviour
  - Example: teaching a dog to lie down by offering a food reward every time it is in a down position
- Negative reinforcement: An increase in the frequency of a behaviour when a negative reinforcer (an aversive stimulus) is removed or avoided at the same time as the behaviour
  - Example: a dog learning to come back to the house when it is raining as it associates being inside with the removal of the unpleasant presence of rain.

- Punishment: The decrease in response probability that results from the presentation of a punisher
- Positive punishment: A decrease in the frequency of a behaviour when a positive punisher (an aversive stimulus) is presented as a consequence of that behaviour
  - Example: a dog learning not to raid a bin because the bin lid falls on the dog's head as it puts its head in
- Negative punishment: A decrease in the frequency of a behaviour when a negative punisher (an appetitive stimulus) is removed or avoided at the same time as the behaviour
  - Example: teaching a dog not to bark for attention by removing all social interaction every time it barks.

In order for reinforcement or punishment to be successful, owners need to be aware of what their pet considers to be an appetitive stimulus and what it considers to be an aversive stimulus. This will be species-specific but there will also be an element of individual variation. For example, some dogs find water appetitive while others would definitely consider it aversive.

Timing, intensity and schedule

Owners need to be made aware of the importance of the timing of delivery of the reinforcer or punisher, the intensity of the stimulus used and schedule by which it is delivered. In order to be effective, reinforcers and punishers need to be delivered at the same time as the behaviour which is to be affected. Inappropriate timing is responsible for the development and the perpetuation of many behavioural problems.

In the case of positive reinforcers the intensity of the stimulus will need to be tailored to the required response. For example, a very intense appetitive stimulus may be needed when teaching a dog to focus on the owner in a very distracting environment but it may induce excitement and therefore be inappropriate when the owner is trying to teach the dog to be calm at home. In the case of positive punishment, the intensity of the aversive stimulus should always be the lowest possible but this is very difficult to achieve and unintentional escalation of the intensity of the punisher is not uncommon.

When considering the schedule of delivery for reinforcers and punishers it is important to explain the principles in terms that the owner can easily understand. There are several regimes which owners may be using, either intentionally or unintentionally, and explaining the implications of their use can be very helpful in motivating owners to interact successfully with their pets.

In the case of positive punishment, the only successful schedule is a continuous one, where the aversive stimulus is presented every time the undesirable behaviour occurs. This is very difficult to achieve and a lack of consistency in the application of punishment adds to the lack of success of this approach.

In the case of positive reinforcement, the most successful schedule for the establishment of a behaviour is a continuous one, where every single desired response is reinforced. However, continuous schedules make behaviours more prone to extinction and, in order to maintain the behaviour, it is important to alter the schedule to a variable ratio. This means that a reinforcement is given after every so many responses, but the number continually varies so that the number of responses required on any one occasion is unpredictable and the animal is more likely to continue to offer the behaviour in expectation of a reward.

Socialization and habituation

The importance of socialization and habituation cannot be over-emphasized. It can be helpful to prepare checklists for new owners (Figure 11.36) which will guide them in their attempts to give their new pet the right sort of experiences in those early weeks. Asking the owner to bring the list with them when they come for the vaccination appointments will also give the nurse the opportunity to make sure that their advice is being followed. It will also emphasize that exposing young animals to a wide variety of people, animals, experiences and situations is not optional but rather an integral part of caring for a new pet.

11.36 Checklist for socialization and habituation

Places to go
Veterinary clinic
Other people's houses
Recreation area
Roadside
Railway stations and bus depots
Rural environment
Towns and cities
Lifts and escalators

People to meet
Men
Women
Children and babies
Elderly people
Disabled people
Delivery people, e.g. milkman, postman
People on bicycles, pushing prams, jogging
People who differ significantly in appearance from the family members
Veterinary practice staff and others in distinctive clothing

Animals to meet
Dogs
Cats
Other domestic pets
Livestock

Things to encounter
Domestic appliances
Vehicles
Children's toys
Pushchairs

Offering advice to owners with problem pets

Prevention of behavioural problems is the preferred approach but the reality is that problems are often already evident before the veterinary practice becomes involved. The owner may have lived with the problem for some considerable time and when a practice starts to provide a behavioural service, and offer advice on existing behavioural problems, it is necessary to bear in mind the varying approaches which owners may have to their pet's 'problem'.

Some owners do not wish to improve their pet's behaviour. Some may find unsociable behaviour amusing and go so far as encouraging it. It is never going to be possible to convince such owners of the benefits of behavioural therapy and it is unlikely that any advice would be successfully applied.

However, these owners are in the minority and far more fall into the category of those who would like to improve their pet's behaviour but do not know where to start.

Many clients would not think of discussing behaviour with their veterinary practice as they view the way in which their pet behaves as something very separate from its health. It is essential that the practice demonstrates its interest in, and commitment to, mental as well as physical health. Some owners will need encouragement and 'permission' to bring up the subject of behavioural problems, as they find the subject difficult to discuss. They may be embarrassed to admit that there is a problem (Figure 11.37). The veterinary nurse is often the first point of contact and therefore needs to respond positively to the behavioural enquiry or encourage the reluctant client to discuss their behavioural concerns.

11.37 Why owners do not seek advice about behaviour

- Do not know where to ask for help
- Do not realize that something can be done to correct unwanted behaviour
- Blame themselves for being poor owners
- Are embarrassed to admit that they have a problem
- Are frightened that others will find the situation amusing and even trivial
- Simply have not thought of asking their veterinary practice for advice

Identifying a problem

Clients may react in a number of ways when their pet begins to display unusual behaviour patterns:

- Accept and even encourage the behaviour
- Tolerate the behaviour
- Consider returning the pet to the breeder
- Consider rehoming
- Consider euthanasia
- Actively seek help from the veterinary practice or other source.

Tolerant owners or those considering rehoming or euthanasia can be identified by the veterinary practice. Through offering advice and assistance, it is often possible to alter their perception of the problem and encourage them to seek appropriate help.

Identifying potential behaviour cases relies on skills of observation and listening. For example, a great deal can be determined about a dog's behaviour by the way in which it enters the waiting room with its owner and by the interaction between owner and pet while they are waiting for an appointment:

- Does a dog charge into the waiting room ahead of the owner?
- Does an owner carry a dog in while partially hiding it under their coat?
- Where does the owner choose to sit ? Is it close to the door for an easy exit or in a quiet corner where they will not be disturbed?

By carefully observing the owner and their pet a lot can be learned about the relationship between them and this information can be used to better understand the problems that may exist within that relationship. Mismatches between

people and their pets may be evident but in most cases it is too late to correct these. The advice that is given to owners needs to be tactful, relevant and practical.

Common behavioural problems of dogs and cats are listed in Figures 11.38 and 11.39.

11.38 Possible behaviour problems in dogs

- Control problems, either at home or out on walks
- Toileting problems
- Destructive behaviours
- Aggression to people and/or animals
- Separation-related problems
- Fears and phobias
- Geriatric behaviour changes
- Medically based behavioural problems
- Behavioural pathologies

11.39 Possible behaviour problems in cats

- Elimination problems
- Inappropriate marking behaviours
- Aggression to people and/or animals
- Pica
- Fears and phobias
- Geriatric behaviour changes
- Medically based behavioural problems
- Behavioural pathologies

Talking to the owner

When dealing with behavioural issues it is essential to avoid the temptation to apportion blame. Behavioural problems in pets often lead their owners to feel guilty and ashamed, and if there is any sign of disapproval or amusement they will be reluctant to give the vital information that is needed to investigate the problem further. Whether the problem is going to be dealt with in the practice, or is going to need referral to someone with more experience in the field, the way in which practice personnel react to the owner on the very first contact can be instrumental in how, or indeed whether, the problem can be resolved.

Once the client has begun to talk about the problem there are vital questions that need to be asked and information that needs to be gleaned. Even if the intention is to refer the case it is important to ask relevant questions when finding out about the problem.

Essential information about the animal:

- Species/breed
- Age
- Sex
- Source
- Age acquired
- Medical history
- Current health status.

Questions to ask about the behaviour:

1. Describe the behaviour in detail
2. When did it start?
3. What were the circumstances of the first occurrence?

4. How has the behaviour developed since the first incident?
5. How often does it occur?
6. When does it occur?
7. Where does it occur?
8. How do the owners rate the severity?
9. What attempts have been made to deal with the behaviour?
10. How do the owners react?

Knowledge of the owner's response to the behaviour will help to determine whether owner involvement has had any effect on the progression of the problem. For example, a dog that growled defensively when someone attempted to remove a valued object from its possession may have been punished by the owner for doing so. The behaviour may subsequently have developed into a more generalized aggression to the owners, rooted in fear of future negative interactions.

Investigating the way in which the behaviour has developed and asking questions about the venue, timing and frequency of the incidents will be useful in order to determine whether there are any easily identifiable triggers for the response. It may also be important in establishing a link between behaviour and disease.

It may seem that for every piece of information given yet another question needs to be asked, but this is the only way to gain all of the relevant details and put together as complete a picture as possible of the problem.

Advice and treatment

The important part of the process is fully understanding the animal's behaviour, its motivation and its purpose and then explaining this information to the owner in a way that is easily understood. The aim of behavioural advice will differ, depending on the problem, the owner and the individual animal. There are a number of possible outcomes, all of which can be considered successful in their own way:

- An alteration in the owner's expectations
- Increasing the owner's understanding of the behaviour – this may enable them to accept behaviour which is normal for the animal, albeit inconvenient
- Redirection of behaviour into an acceptable form
- Total resolution of the inappropriate behaviour
- Rehoming – where there is incompatibility between owner and pet or environment and pet
- Euthanasia – after lengthy discussion with the veterinary surgeon.

Treating behaviour problems is a complex process and requires an understanding of ethology, learning theory, human psychology, psychopharmacology, animal welfare and even the law! Every case is individual and it can be dangerous to offer recipe book approaches to problems. Expanding the behavioural service within the practice to include the provision of behavioural consultations lasting between one and a half and two hours adds another dimension to the service that the practice can offer to its clients and anyone wanting to progress to this level of behavioural service will find relevant information in behavioural textbooks and will find it helpful to attend relevant courses on behavioural therapy. However, where in-house behavioural consultations are not feasible, the careful use of referral can enable all practices to offer a comprehensive behavioural service to their clients.

Whatever the outcome of individual cases it is essential that veterinary practices take behavioural problems seriously and make the effort to provide the service that owners of problem pets are looking for. If veterinary nurses take the time to offer behavioural advice to clients they will increase the holistic image of the practice and encourage clients to visit the practice frequently.

Further reading

Diet

Burger I (1993) *The Waltham Book of Companion Animal Nutrition*. Pergamon Press, Oxford

Edney ATB (1982) *Dog and Cat Nutrition*. Pergamon Press, Oxford

Lewis LD, Morris, ML and Hand MS (1987) *Small Animal Clinical Nutrition III*. Mark Morris Associates, Kansas

Wills JM and Simpson KW (1994) *The Waltham Book of Clinical Nutrition in the Dog and Cat*. Pergamon Press, Oxford

Bereavement

- The BSAVA produces a short leaflet, 'Coping with the Loss of your Pet', which can be given to clients to read
- The Pet Bereavement Support Service (0800 0966606) offers help and a sympathetic ear.

Butler C and Lagoni L (1995) Facilitating owner-present euthanasia. In: Bonagura J (ed.) *Kirk's Current Veterinary Therapy XII*. WB Saunders, Philadelphia, pp. 87–91

Howell J (1998) Euthanasia: how to support clients. *Veterinary Nursing* 13, 175–178

Ironside, Virginia (1994) *Goodbye, Dear Friend*. Robson Books,

Lee, Laura and Martin (1992) *Absent Friends*. Henston, Bucks

McCulloch MJ, Harris JM and McCulloch WF (1989) Human–animal bond and euthanasia – a special problem. In: Ettinger SJ (ed.) *Textbook of Veterinary Medicine*. WB Saunders, Philadelphia, pp. 243–244

SCAS (1990) *Death of an Animal Friend*. Society for Companion Animal Studies, Perthshire

Stewart M (1994) Coping with client grief. *Veterinary Nursing* 9, 170–172

Stewart M, Docherty A and Brown A (1996) *When a Pet Dies A Learning Pack for people who support owners when their pet dies*. SCAS, Perthshire

Stewart M (1999) *Companion Animal Death*. Butterworth Heinemann

Behaviour

Askew H (1996) *Treatment of Behaviour Problems in Dogs and Cats*. Blackwell Science, Oxford

Beaver B (1992) *Feline Behaviour – a Guide for Veterinarians*. WB Saunders, Philadelphia

Jevring C and Catanzaro T (1999) *Healthcare of the Well Pet*. WB Saunders, Philadelphia

Landsberg G, Hunthausen W and Ackerman L (1997) *Handbook of Behavioural Problems of the Dog and Cat*. Butterworth-Heinemann, Oxford

Neville PF and O'Farrell V (1994) *Manual of Feline Behaviour*, 2nd edn. BSAVA, Cheltenham

O'Farrell V (1992) *Manual of Canine Behaviour*. BSAVA, Cheltenham

Overall K (1997) *Clinical Behavioural Medicine for Small Animals*. Mosby, St Louis

Peachey E *Running Puppy Classes*. APBC, Worcester

Recommenced reading for clients:

Appleby D *How to have a Happy Puppy*. APBC, Worcester

Appleby D *How to have a Contented Cat*. APBC, Worcester

Appleby D (1998) *Ain't MisBehavin'*. Broadcast Books, Bristol

Bailey G (1995) *Perfect Puppy*. Hamlyn, London

Dunbar I (1991) *Doctor Dunbar's Good Little Dog Book*. James and Kenneth Publishers, Berkeley, California

Dunbar I (1996) *How to Teach a New Dog Old Tricks*. James and Kenneth Publishers, Berkeley, California

Evans M (1996) *The Complete Guide to Kitten Care*. Mitchell Beazley, London

Evans M (1996) *The Complete Guide to Puppy Care*. Mitchell Beazley, London

Fisher J (1993) *Why Does My Dog....?* Souvenir Press, London

Heath S (1995) *Why Does My Cat....?* Souvenir Press, London

Neville P and Bessant C (1997) *Perfect Kitten*. Hamlyn, London

Patmore K (1991) *So Your Children want a Dog*. Popular Dogs, London

Useful addresses

Companion Animal Behaviour Therapy Study Group
c/o Miss S.E. Heath BVSc MRCVS
CABTSG Secretary
11 Cotebrook Drive
Upton
Chester
CH2 1RA
Tel: 01244 377365
Fax: 01244 399228
Email: heath@vetethol.demon.co.uk

European Society of Veterinary Clinical Ethology
c/o Dr. J. Dehasse DVM,
3 Avenue du Cosmonaute
B-1150
Brussels
Belgium.
Tel/Fax: 00 32 2 770 4008
E-mail: joel.dehasse@advalvas.be

Association of Pet Behaviour Counsellors (APBC)
PO Box 46
Worcester
WR8 9YS
Tel/Fax: 01386 751151
E-mail : apbc@petbcent.demon.co.uk.

American Veterinary Society of Animal Behaviour
c/o Dr Debra Horwitz
AVSAB Secretary/Treasurer
Veterinary Behaviour Consultations
253 S. Graeser Rd
St Louis
MO 63141
USA

Animal Behaviour Society
c/o Dr Ira Perelle
ABS
Mercy College
Dobbs Ferry
NY 10522
USA.

Society for Companion Animal Studies
10(b) Leny Road
Callander
FK17 8BA

12 Veterinary nursing and the law

George Malynicz

This chapter is designed to give information on:

- Ethics and the law relating to the practice of small animal veterinary nursing
- The relationship between veterinary nursing and veterinary surgery

Brief history of veterinary nursing in the UK

Veterinary nursing in Britain was launched in 1961 when the Royal College of Veterinary Surgeons (RCVS, 1961) 'introduced a scheme for the recruitment, training and registration of (Registered) Animal Nursing Auxiliaries' (RANAs). This initiative, known as the Veterinary Nursing Scheme, was the responsibility of the Veterinary Nursing Committee (VNC) of the College.

At that time the Veterinary Surgeons Act 1966 (VSA) treated RANAs as no different from other members of the public. However, it became apparent that a body of people had emerged who were skilled at caring for sick and injured animals but were not vets. The title was changed to Veterinary Nurse (VN) in 1984 and by 1990 the RCVS accepted that 'the eventual aim should be the establishment of a College of Veterinary Nursing with a council consisting of equal numbers of veterinary nurses and veterinary surgeons plus representatives of educational institutes offering full time courses' (RCVS, 1990).

In 1991, amendments were made to Schedule 3 of the VSA which allowed listed veterinary nurses to 'carry out any treatment or minor surgery ... to a companion animal provided that [this] ... is carried out ... at his [the employing veterinary surgeon's] direction' (VSA 1966 (Schedule 3 Amendment Order) 1991). This represented the first recognition that veterinary nurses could be delegated some aspects of the work of veterinary surgeons. In 1994 the RCVS published a List of Veterinary Nurses, membership of which (through examination and payment of the retention fee) entitled veterinary nurses to perform the procedures delegated under Schedule 3 and more recently to train, assess and verify veterinary nurse students undertaking the NVQ scheme for VN training (RCVS, 1999).

The RCVS has since accepted that 'the legislation has quite clearly become out of line with the procedures which veterinary nurses are and should be enabled to perform' and

was 'unnecessarily restrictive' (RCVS, 1998a). New or amended legislation will be introduced with the following objectives:

- To define veterinary nursing as a profession in its own right and protect the title
- To define the qualifications necessary to be described as a veterinary nurse
- To allow for student veterinary nurses to undertake procedures under the supervision of a veterinary surgeon or a qualified veterinary nurse in order to acquire pre-qualification experience
- To determine what procedures veterinary nurses can undertake – under the direction or supervision of a veterinary surgeon
- To provide a means of regulating the professional conduct of veterinary nurses, perhaps by maintaining a Register and a disciplinary body.

The British Animal Nursing Auxiliary Association (later the BVNA) was established in 1965 and its aims were to 'foster and promote the standard of veterinary nursing and the interest and status of the RANA' (Turner, 1986). The BVNA now has 3000 members and has worked tirelessly in attending the VNC, fostering its members' interests, arranging annual congresses and participating in training of its members through schemes such as the S/NVQ Training Scheme.

Relationship between veterinary nursing and veterinary surgery

'Under the Veterinary Surgeons Act 1966 the Royal College of Veterinary Surgeons is responsible for all matters relating to the ethical conduct of those involved in veterinary practice within the United Kingdom. That responsibility encompasses the work of both veterinary surgeons and veterinary nurses.'

This statement (RCVS, 1998b) encapsulates the current legal position on the ethics of veterinary nursing. The RCVS is responsible for two professions: veterinary surgeons and veterinary nurses.

Control of its professional standards, education and membership are the three basic privileges that any profession enjoys. To assist members in meeting standards and avoiding misconduct, it is usual for a professional body to have a code of conduct. The RCVS has published a *Guide to Professional Conduct for Veterinary Nurses* (GPCVN) (RCVS, 1998b) which lays out the professional standards expected of the veterinary nursing profession. Misconduct covers a very wide range of acts that could bring veterinary practice into disrepute. Removal from the List of Veterinary Nurses is the ultimate sanction available to the College in cases of misconduct.

Some of the more important points in the GPCVN include:

- Nurses are 'only permitted to act under the supervision or direction of a veterinary surgeon'
- They are 'personally responsible for their own professional standards and negligence'
- They shall 'act at all times in the best interest of the animal while taking into consideration the wishes of the owner/keeper and employer and in such a manner as to justify the trust and confidence of the public and to uphold the good standing of the veterinary profession'.

These guidelines are consistent with the view of the College that the veterinary nursing profession exists to serve and maintain the good standing of veterinary practice as a whole.

The responsibility for 'the animal' is interesting. Domesticated animals are considered to be chattels (moveable possessions) and therefore it would appear that, once a veterinary practice has agreed to care for an animal, it is to the owner that the practice and its employees – including any veterinary nurses – are liable and not the animal. There would of course be overriding statutory considerations such as the prevention of cruelty under the Protection of Animals Act 1911, which would, for example, be a defence if a practice was to destroy a suffering animal against the owner's wishes.

The veterinary practice owes a duty of care to its clients and will be liable for acts and omissions carried out negligently by any of its employees, including veterinary surgeons and veterinary nurses. This will be so unless it can be said that the negligent act was carried out independently from their employment. In fact almost all acts carried out by veterinary nurses to do with their work will be considered to have been carried out in the course of their employment, leaving the practice and not the nurse liable. The practice, of course, might take disciplinary action against a nurse who acted negligently.

Parliament has recently passed what has become known as the 'Whistleblowers Act'. The Public Interest Disclosure Act 1998 is designed to protect from victimization employees who report irregular workplace practices to an outside body. Disclosures cover crimes, breaches of legal obligation, and environmental and health and safety issues. Workers who suffer as a result of such disclosures are eligible to take their cases to an industrial tribunal and seek unlimited compensation. This Act may protect nurses from their employing veterinary surgeon if they should disclose transgressions to an appropriate body such as the RCVS, Police, RSPCA or the Health and Safety Executive.

The role of veterinary nurses

The question of what veterinary nurses can actually do under the present legislation was exhaustively analysed in the Deregulation Paper (RCVS, 1996). While accepting that 'interpretation of an Act [the VSA] drafted over 30 years ago and which still largely reflects the provisions of the earlier Act of 1948 is no simple matter', a set of tests was proposed for defining acts of veterinary surgery, which unless specifically delegated were the unique preserve of veterinary surgeons. These tests were to be used on matters that were not already defined as acts of veterinary surgery in the VSA and could be taken to fall within the scope of the phrase 'art and science of veterinary medicine'.

Veterinary surgery is defined in the VSA to include 'the diagnosis of diseases in, and injuries to animals including tests performed on animals for diagnostic purposes; the giving of advice based upon such diagnosis; the medical or surgical treatment of animals; and the performance of surgical operations upon animals'. This has been reinforced by the Veterinary Training Directive of the European Union to further restrict practices to veterinary surgeons (RCVS, 1996).

The principal test of whether a procedure is an act of veterinary surgery was whether it required a full veterinary education to understand what was being done and why. Having defined what constituted 'veterinary surgery', the Deregulation Report recognized that a number of acts of veterinary surgery had already been delegated and went on to set criteria for further delegation. The only new procedure in small animals which the report was able to recommend for delegation to listed veterinary nurses was the collection of blood for diagnostic purposes. To quote from GPCVN (RCVS, 1998b):

'The 1991 Amendment of the Veterinary Surgeons Act 1966 provides that a Veterinary Nurse whose name is entered in the List of Veterinary Nurses maintained by the Royal College of Veterinary Surgeons may carry out any medical treatment or minor surgery (not involving entry into a body cavity) to a companion animal provided the conditions set out in paragraph 4 in the interpretation of the amendment ... are complied with.'

The paragraph 4 referred to is included in (unattributed) legal advice on the interpretation of the relevant section of the VSA and attempts to define what a veterinary nurse can and cannot do, while making the caveat that what constitutes medical treatment or surgery is left to the 'directing veterinary surgeon to interpret ... with common sense, allied to professional judgement'.

The scope of veterinary nursing has more recently been addressed within the context of 'occupational standards' for veterinary nursing integral to the new Veterinary Nurse S/NVQ Training Scheme, which has superseded the VN Scheme in 1999. This programme is part of a national initiative by the Department for Education and Employment aimed at introducing a system of vocational qualifications (DfEE, 1985). The occupational standards for veterinary nurses have been developed primarily by the RCVS and are consistent with the College's existing views on deregulation.

The argument for greater deregulation

In discussing the relationship between veterinary surgeons and veterinary nurses, the critical question that has to be addressed is: should everything to do with the care of sick animals be contained within the legal domain of veterinary surgeons? If not, what should be the boundaries of veterinary surgery and what other domains should legally coexist? Ultimately it is up to Parliament and the courts to set these boundaries but both are subject to pressure from the media and interested parties. The British Veterinary Association acts as the veterinary surgeons' main lobby group. However, the RCVS, nominally a part of the Government's executive branch, is also a powerful force for change or stasis in its own right.

Recent governments have felt that statutory monopolies, such as that accorded to veterinary surgeons, may not be in the best interest of the public and have called for deregulation. The RCVS recognized that 'the Government wants to curb monopolies, remove what it sees as petty restrictions and reduce expenditure by delegating certain tasks to non-veterinarians' and furthermore 'that the public ... tend to be suspicious of professional monopolies'. While disclaiming any self-interest in the outcome of the debate, the College stated that it 'places its duty to animals and the public as its first priority' and took the view that deregulation would 'mean the removal of or replacement of controls or other effective measures which were established to protect animals, their owners or the public at large from unsatisfactory standards of practice' (RCVS, 1996). From this it is clear that the College considers that deregulation would threaten standards. Not everyone would agree.

Recent statements from nurses and veterinary surgeons have suggested a more integrated team approach to the care of animals where veterinary surgeons, while enjoying a powerful voice, would not play a commanding role (Cooper *et al.*, 1998). This model was first suggested by Pepper (1993), who considered that veterinary para-professionals would, after 2000, be conducting a wide range of supporting roles to veterinary surgeons

> 'as part of the animal care team ... They will be running vaccine clinics ... dietary management clinics, well-animal clinics, primary examination screening, and emergency first aid for all the admissions to veterinary clinics. They will also make domiciliary visits under the same categories.'

Although the year 2000 now seems optimistic, nurse clinics are already held in some more progressive practices where they are advising on various aspects of health maintenance.

Pharmacy ethics and law

The two pieces of legislation affecting medicinal products used in animals are the European Directives and the Medicines Act 1968 (Appleby and Wingfield, 1997). The veterinary aspects of this legislation are administered by the Veterinary Medicines Directorate of the Ministry of Agriculture, Fisheries and Food, which is politically accountable to the Minister for Agriculture. A medicinal product is any substance used for treating or preventing diseases in animals or which may be administered to make a diagnosis or modify a normal physiological function.

The legislation deals with the steps required for medicinal products to be manufactured, marketed, advertised, distributed and sold. Advertising of controlled and prescription-only drugs to the public is prohibited – except, curiously, in the case of animal medicines.

Classification of medicinal products

Medicinal products fall into a number of classes, described in more detail in Chapter 2:

- General sales medicines can be sold without the supervision of a pharmacist
- Prescription-only medicines can only be supplied by veterinary surgeons to animals under their care or sold by pharmacies on receipt of a prescription by an appropriate practitioner
- Pharmacy medicines are those that do not fall into either of the two above categories; they include all preparations prepared and dispensed by pharmacists
- Pharmacy and merchants list medicines are unique to animal medicines and may be sold by veterinary surgeons, pharmacists and registered agricultural merchants
- Controlled drugs are prescription-only drugs that are dangerous and addictive and over which much stricter controls are exerted to prevent misuse. They are grouped into five schedules according to the degree of security over them (Chapter 2).

Exemptions from licensing are in place enabling practising doctors, dentists, veterinarians, pharmacists and certain registered nurses, health visitors and midwives to hold a stock of and dispense certain medicines for administration to patients in their care. The inclusion of nurses in this exemption should be noted, because it does suggest that in the future veterinary nurses might enjoy similar dispensations.

References

Appleby GE and Wingfield J (1997) *Pharmacy Law and Ethics*. Pharmaceutical Press, London

BVNA (1999) Mission Statement. In: *A Career in Veterinary Nursing*. British Veterinary Nursing Association, Harlow

Cooper B, Dyson S, Michell B, Pepper D and Turner T (1998) Animals under our care – whose care and for how long? *Veterinary Record* **142**, 172–173

DfEE (1985) *Education and Training for Young People*. White Paper, Command No. 9482, Department for Education and Employment

Pepper DB (1993) The future structuring of veterinary expertise: professionals and para-professionals. In: Michell AR (ed.) *Veterinary Medicine beyond 2000*. CAB, Wallingford

RCVS (1961) A Register of Animal Nursing Auxiliaries. *Veterinary Record* **73**, 1320

RCVS (1985) Veterinary Nurses: new badges and certificates. *Veterinary Record* **117**, 618

RCVS (1990) June Meeting of Council. *Veterinary Record* **126**, 643

RCVS (1996) Deregulation – implications for animal welfare, consumer protection and the Veterinary Surgeons Act. *Veterinary Record* **139**, 610

RCVS (1998a) Bringing the VN rules up to date. *Veterinary Record* **142**, 708–709

RCVS (1998b) *List of Veterinary Nurses*. [includes Guide to Professional Conduct for Veterinary Nurses]

RCVS (1999) *Veterinary Nurse Training Scheme. Training Centre Handbook*, 2nd edn.

Turner T (1986) Veterinary Nursing History. In: *Veterinary Nursing, the First Twenty-Five Years*. BVNA, Harlow

Index

Ovaries, surgical conditions 158, 228
Ovariohysterectomy 157, 228
Ovulation
    bitch 226
    queen 230
Oxygen therapy 42–3
Oxytocin 239

Packed cell volume 111
Palate, surgical conditions 148
Pancreatic diseases 70–1
Pancreatitis 70–1
Paracentesis 120
Parallel Lack circuit 181, 183
Paralysis 44, 74
Paraplegia 7, 44
Parasites
    control 259–63
    detection in faeces 119
Parasitic skin diseases 79–80
Parenteral feeding 88, 94
Paresis 74
Parturition
    hormonal changes 239
    postpartum care 243
    signs 239
    stages 239–40
Passive exercise 97–8
Patent ductus arteriosus 66
Pathogens 250, 252
PCV 111
PEG tubes 92–3
Penis, abnormalities 156, 232
Percussions 95
Percutaneous endoscopically placed
        gastrostomy (PEG) tubes 92–3
Periodontitis 151
Persistent right aortic arch 66
Petrissage 97
Phagocytosis 253
Phantom pregnancy see
        Pseudopregnancy
Pharmacodynamics 21
Pharmacokinetics 21
Pharmacology 21–30
Pharmacy 31–7
Pharyngostomy tube feeding 91–2
Physiotherapy 94–9
    hydrotherapy 99
    respiratory 94–5
    orthopaedic and neurological 95-9
Pica 8
Placental retention 243
Plasma samples 106, 107, 111
Platelet staining 115
Play 247
Pneumothorax 43–4
Poisoning 49–50
Polydipsia 8
Polyuria 8
Postmortem, cadaver preparation 126
Postoperative care
    after Caesarean 158–9
    after castration 157

after ear surgery 161
after eye surgery 161
after gastric surgery 152
after intestinal surgery 154
after respiratory tract surgery 150
after urinary tract surgery
        154–5, 156
Postoperative problems 134–6
Postpartum problems 243–4
Postural drainage 94
Posture 7
Pregnancy
    abnormalities 238–9
    bitch 236–8
    queen 238
Premedication 185–7
Preparation/triage area 3–4
Prescribing
    cascade 34–5
    prescription writing 35
Pressure bandages 16–17
Professional standards 284
Progesterone 226, 230, 239
Prolactin 239
Prostate gland, surgical conditions
        157, 232
Pseudopregnancy, bitch 229
Puberty, bitch 225
Pulmonary osteopathy 78
Pulmonary stenosis 66
Pulse
    abnormalities 7, 200
    monitoring 6, 51
    normal, cats/dogs 6, 40, 200
Puppies
    dewclaw removal 246
    fading puppy syndrome 246
    feeding 247
    neonatal characteristics 245
    socialization 247
    vaccination 257–8
    worming 247
Pyoderma 80
Pyometra 158
    bitch 229–30
    queen 231
Pyrexia 6

Quadriplegia 7, 44
Queen
    dystocia 240
    gestation period 238
    mammary glands 244
    oestrous cycle 230–1
    ovulation 230
    pregnancy 238
    pyometra 231

Rabies 25, 64, 256
Radiation
    hazards 223–4
    use for sterilization 168
Radiography
    basic principles 203–10

care of equipment 214–17
centring 213
collimation 206–7, 213
control panel 207
distortion 212
exposure factors 210
film
    cassettes 207, 215
    faults 215, 220–3
    processing 218–19
    storage 216
    types 208
film–focus distance 211
filtration 206
grids 209–10, 214, 216
image formation 207
image quality 220–3
image receptors 207–9
labelling 214
patient preparation 210
patient restraint 211–2
positioning 212
aids 213, 216
pregnancy diagnosis 237, 238
protective clothing 217
regulations and safety 219, 223–4
scattered radiation 209
screens 207–8, 216
views 213–14
RCVS 283, 284
Recovery area 4
Rectum, surgical conditions 153, 154
Recumbent patients 85–7
Red blood cell count 111
Reflexes, monitoring 200–1
Regurgitation 8
Relaxin 239
Renal diseases 71–2, 155, 268
Reovirus 63
Reproductive system
    drugs for 28, 29
    surgical conditions 156–9
Respiration
    abnormalities 7
    monitoring 7, 51–2
    rate, cats/dogs 7, 40, 199
Respiratory physiotherapy
Respiratory system
    diseases 65–6
    drugs for 26, 27
    emergencies 42–4
    postoperative care 150
    surgical conditions 147–50
Restraint 9–11
Resuscitation 41, 42, 194
Retrovirus 64
Rhabdovirus 64
Rickets 78
Ringworm see Dermatophytosis
Robert Jones bandage 12–13
Ruptures 139–40

Saliva, in anaesthesia 201
Salmonella 65, 69